ATLAS OF EMERGENCY MEDICINE

ATLAS OF EMERGENCY MEDICINE

Kevin J. Knoop

Assistant Program Director
Emergency Medicine Residency, Naval Medical Center
Portsmouth, Virginia

Lawrence B. Stack

Assistant Professor of Emergency Medicine
Vanderbilt University Medical Center
Nashville, Tennessee

Alan B. Storrow

Staff Attending and Research Director
Joint Military Medical Centers Emergency Medicine Residency
San Antonio, Texas

McGraw-Hill
HEALTH PROFESSIONS DIVISION

New York   St. Louis   San Francisco   Auckland   Bogota   Caracas   Lisbon   London   Madrid
Mexico City   Milan   Montreal   New Delhi   San Juan   Singapore   Sydney   Tokyo   Toronto

McGraw-Hill

*A Division of The **McGraw·Hill** Companies*

ATLAS OF EMERGENCY MEDICINE

1 2 3 4 5 6 7 8 9 0 Q P K / Q P K 9 9 8 7

ISBN 0-07-035202-X

This book was set in Friz Quadrata by York Graphic Services, Inc. The editors were John Dolan and Pamela Touboul; the production supervisor was Rick Ruzycka; the cover and text designer was Marsha Cohen. The indexer was Dr. Tony Greenberg. Quebecor Printing/Kingsport was printer and binder.

Library of Congress Cataloging-in-Publication Data

Atlas of emergency medicine / [edited by] Kevin J. Knoop, Lawrence
    Stack, Alan B. Storrow.
       p.   cm.
    Includes bibliographical references and index.
    ISBN 0-07-035202-X
    International Edition ISBN 0-07-114419-6
    1. Emergency medicine—Atlases. I. Knoop, Kevin J. II. Stack,
Lawrence. III. Storrow, Alan B.
    [DNLM: 1. Emergency Medicine—methods—atlases. 2. Emergencies—
atlases. 3. Critical Care—methods—atlases. WB 17 A8817 1997]
RC86.7.A85 1997
616.02′5—DC21
DNLM/DLC
for Library of Congress   97-1279
                                            CIP

DEDICATION

To the outstanding Emergency Medicine residents
of the Naval Medical Center Portsmouth,
Joint Military Medical Centers, and Vanderbilt University Medical Center,
who teach us something new every day.
Kevin J. Knoop
Lawrence B. Stack
Alan B. Storrow

To my children, Amelia and Stephen,
who are my greatest joy,
and
To my wife, Mary Jo,
for her unending support, love, and friendship.
Kevin J. Knoop

To my children, Laura, Andrew, and Emily,
God's greatest blessing to me,
and
To my wife Venette,
God's gift to me, for her patience and support
during the development of this project.
Lawrence B. Stack

To my children, Robert Leslie and Allison Marie,
who are the highlight of my life,
and, most importantly,
To my wife, Julia Ann,
for her cheerful spirit, encouragement, and devotion to a loving family.
Without her patience and many sacrifices this work
would never have been completed.
Alan B. Storrow

CONTENTS

Part 1
REGIONAL ANATOMY

Chapter 1

HEAD AND FACIAL TRAUMA

David W. Munter
Timothy D. McGuirk

Chapter 2

OPHTHALMIC CONDITIONS

Frank Birinyi
Thomas F. Mauger

FUNDUSCOPIC FINDINGS   Chapter 3

David Effron
Beverly C. Forcier
Richard E. Wyszynski

OPHTHALMIC TRAUMA   Chapter 4

Dallas E. Peak
Carey D. Chisholm
Kevin J. Knoop

Chapter 5	ENT CONDITIONS

Edward C. Jauch
Alexander T. Trott
Kevin J. Knoop

Chapter 6	MOUTH

Edwin Turner
Edward C. Jauch
Sara-Jo Gahm

Oral Trauma

Odontogenic Infections

Oral Conditions

CHEST AND ABDOMEN   Chapter 7

Stephen Corbett
Lawrence B. Stack
Kevin J. Knoop

Chest and Abdominal Trauma

Chest and Abdominal Conditions

Chapter 8   UROLOGICAL CONDITIONS

Jeffery D. Bondesson

Chapter 9   SEXUALLY TRANSMITTED DISEASES AND ANORECTAL CONDITIONS

Diane M. Birnbaumer
Lynn K. Flowers

Sexually Transmitted Disease

Anorectal Conditions

GYNECOLOGIC AND OBSTETRIC CONDITIONS   Chapter 10

Robert G. Buckley
Kevin J. Knoop

Gynecologic Conditions

Obstetric Conditions

| Chapter 11 | EXTREMITY TRAUMA |

Kathleen M. Vossler
Daniel L. Savitt
Alan B. Storrow

Upper Extremity

Pelvis and Hip

Lower Extremity

EXTREMITY CONDITIONS   Chapter 12

Selim Suner
Daniel L. Savitt

CUTANEOUS CONDITIONS   Chapter 13

Christopher R. Sartori
Michael B. Brooks

Part 2
SPECIALTY AREAS

| Chapter 14 | PEDIATRIC CONDITIONS |

Javier A. Gonzalez del Rey
Richard M. Ruddy

Newborn Conditions

Rashes and Lesions

General Conditions

CHILD ABUSE

Chapter 15

Robert A. Shapiro
Charles J. Shubert

Physical Abuse

Sexual Abuse

Findings Mistaken for Sexual Abuse

Chapter 16   ENVIRONMENTAL CONDITIONS

Ken Zafren
Alan B. Storrow
Joseph C. Schmidt
Lawrence B. Stack

MICROSCOPIC FINDINGS   Chapter 17

Diane M. Birnbaumer

FRANK BIRINYI, M.D., FACEP
Clinical Assistant Professor of Emergency Medicine
The Ohio State University
Attending Physician
Mount Carmel Medical Center
Mount Carmel East Hospital
Columbus, Ohio (2)

DIANE M. BIRNBAUMER, M.D., FACEP
Associate Residency Director
Department of Emergency Medicine
Harbor-UCLA Medical Center
Torrence, California (9, 17)

JEFFERY D. BONDESSON, M.D.
Medical Director
Emergency Medicine Department
Menorah Medical Center
Overland Park, Kansas (8)

MICHAEL B. BROOKS, M.D.
Attending Physician
Joint Military Medical Centers Emergency Medicine
Residency
Brooke Army Medical Center
San Antonio, Texas (13)

ROBERT G. BUCKLEY, M.D., FACEP
LCDR, MC, USNR
Research Director
Department of Emergency Medicine
Naval Medical Center
San Diego, California (10)

CAREY D. CHISHOLM, M.D., FACEP
Emergency Medicine Residency Director
Clinical Associate Professor of Emergency Medicine
Methodist-Indiana University
Indianapolis, Indiana (4)

STEPHEN CORBETT, M.D.
Department of Emergency Medicine
Loma Linda University Medical Center
Loma Linda, California (7)

DAVID EFFRON, M.D., FACEP
Department of Emergency Medicine
MetroHealth Medical Center
Cleveland, Ohio (3)

LYNN K. FLOWERS, M.D.
LCDR(s) MC, USNR
Emergency Medicine Department
Naval Medical Center
Portmouth, Virginia
Assistant Professor of Emergency Medicine
Eastern Virginia Medical School
Norfolk, Virginia (9)

BEVERLY C. FORCIER, M.D.
Department of Emergency Medicine
MetroHealth Medical Center
Cleveland, Ohio (3)

SARA-JO GAHM, M.D.
Resident
Department of Emergency Medicine
Medical College of Pennsylvania
Philadelphia, Pennsylvania (6)

JAVIER A. GONZALEZ DEL REY, M.D., FAAP
Assistant Professor of Clinical Pediatrics and
Emergency Medicine
University of Cincinnati College of Medicine
Attending Physician, Division of Emergency Medicine
Children's Hospital Medical Center, Cincinnati, Ohio
(14)

EDWARD C. JAUCH, M.D., M.S.
Chief Resident
Department of Emergency Medicine
University of Cincinnati Medical Center
Cincinnati, Ohio (5, 6)

KEVIN J. KNOOP, M.D., M.S., FACEP
CDR, MC, USNR
Assistant Program Director
Emergency Medicine Residency
Naval Medical Center
Portsmouth, Virginia (4, 5, 7, 10)

THOMAS F. MAUGER, M.D.
Associate Professor of Ophthalmology
Department of Ophthalmology
William H. Havener Eye Center
The Ohio State University
Columbus, Ohio (2)

TIMOTHY D. McGUIRK, D.O., FACEP
CDR, MC, USN
Research Coordinator
Emergency Medicine Residency
Naval Medical Center
Portsmouth, Virginia (1)

DAVID W. MUNTER, M.D., FACEP
CDR, MC, USN
Program Director
Emergency Medicine Residency
Naval Medical Center
Portsmouth, Virginia (1)

DALLAS E. PEAK, M.D.
Attending Physician
Department of Emergency Medicine
Methodist Hospital of Indiana
Indianapolis, Indiana (4)

RICHARD M. RUDDY, M.D., FAAP

Professor of Clinical Pediatrics and Emergency
Medicine
University of Cincinnati College of Medicine
Director, Division of Emergency Medicine
Children's Hospital Medical Center
Cincinnati, Ohio   (14)

CHRISTOPHER R. SARTORI, M.D.

Chief, Outpatient Dermatology
Wilford Hall Medical Center
San Antonio, Texas   (13)

DANIEL L. SAVITT, M.D.

Attending Physician and Residency Director
Department of Emergency Medicine
Rhode Island Hospital
Assistant Professor of Medicine
Brown University
Providence, Rhode Island   (11, 12)

JOSEPH C. SCHMIDT, M.D.

Chief Resident
Joint Military Medical Centers Emergency
Medicine Residency
Wilford Hall Medical Center
San Antonio, Texas   (16)

CHARLES J. SCHUBERT, M.D., FAAP

Assistant Professor of Pediatrics
University of Cincinnati College of Medicine
Attending Physician, Division of Emergency
Medicine
Children's Hospital Medical Center
Cincinnati, Ohio   (14)

ROBERT A. SHAPIRO, M.D., FAAP

Associate Professor of Pediatrics
University of Cincinnati College of Medicine
Medical Director, Child Abuse Program
Attending Physician, Division of Emergency
Medicine
Children's Hospital Medical Center
Cincinnati, Ohio   (14)

LAWRENCE B. STACK, M.D., FACEP

Assistant Professor
Department of Emergency Medicine
Vanderbilt University Medical Center
Nashville, Tennessee   (7, 16)

ALAN B. STORROW, M.D., FACEP

Research Director and Attending Physician
Joint Military Medical Centers Emergency Medicine
Residency
Wilford Hall Medical Center
San Antonio, Texas   (11, 16)

SELIM SUNER, M.D., M.S.

Resident
Department of Emergency Medicine
Rhode Island Hospital and Brown University
Providence, Rhode Island   (12)

ALEXANDER T. TROTT, M.D.

Professor of Emergency Medicine
University of Cincinnati
College of Medicine
Cincinnati, Ohio   (5)

EDWIN TURNER, M.D.

LCDR, MC, USNR
Attending Physician
Emergency Medicine Department
Naval Hospital
Great Lakes, Illinois   (6)

CATHLEEN M. VOSSLER, M.D.

Resident
Department of Emergency Medicine
Rhode Island Hospital and Brown University
Providence, Rhode Island   (11)

RICHARD E. WYSZYNSKI, M.D.

Department of Emergency Medicine
MetroHealth Medical Center
Cleveland, Ohio   (3)

KEN ZAFREN, M.D., FACEP, FAAEM

Alaska Regional Hospital
Anchorage, Alaska
Medical Director
Denali National Park Mountaineering Rangers and
Lake Clark National Park, Alaska
Associate Medical Director (USA), Himalayan Rescue
Association   (16)

American Academy of Ophthalamology
San Francisco, California

American Academy of Pediatrics
Elk Grove Village, Illinois

American Society of Colon and Rectal Surgeons
Arlington Heights, Illinois

PAMELA AMBROZ, M.D.
LT, MC, USNR
Resident
Department of Obstetrics and Gynecology
Naval Medical Center
San Diego, California

EDWARD S. AMRHEIN, D.D.S.
CAPT, DC, USN
Head, Dental Department
Director, Oral & Maxillofacial Surgery Residency
Naval Medical Center
Portsmouth, Virginia

Armed Forces Institute of Pathology
Bethesda, Maryland

MATTHEW BACKER JR., M.D.
RADM, MC, USNR (ret)
Attending Physician
Department of Obstetrics and Gynecology
Naval Medical Center
San Diego, California

RAYMOND C. BAKER, M.D.
Professor of Pediatrics
University of Cincinnati College of Medicine
Pediatrician, Division of Pediatrics
Children's Hospital Medical Center
Cincinnati, Ohio

WILLIAM S. BALL JR., M.D.
Professor of Radiology and Pediatrics
Chief, Section Neuroradiology and Staff Radiologist
Medical Director Imaging Research Center
Children's Hospital Medical Center
Cincinnati, Ohio

KEITH F. BATTS, M.D.
LCDR, MC, USNR
Attending Physician
Emergency Medicine Department
Naval Medical Center
Portsmouth, Virginia

JUDITH C. BAUSHER, M.D.
Associate Professor of Pediatrics and Emergency
Medicine
University of Cincinnati College of Medicine
Attending Physician, Division of Emergency Medicine
Children's Hospital Medical Center
Cincinnati, Ohio

BILL BECK, CRA
Clinic Photographer, Florida Eye Clinic
Altamonte Springs, FL

FRANK BIRINYI, M.D., FACEP
Clinical Assistant Professor of Emergency Medicine
The Ohio State University
Attending Physician
Mount Carmel Medical Center
Mount Carmel East Hospital
Columbus, Ohio

DIANE M. BIRNBAUMER, M.D., FACEP
Associate Residency Director
Department of Emergency Medicine
Harbor-UCLA Medical Center
Torrance, California

JEFFERY D. BONDESSON, M.D.
Medical Director
Emergency Medicine Department
Menorah Medical Center
Overland Park, Kansas

JOHN BOYLE, M.D.
LT, MC, USNR
Resident
Department of Obstetrics and Gynecology
Naval Medical Center
San Diego, California

MICHAEL B. BROOKS, M.D.
Attending Physician
Joint Military Medical Centers Emergency Medicine
Residency
Brooke Army Medical Center
San Antonio, Texas

ALAN S. BRODY, M.D.
Staff Radiologist
Children's Hospital Medical Center
Cincinnati, Ohio

ROBERT G. BUCKLEY, M.D. FACEP
LCDR, MC, USNR
Research Director
Department of Emergency Medicine
Naval Medical Center
San Diego, California

WILLIAM E. CAPPAERT, M.D.
Department of Emergency Medicine
MetroHealth Medical Center
2500 MetroHealth Drive
Cleveland, OH

CAREY D. CHISHOLM, M.D., FACEP

Emergency Medicine Residency Director
Clinical Associate Professor of Emergency Medicine
Methodist-Indiana University
Indianapolis, Indiana

RICHARD A. CHOLE, M.D., PhD

Professor and Chair, Department of Otolaryngology
School of Medicine, University of California, Davis,
Medical Center

JUDY CHRISTIANSON

Medical Illustrator
Graphics Division
Staff Education and Training
Naval Medical Center
San Diego, California

MARCO COPOLLA, D.O., FACEP

Major, USA, Medical Corps
Program Director, Emergency Medicine Residency
Darnall Army Community Hospital
Fort Hood, Texas
Assistant Professor of Emergency Medicine
Texas A&M University Health Science Center
College Station, Texas

STEPHEN CORBETT, M.D.

Department of Emergency Medicine
Loma Linda University Medical Center
Loma Linda, California

ROBIN T. COTTON, MD

Professor
Department of Otolaryngology and Maxillofacial
Surgery
Childrens Hospital Medical Center
Cincinnati, Ohio

RICHARD A. CLINCHY, III, PhD, NREMT-P

American College of Prehospital Medicine
Ft. Walton Beach, FL

BARBARA R. CRAIG, M.D.

CAPT, MC, USN
Medical Consultant for Child Abuse and Neglect
National Naval Medical Center
Bethesda, Maryland

Curatek Pharmacuticals
Elk Grove Village, Illinois

Departments of Dermatology
Collective Files,
Brooke Army Medical Center
Wilford Hall USAF Medical Center
San Antonio, Texas

Department of Dermatology
Naval Medical Center
Portsmouth, Virginia

Department of Ophthalmology
Naval Medical Center
Portsmouth, Virginia

Department of Otolaryngology
Children's Hospital Medical Center
Cincinnati, Ohio

HERBERT L. DuPONT, M.D.

Chief, Internal Medicine Service
St. Luke's Episcopal Hospital
Houston, Texas

LEE E. EDSTROM, M.D.

Surgeon in Chief
Division of Plastic Surgery
Rhode Island Hospital
Assistant Professor of Surgery
Brown University
Providence, Rhode Island

DAVID EFFRON, M.D., FACEP

Department of Emergency Medicine
MetroHelath Medical Center
Cleveland, Ohio

ERIC EINFALT, M.D.

LCDR, MC, USNR
Staff Physician
Emergency Medicine Department
Naval Medical Center
Jacksonville, Florida

EDWARD M. EITZEN, JR., M.D., MPH

Chief, Preventive Medicine Department
US Army Medical Research Institute of Infectious
Diseases
Fort Detrick, Maryland

KIM MARIE FELDHAUS, M.D.

Emergency Medical Services
Denver General Hospital
Denver, Colorado

JOHN FILDES, M.D., FACS

Attending Surgeon
Division of Trauma
Department of Surgery
Cook County Hospital
Chicago, Illinois

JEFFREY FINKELSTEIN, M.D., FACEP

Chief, Division of Acute Care
Chairman, Department of Emergency Medicine
Wilford Hall Medical Center
Attending Physician
Joint Military Medical Centers
Emergency Medicine Residency
San Antonio, TX

LYNN K. FLOWERS, M.D.
LCDR(s), MC, USNR
Emergency Medicine Department
Naval Medical Center
Portsmouth, Virginia
Assistant Professor of Emergency Medicine
Eastern Virginia Medical School
Norfolk, Virginia

BEVERLY C. FORCIER, M.D.
Department of Emergency Medicine
MetroHealth Medical Center
Cleveland, OH

SARA-JO GAHM, M.D.
Resident
Department of Emergency Medicine
Medical College of Pennsylvania
Philadelphia, PA

Geisinger Medical Center
Department of Emergency Medicine
Danville, PA

W. BRIAN GIBLER, M.D.
Professor and Chair
Department of Emergency Medicine
University of Cincinnati College of Medicine
Cincinnati, Ohio

JEFFREY S. GIBSON, M.D.
LCDR, MC, USNR
Staff Physician
Emergency Medicine Department
Naval Medical Center
Jacksonville, Florida

JAVIER A. GONZALEZ DEL REY, M.D., FAAP
Assistant Professor of Clinical Pediatrics and
Emergency Medicine
University of Cincinnati College of Medicine
Attending Physician, Division of Emergency Medicine
Children's Hospital Medical Center, Cincinnati, Ohio

RALPH A. GRUPPO, M.D.
Professor of Pediatrics
University of Cincinnati College of Medicine
Director, Hemophilia Treatment Center
Children's Hospital Medical Center
Cincinnati, Ohio

PETER HACKETT, M.D., FACEP
St. Mary's Hospital
Grand Junction, Colorado

H. HUNTER HANDSFIELD, M.D.
Professor of Medicine
University of Washington
Director, STD Control Program
Seattle-King County Department of Public Health
Seattle, Washington

ROBERT S. HOFFMAN, M.D., FACEP
Assistant Professor, Clinical Surgery and Emergency
Medicine
NYU School of Medicine
Director, NYC Poison Control Center
New York City, New York

STEPHEN HOLT, M.D.
San Antonio, Texas

KING K. HOLMES, M.D., PhD
Director, University of Washington Center for AIDS
and STD
Professor of Medicine
University of Washington
Seattle, Washington

GERALD VAN HOUDT, M.D.
CDR, MC, USN
Resident
Department of Emergency Medicine
Naval Medical Center
San Diego

CURTIS HUNTER, M.D.
Chief, Emergency Medical Services
General Leonard Wood Army Community Hospital
Fort Leonard Wood, Missouri

LIUDVIKAS JAGMINAS, M.D.
Attending Physician
Department of Emergency Medicine
Rhode Island Hospital
Assistant Professor of Medicine
Brown University
Providence, Rhode Island

JENNIFER JAGOE, M.D.
LT, MC, USNR
Resident
Department of Obstetrics and Gynecology
Naval Medical Center
San Diego

TIMOTHY JAHN, M.D.
LCDR, MC, USNR
Attending Physician
Department of Emergency Medicine
Naval Hospital
Great Lakes, Illinois

EDWARD C. JAUCH, M.D. M.S.
Chief Resident
Department of Emergency Medicine
University of Cincinnati Medical Center
Cincinnati, Ohio

ARTHUR M. KAHN, M.D., FACS
Assistant Professor of Surgery
UCLA School of Medicine
Attending Surgeon
Cedars-Sinai Medical Center
Los Angeles, California

LEE KAPLAN, M.D.
Chief of Dermatology
VA Medical Center; San Diego, California
Associate Clinical Professor of Medicine and
Dermatology
University of California, San Diego

MARGARET J. KARNES, D.O.
Assistant Professor of Emergency Medicine
Texas A&M University Health Science Center
College Station, Texas
Senior Staff Physician
Department of Emergency Medicine
Scott and White Memorial Hospital and Clinic
Temple, Texas

KEVIN J. KNOOP, M.D., M.S., FACEP
CDR, MC, USNR
Assistant Program Director
Emergency Medicine Residency
Naval Medical Center
Portsmouth, Virginia

PAUL J. KOVALCHIK, M.D., FACS
Colorectal Surgeon
Chesapeake, Virginia

DAVID P. KRETZSCHMAR, D.D.S., M.S.
Chief, Department of Oral and Maxillofacial Surgery
2nd Medical Group
Barksdale AFB, Louisiana
Assistant Professor
Department of Surgery
Louisiana State University Medical Center

JAMES L. KRETZSCHMAR, D.D.S., M.S.
LTCOL, USAF
OIC Flight Dental Clinic
Holloman AFB, New Mexico

JEFFERY KUHN, M.D.
LCDR, MC, USNR
Department of Otolaryngology—Head and Neck
Surgery
Naval Medical Center
Portsmouth, Virginia

DOUGLAS R. LANDRY, M.D.
LCDR, MC, USNR
Resident
Emergency Medicine Department
Naval Medical Center
Portsmouth, Virginia

PATRICK W. LAPPERT, M.D.
CDR, MC, USN
Naval Medical Center, Portsmouth VA
Clinical Assistant Professor, Department of Surgery
Uniformed Services University of the Health Sciences
Bethesda, MD

HILLARY J. LARKIN, PA-C
Director, Medical Sexual Assault Services
Department of Emergency Medicine
Alameda Sexual Assault Response Team
Highland General Hospital
Oakland, California

LORENZ F. LASSEN, M.D.
CAPT, MC, USN
Assistant Professor of Otolaryngology—Head and
Neck Surgery
Eastern Virginia Medical School
Chairman and Residency Program Director
Otolaryngology—Head and Neck Surgery
Naval Medical Center
Portsmouth, VA

WILLIAM LENINGER, M.D.
LT, MC, USNR
Resident
Department of Obstetrics and Gynecology
Naval Medical Center
San Diego

ANNE W. LUCKY, M.D.
Volunteer Professor of Dermatology and Pediatrics
University of Cincinnati College of Medicine
Director, Dermatology Clinic
Children's Hospital Medical Center, Cincinnati

C. BRUCE MACDONALD, M.D.
Assistant Professor, Department of Otolaryngology
Boston University School of Medicine
Boston, Massachusetts

MARK L. MADENWALD, M.D.
LT, MC, USNR
Chief Resident
Emergency Medicine Department
Naval Medical Center
Portsmouth, Virginia

WILLIAM K. MALLON, M.D., FACEP
Associate Director of Residency Training
Assistant Professor of Medicine
University of Southern California School of Medicine
Los Angeles, California

THOMAS F. MAUGER, M.D.
Associate Professor of Ophthalmology
Department of Ophthalmology
William H. Havener Eye Center
The Ohio State University
Columbus, OH

TIMOTHY D. MCGUIRK, D.O., FACEP
CDR, MC, USN
Research Coordinator
Emergency Medicine Residency
Naval Medical Center
Portsmouth, Virginia

PATRICK H. MCKENNA, M.D., FACS, FAAP
Assistant Clinical Professor of Urology and Pediatrics
University of Connecticut Health Center
Hartford, Connecticut

AURORA MENDEZ, RN
Sexual Assault Response Team Coordinator
Villavu Community Hospital, San Diego

JAMES MENSCHING, M.D.
LCDR, MC, USN
Attending Physician
Emergency Medicine Department
Naval Hospital
Okinawa, Japan

SHERMAN MINTON, M.D.
Professor Emeritus
Department of Microbiology and Immunology
Indiana University School of Medicine
Indianapolis, Indiana

MARGARET P. MUELLER, M.D.
Department of Emergency Medicine
Rhode Island Hospital and Brown University
Providence, Rhode Island

DAVID W. MUNTER, M.D., FACEP
CDR, MC, USN
Program Director
Emergency Medicine Residency
Naval Medical Center
Portsmouth, Virginia

GEORGE L. MURRELL, M.D.
LCDR, MC, USN
Department of Otolaryngology—Head and Neck
Surgery
Naval Medical Center, Portsmouth VA
Assistant Professor of Clinical Otolaryngology Head
and Neck Surgery,
Eastern Virginia Medical School, Norfolk, VA

MICHAEL J. NOWICKI, M.D.
CDR, MC, USN
Division of Pediatric Gastroenterology
Department of Pediatrics
Naval Medical Center
Portsmouth, Virginia

ALAN E. OESTREICH, M.D.
Professor of Radiology and Pediatrics
University of Cincinnati College of Medicine
Chief, Section of Diagnostic Radiology
Staff Radiologist
Children's Hospital Medical Center
Cincinnati, Ohio

JAMES O'MALLEY, M.D.
Alaska Regional Hospital
Anchorage, Alaska

EDWARD J. OTTEN, M.D.
Professor of Emergency Medicine and Pediatrics
Director, Division of Toxicology
University of Cincinnati College of Medicine
Cincinnati, Ohio

JAMES PALOMBARO M.D.
LCDR, MC, USNR
Attending Physician
Department of Obstetrics and Gynecology
Naval Medical Center
San Diego

LAURI PAOLINETTE, PA-C
Sexual Assault Examiner
Department of Emergency Medicine
Alameda Sexual Assault Response Team
Highland General Hospital
Oakland, California

DALLAS E. PEAK, M.D.
Attending Physician
Department of Emergency Medicine
Methodist Hospital of Indiana
Indianapolis, Indiana

MICHAEL P. POIRIER, M.D.

Assistant Professor of Pediatrics
Eastern Virginia Medical School
Division of Pediatric Emergency Medicine
Children's Hospital of the King's Daughters
Norfolk, Virginia

MICHAEL REDMAN, PA-C

Staff, Emergency Medicine
Fort Leonard Wood Army Community Hospital
Fort Leonard Wood, Missouri

SUE RIST, FNP

CAPT, NC, USN (ret)
Naval Training Center
San Diego, California

HAROLD RIVERA, HM1, USN

Optician
Department of Ophthalmology
Naval Medical Center
Portsmouth, Virginia

Roche Laboratories

DONALD L. RUCKNAGEL, M.D., PhD

Professor of Pediatrics and Internal Medicine
University of Cincinnati College of Medicine
Comprehensive Sickle Cell Center
Children's Hospital Medical Center
Cincinnati, Ohio

RICHARD M. RUDDY, M.D., FAAP

Professor of Clinical Pediatrics and Emergency
Medicine
University of Cincinnati College of Medicine
Director, Division of Emergency Medicine
Children's Hospital Medical Center
Cincinnati, Ohio

WARREN K. RUSSELL, M.D.

LCDR, MC, USNR
Head, Emergency Medicine Department
Naval Hospital
Roosevelt Roads, Puerto Rico

KATRINA C. SANTOS, HM3, USN

Ocular Technician
Department of Ophthalmology
Naval Medical Center
Portsmouth, Virginia

SALLY SANTEN, M.D.

Assistant Professor
Department of Emergency Medicine
Vanderbilt University Medical Center
Nashville, Tennessee

CHRISTOPHER R. SARTORI, M.D.

Chief, Outpatient Dermatology
Wilford Hall Medical Center
San Antonio, Texas

ADAM R. SAPERSTON, M.D., M.S.

LCDR, MC, USN
Resident
Emergency Medicine Residency
Naval Medical Center
Portsmouth, Virginia

DANIEL L. SAVITT, M.D.

Attending Physician and Residency Director
Department of Emergency Medicine
Rhode Island Hospital
Assistant Professor of Medicine
Brown University
Providence, Rhode Island

JOSEPH C. SCHMIDT, M.D.

Chief Resident
Joint Military Medical Centers Emergency Medicine
Residency
Wilford Hall Medical Center
San Antonio, Texas

ROBERT SCHNARRS, M.D.

Staff Physician
Department of Plastic Surgery
Sentara Norfolk General Hospital
Norfolk, VA

CHARLES J. SCHUBERT, M.D.

Assistant Professor of Pediatrics and Emergency
Medicine
University of Cincinnati College of Medicine
Attending Physician, Division of Emergency Medicine
Children's Hospital Medical Center
Cincinnati, Ohio

GARY SCHWARTZ, M.D.

Assistant Professor
Department of Emergency Medicine
Vanderbilt University Medical Center
Nashville, Tennessee

ROBERT A. SHAPIRO, M.D.

Associate Professor of Pediatrics and Emergency
Medicine
University of Cincinnati College of Medicine
Attending Physician, Division of Emergency Medicine
Children's Hospital Medical Center
Cincinnati, Ohio

VIRENDER K. SHARMA, M.D.
Fellow
Division of Digestive Disease and Nutrition
University of South Carolina School of Medicine
Columbia, South Carolina

REES W. SHEPPARD, M.D., FACS
Assistant Director of Pediatric Ophthalmology
Children's Hospital Medical Center
Volunteer Associate Professor
University of Cincinnati College of Medicine
Cincinnati, Ohio

TIMOTHY L. SMITH, M.D.
Assistant Professor
Department of Otolaryngology—Head and Neck
Surgery
Vanderbilt University Medical Center
Nashville, Tennessee

D. J. SPALTON FRCS, MRCP
Consultant Ophthalmic Surgeon
Medical Eye Unit
St. Thomas's Hospital
London, UK

LAWRENCE B. STACK, M.D., FACEP
Assistant Professor
Department of Emergency Medicine
Vanderbilt University Medical Center
Nashville, Tennessee

WALTER STAMM, M.D.
Professor of Medicine
Head, Infectious Diseases Division
Harborview Medical Center
Seattle, Washington

JAMES F. STEINER, D.D.S.
Professor of Pediatrics
University of Cincinnati College of Medicine
Pediatric Dentistry
Children's Hospital Medical Center
Cincinnati, Ohio

ALAN B. STORROW, M.D., FACEP
Research Director and Attending Physician
Joint Military Medical Centers Emergency Medicine
Residency
Wilford Hall Medical Center
San Antonio, Texas

SELIM SUNER, M.D., M.S.
Resident
Department of Emergency Medicine
Rhode Island Hospital and Brown University
Providence, Rhode Island

GARY TANNER, M.D.
CDR, MC, USN
Staff Physician
Department of Ophthalmology
Naval Medical Center
Portsmouth, Virginia

ALEXANDER T. TROTT, M.D.
Professor, Department of Emergency Medicine
University of Cincinnati College of Medicine
Cincinnati, Ohio

EDWIN TURNER, M.D.
LCDR, MC, USNR
Attending Physician
Emergency Medicine Department
Naval Hospital
Great Lakes, Illinois

CATHLEEN M. VOSSLER, M.D.
Resident
Department of Emergency Medicine
Rhode Island Hospital and Brown University
Providence, Rhode Island

JANICE E. UNDERWOOD, RDMS
Advanced Health Education Center, Inc.
Houston, Texas

US Government Printing Office
Washington, DC

RICHARD E. WYSZYNSKI, M.D.
Department of Emergency Medicine
MetroHealth Medical Center
Cleveland, OH

SCOTT W. ZACKOWSKI, M.D.
Attending Physician
Emergency Medicine Residency
Naval Medical Center
Portsmouth, VA

KEN ZAFREN, M.D., FACEP, FAAEM
Alaska Regional Hospital
Anchorage, Alaska
Medical Director
Denali National Park Mountaineering Rangers and
Lake Clark National Park, Alaska
Associate Medical Director (USA), Himalayan Rescue
Association

RICHARD ZIENOWICZ, M.D.
Attending Physician
Division of Plastic Surgery
Rhode Island Hospital
Assistant Professor of Surgery
Brown University
Providence, Rhode Island

FOREWORD

The emergency physician represents the buffer between the "high technology" of the medical center and the "high touch" needs of the patient. Given an increasing emphasis on reducing costs, the emergency physician will be expected to demonstrate a more cost-effective practice. While achieving this goal will depend in part upon sensible therapeutics, more importantly, the emergency physician will need to become increasingly facile at clinical diagnosis. This latter skill will lead to less common use of expensive diagnostic studies.

While establishment of a clinical diagnosis depends in large part upon the patient's description of symptomology, the physical examination remains crucial for confirmation of many clinical illnesses. Although physical findings may be detected using our tactile and auditory senses, most physical findings are detected visually. This text by Knoop, Stack, and Storrow, provides a unique resource to the clinician who seeks to link visual cues with clinical diagnosis. The text also incorporates plain film, ultrasound, and computed tomographic findings of unique importance to emergency physicians.

The authors are well known in emergency medicine for their ability to combine photographic technique with clinical education and have taught medical photography as an educational tool at national forums. The authors seek to extend their linkage of visual cues and clinical education with this text. While the text will aid many novice clinicians, others will gain from this tool. The practicing emergency physician seldom has the opportunity to obtain immediate consultation regarding visual findings. Often the clinician's prior experience with a visual cue as a student or resident may be "fuzzy" or perhaps was incorrect. This text offers the clinician an opportunity for immediate feedback regarding visual cues for injury and illness. The wise clinician will accept that opportunity.

Jerris R. Hedges, MD, MS

PREFACE

Medical diagnosis is an extremely visual discipline. Volumes of accurate and well written text simply cannot replace what our eyes experience. In few specialities is this so true as Emergency Medicine. We are constantly reminded of how a visual image is one of the most powerful teaching educational tools in medicine. In Emergency Medicine, it is commonplace to evaluate that "great case", then quickly have the patient taken to an inpatient bed or operating room. A good photograph allows for sharing the salient visual clues with our colleagues, residents, and medical students. It is simply the next best experience to going to the bedside.

Purpose

Atlas of Emergency Medicine is designed to serve as a reference and teaching guide to the visual clues seen in Emergency Medicine. While many different atlases and color guides are currently available, none are comprehensive enough as a single reference for use in the emergency department or acute care clinic. We have collected images representing the scope and breadth of emergency practice and have asked experts to collect, catalog, and write about these images. The "Atlas" is *not* meant to be a comprehensive text nor treatise on diagnosis. That is left to the many excellent references currently available. It *is* however, meant to be the most comprehensive collection of excellent emergency clinical images. Such a book does not currently exist and we envision this text to fill a significant void.

Intended Audience

The primary audience for this text is emergency medicine clinicians, educators, residents, and medical students who provide emergency care. We hope it will aid the clinician in making the diagnosis and help the teacher take the student "to the bedside". Other groups of physicians may find *Atlas of Emergency Medicine* a useful guide in identifying and treating the many conditions for which visual cues significantly guide or expedite diagnosis and treatment. These include those involved in primary care, including family physicians, internists, and pediatricians. Physician extenders such as Nurse Practictioners and Physician Assistants may also appreciate the "clinical experience" this text can add to their training and practice. Finally, interested medical students can augment their clinical repertoire early in their training from the "visual discoveries" they will encounter in this text. We would like all readers to appreciate and understand the important clues inherent in these clinical images, and perhaps more importantly, to share these with physicians in training.

Organization

The organization of the *Atlas of Emergency Medicine* is based upon regional anatomy for part I, with part II composed of selected areas which deserve special attention (Pediatric Conditions, Child Abuse, Environmental Conditions and Microscopic Findings). A review of the Table of Contents shows the individual diagnosis displayed in each chapter. A brief text accompanies each diagnosis and includes the following sections: Associated Clinical Features, Differential Diagnosis, ED Treatment and Disposition, and Clinical Pearls. The final chapter (Microscopic Findings) varies from this format and instead includes a brief text accompanying each microscopic technique: Uses, Materials, and Methods. Approximately 570 color clinical photographs, 67 radiographs and 55 line drawings are referenced throughout the text and contain pertinent captions.

KJK
LBS
ABS

ACKNOWLEDGMENTS

As for any text of this nature, it could never have been completed without the sacrifices, time, and help of many people. Unfortunately, space does not allow a recounting of the numerous individuals who have contributed to this project over the five years since its inception. The inspiration at the beginning, and the encouragement throughout the project from W. Brian Gilber, M.D. was invaluable and greatly appreciated. Special thanks also go to each of the four McGraw-Hill editors that guided the project through its various stages during its long journey. They include William J. Lamsback, Jamie Kircher, Martin Wonsiewicz, and John J. Dolan. They provided invaluable assistance, guidance and motivation in completing each phase of the project. Thomas Xenakis was especially helpful with providing numerous excellent illustrations within our hurried time constraints. Special acknowledgement is due to all the photograph contributors who lent their photographs in support of this text. Finally, and most importantly, we are grateful to the many patients who contributed; without them this book would not have been possible.

PART I

REGIONAL ANATOMY

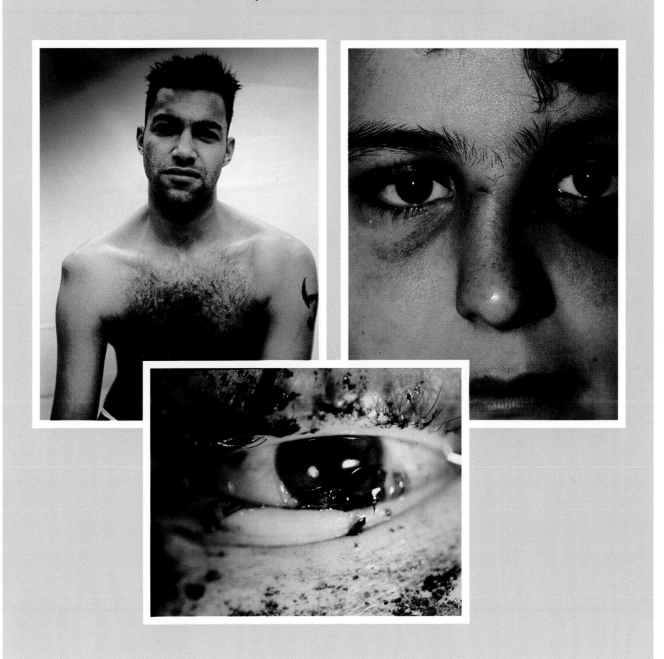

CHAPTER 1

HEAD AND FACIAL TRAUMA

David W. Munter
Timothy D. McGuirk

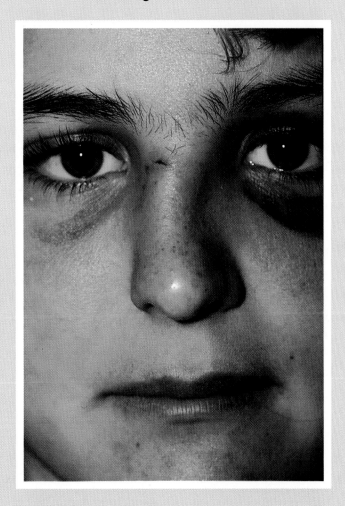

Associated Clinical Features

The skull base comprises the floors of the anterior, middle, and posterior cranial fossae. Trauma resulting in fractures to this basilar area typically do not have localizing symptoms. Plain skull radiographs are poor in identifying these fractures. Indirect signs of the injury may include visible evidence of bleeding from the fracture into surrounding soft tissue such as a Battle's sign or raccoon eyes (Figs. 1.1, 1.2). Bleeding into other structures including hemotympanum (Fig. 1.3) or blood in the sphenoid sinus seen as an air-fluid level may also be seen. Cerebrospinal fluid (CSF) leaks may also be evident and noted as clear or pink rhinorrhea. If CSF is present, a dextrose stick test may be positive. The fluid can be placed on filter paper and a "halo" or double ring may be seen (Fig. 1.4).

Differential Diagnosis

Direct trauma without skull fracture can result in external ecchymosis. Barotrauma can cause hemotympanum. Facial injuries and fractures can cause facial ecchymosis.

ED Treatment and Disposition

The mainstay of therapy is to identify underlying brain injury, which is best accomplished by CT. CT is also the best diagnostic tool for identifying the fracture site, but fractures may not always be evident. Evidence of open communication such as a CSF leak mandates neurosurgical consultation and admission. Otherwise, the decision for admission is based on the patient's clinical condition, other associated injuries, and evidence of underlying brain injury as seen on CT. The use of antibiotics in the presence of a CSF leak is controversial because of the possibility of selecting resistant organisms.

Clinical Pearls

1. The clinical manifestations of basilar skull fracture may take several hours to fully develop.
2. Since plain films are unhelpful, there should be a low threshold for head CT in any patient with head trauma, loss of consciousness, obtundation, severe headache, visual changes, or nausea or vomiting.
3. The use of filter paper or dextrose stick test to determine if CSF is present in rhinorrhea is not 100% reliable.

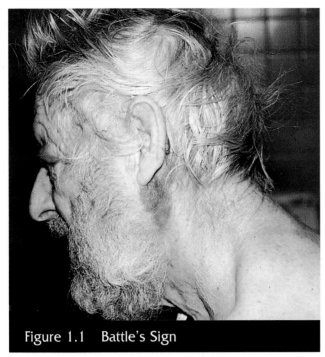

Figure 1.1 Battle's Sign

Ecchymosis in the postauricular area develops when the fracture line communicates with the mastoid air cells, resulting in blood accumulating in the cutaneous tissue. This sign may take several hours to fully develop. (Courtesy of Daniel L. Savitt, MD.)

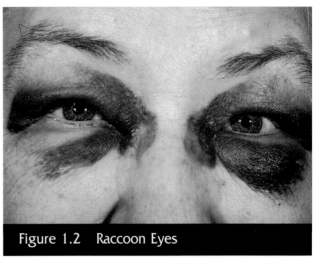

Figure 1.2 Raccoon Eyes

Ecchymosis in the periorbital area, resulting from bleeding from a fracture site in the anterior portion of the skull base. May also be caused by facial fractures. (Courtesy of Frank Birinyi, MD.)

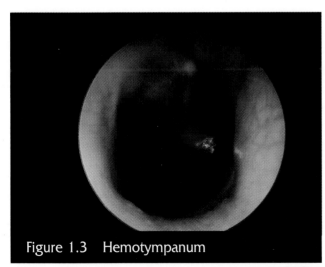

Figure 1.3 Hemotympanum

Seen in a basilar skull fracture when the fracture line communicates with the auditory canal, resulting in bleeding into the middle ear. Blood can be seen behind the tympanic membrane. (Courtesy of Richard A. Chole, MD, PhD.)

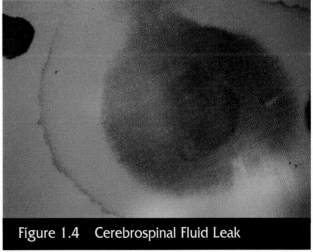

Figure 1.4 Cerebrospinal Fluid Leak

This example, from the nose, can be difficult to distinguish from blood or mucus. The distinctive double-ring sign, seen here, comprises blood *(inner ring)* and CSF *(outer ring)*. The reliability of this test has been questioned. (Courtesy of David W. Munter, MD.)

Associated Clinical Features

Depressed skull fractures typically occur when a large force is applied over a small area. They are classified as open if the skin above them is lacerated (Fig. 1.5) and closed if the overlying skin is intact. Abrasions, contusions, and hematomas may also be present over the fracture site. The patient's mental status can range from comatose to fully alert depending on the extent of the associated brain injury. Soft tissue bleeding and swelling may be present. Evidence of other injuries such as a basilar fracture or facial fractures may also be present.

Differential Diagnosis

Direct trauma can cause abrasions, contusions, hematomas, and lacerations without an underlying depressed skull fracture. Every laceration to the scalp should be explored and palpated to rule out depression of a fracture. Alterations in mental status may occur with or without fracture. Penetrating injuries to the skull and brain can produce a similar clinical picture.

ED Treatment and Disposition

Plain films have been suggested for suspected depressed skull fractures and if positive should be followed by CT, which will more accurately demonstrate the degree of depression as well as any underlying brain injury (Fig. 1.6). Others suggest that plain films offer little diagnostic utility and recommend CT with its more accurate bone windows for any suspected depressed skull fracture. When depressed skull fractures are noted on plain films or CT, immediate neurosurgical consultation is required. Open fractures also require antibiotics and tetanus prophylaxis as indicated. The decision to observe or operate immediately is made by the neurosurgeon. Children younger than 2 years with skull fractures can develop leptomeningeal cysts. These cysts, which are extrusion of CSF or brain through dural defects, are associated with skull fractures. For this reason, children younger than 2 years with skull fractures require follow-up or admission.

Clinical Pearls

1. Gently palpate all scalp injuries including lacerations for evidence of fractures or depression. When fragments are depressed more than 3 to 5 mm below the inner table, penetration of the dura and injury to the cortex are more likely.
2. Children with depressed skull fractures are more likely to develop epilepsy.
3. The index of suspicion for nonaccidental trauma should be raised for children younger than 2 years with depressed skull fractures.

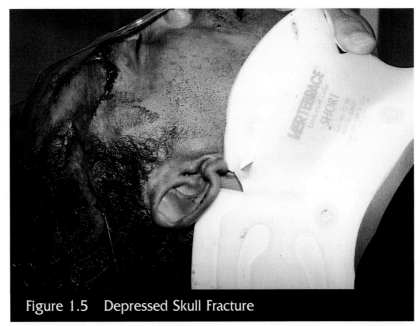

Figure 1.5 Depressed Skull Fracture

A scalp laceration overlying a depressed skull fracture. Wearing a sterile glove, digitally explore all scalp lacerations for evidence of fracture or depression. (Courtesy of David W. Munter, MD.)

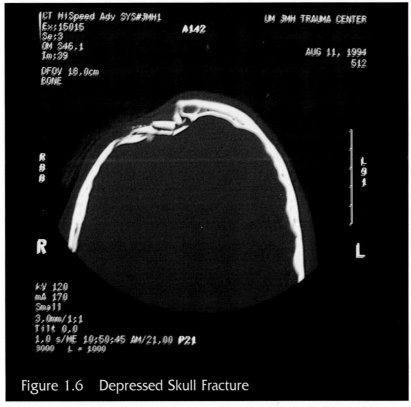

Figure 1.6 Depressed Skull Fracture

CT demonstrating depressed skull fracture. (Courtesy of David W. Munter, MD.)

Associated Clinical Features

Clinically significant nasal fractures are almost always evident on examination, with deformity, swelling, and ecchymosis present (Fig. 1.7). Injuries may occur to other surrounding bony structures, including fractures of the orbit, frontal sinus, or cribriform plate. A history of a mechanism with significant force, loss of consciousness, or findings of facial bone injury or CSF leak should alert the clinician to look for these associated injuries. Epistaxis may be due to a septal or turbinate laceration, but can also be seen with fractures of surrounding bones including the cribriform plate. Septal hematoma (Fig. 1.8) is a rare but important complication that, if untreated, may result in necrosis of the septal cartilage and a resultant "saddlenose" deformity.

Differential Diagnosis

Nasal fractures may have associated facial injuries such as orbital, frontal sinus, or cribriform plate fractures, and these more serious injuries must be ruled out. A simple nasal contusion may present identically to a simple nasal fracture with pain, swelling, and ecchymosis. A frontonasoethmoid fracture has nasal or frontal crepitus and may have associated telecanthus or obstruction of the nasolacrimal duct.

ED Treatment and Disposition

Look for more serious injuries first. Patients with associated facial bone deformity or tenderness may require radiographs to rule out facial fractures. Nasal fractures rarely require radiographs (Fig. 1.9). Obvious deformities are referred within 2 to 5 days for reduction after the swelling has subsided. Nasal injuries without deformity need only conservative therapy with an analgesic and possibly a nasal decongestant. Septal hematomas must be immediately drained, with packing placed to prevent reaccumulation. In some cases, epistaxis may not be controlled by pressure alone and may require nasal packing. Lacerations overlying a simple nasal fracture should be vigorously irrigated and primarily closed with the patient placed on antibiotic coverage. Complex nasal lacerations with underlying fractures should be referred for closure. Nasal fractures with mild angulation and without displacement may be reduced in the ED by manipulating the nose with the examiner's thumbs into the correct alignment.

Clinical Pearls

1. Rule out any life threats or serious associated injuries.
2. Control epistaxis to perform a good intranasal examination. If there is no epistaxis or deformity, treat the patient with ice and analgesics. If obvious deformity is present, including a new septal deviation or deformity, treat with ice and analgesics and refer to ENT in 2 to 5 days for reduction.
3. Although the effectiveness of prophylactic antibiotics to prevent toxic shock syndrome is unproved, every patient discharged with nasal packing should be placed on antistaphylococcal antibiotics and referred to ENT in 2 to 3 days.
4. Consider cribriform plate fractures in patients with clear rhinorrhea after nasal injury, with the understanding that this finding may be delayed.
5. Check every patient for a septal hematoma.

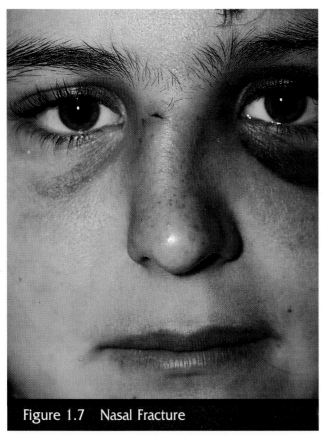

Figure 1.7   Nasal Fracture

Deformity is evident on examination. Note periocular ecchymosis indicating the possibility of other facial fractures (or injuries). The decision to obtain radiographs is based on clinical findings. A radiograph is not indicated for an isolated simple nasal fracture. (Courtesy of David W. Munter, MD.)

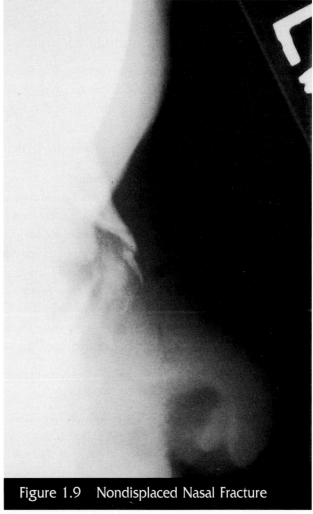

Figure 1.9   Nondisplaced Nasal Fracture

Radiograph of a fracture of the nasal spine, for which no treatment other than ice and analgesics is needed. This radiograph did not change the treatment or disposition of the patient. (Courtesy of Lorenz F. Lassen, MD.)

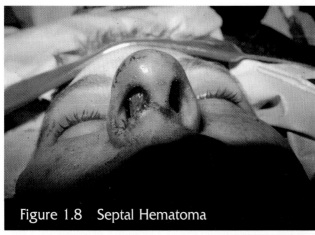

Figure 1.8   Septal Hematoma

A bluish, grapelike mass on the nasal septum. If untreated, this can result in septal necrosis and a saddle-nose deformity. An incision, drainage, and packing are indicated. (Courtesy of Lawrence B. Stack, MD.)

Associated Clinical Features

The zygoma bone has two major components, the zygomatic arch and the body. The arch forms the inferior and lateral orbit, and the body forms the malar eminence of the face. Fractures to the zygoma are usually the result of blunt trauma. Direct blows to the arch can result in isolated arch fractures (Figs. 1.10). These present clinically with pain on opening the mouth secondary to the insertion of the temporalis muscle at the arch or impingement on the coronoid process. More extensive trauma can result in the "tripod fracture," which consists of fractures through three structures: the frontozygomatic suture; the maxillary process of the zygoma including the inferior orbital floor, inferior orbital rim, and lateral wall of the maxillary sinus; and the zygomatic arch (Figs. 1.11, 1.12). Clinically, patients present with a flattened malar eminence and edema and ecchymosis to the area, with a palpable step-off on examination. Injury to the infraorbital nerve may result in infraorbital paresthesia, and gaze disturbances may result from injury to orbital contents. Subcutaneous emphysema may be caused by a fracture of the antral wall at the zygomatic buttress.

Differential Diagnosis

Other facial fractures, including LeFort II and III fractures, may involve the zygoma bone or orbit. These fractures typically have more extensive facial trauma. Orbital blowout fractures may present with eye findings, but the malar eminence appears normal.

ED Treatment and Disposition

Plain films, including a Waters view and "jughandle" view (a submental-vertex view of the zygomatic arches), demonstrate the fracture and evaluate the zygomaticomaxillary complex. In the case of a tripod fracture, facial CT will best show the involvement and degree of displacement. Since plain films often do not adequately demonstrate all elements of the fracture, patients with evidence of a tripod fracture should have CT on an urgent basis to help identify the extent of bony injuries. The CT results guide the need for urgent referral. Simple zygomatic arch or tripod fractures without eye injury can be treated with ice and analgesics, and referred for delayed operative consideration in 5 to 7 days. More extensive tripod fractures, or those with eye injuries, should be referred more urgently. Decongestants and broad spectrum antibiotics are generally recommended for tripod fractures, since the fracture crosses into the maxillary sinus.

Clinical Pearls

1. Tripod fractures are often associated with orbital and ocular trauma. Palpate the zygomatic arch and orbital rims carefully for a step-off deformity.
2. Examine for eye findings such as diplopia, hyphema, or retinal detachment. Check for infraorbital paresthesia indicating injury or impingement of the second division of cranial nerve V.
3. Visual inspection of the malar eminence from several angles (especially by viewing the area from over the head of the patient in the coronal plane Fig. 1.11) allows detection of a subtle abnormality.
4. Insist on adequate radiographs of the zygomatic arches, which require good positioning of the patient to obtain.

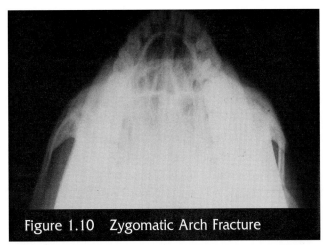

Figure 1.10 Zygomatic Arch Fracture

Jughandle view of the zygomatic arch demonstrating a depressed fracture. Operative reduction can be delayed for several days. (Courtesy of Timothy D. McGuirk, DO.)

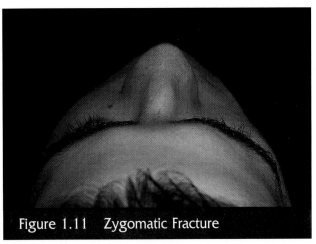

Figure 1.11 Zygomatic Fracture

Patient with blunt trauma to the zygoma. Flattening of the right malar eminence is evident. (Courtesy of Amchein, DDS.)

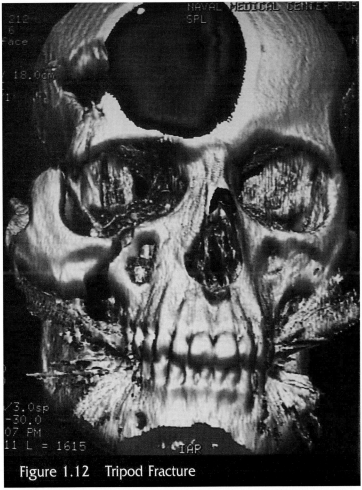

Figure 1.12 Tripod Fracture

The fracture lines involved in a tripod fracture are demonstrated in this three-dimensional CT reconstruction. The large defect in the frontal area is artifact from the reconstruction. (Courtesy of Patrick W. Lappert, MD.)

Associated Clinical Features

All LeFort facial fractures involve the maxilla (Fig. 1.13). Clinically, the patient has facial injuries, swelling, and ecchymosis (Figs. 1.14, 1.15). LeFort I fractures are those involving an area under the nasal fossa. LeFort II fractures involve a pyramidal area including the maxilla, nasal bones, and medial orbits. LeFort III fractures, sometimes described as craniofacial dissociation, involve the maxilla, zygoma, nasal and ethmoid bones, and the bones of the base of the skull. Airway compromise may be associated with LeFort II and III fractures. Physical examination is sometimes helpful in distinguishing the three. The examiner places fingers on the bridge of the nose, and tries to move the central maxillary incisors with the other hand. If only the maxilla moves, a LeFort I is present, movement of the upper jaw and nose indicates a LeFort II, and movement of the entire midface and zygoma indicates a LeFort III. Because of the extent of LeFort II and III fractures, they may be associated with cribriform plate fractures and CSF rhinorrhea. The force required to sustain a LeFort II or III fracture is considerable, and associated brain or cervical spine injuries are common.

Differential Diagnosis

LeFort II and III fractures can be difficult to distinguish, and combination LeFort fractures (e.g., LeFort II on one side and LeFort III on the other) are common. Tripod and frontonasoethmoid fractures may be present in blunt facial trauma as well.

ED Treatment and Disposition

Patients with associated facial bone deformity or tenderness may require radiographs to rule out facial fractures. Plain facial films will reveal the presence of facial fractures, but are less helpful in determining the type or extent. Head and facial CT, including three-dimensional re-creations, offer much more useful information. Management of LeFort I fractures may involve only dental splinting and oral surgery referral, but management of LeFort II and III fractures normally requires admission because of associated injuries, as well as definitive operative repair. Epistaxis may be difficult to control in LeFort II and III fractures, in rare cases requiring intraoperative arterial ligation.

Clinical Pearls

1. Attention should be focused on immediate airway management, since the massive edema associated with LeFort II and III fractures may quickly lead to airway compromise.
2. Nasotracheal intubation should be avoided because of the possibility of intracranial passage.
3. Any serious facial trauma may also be associated with cervical spine injuries.
4. Associated cranial injuries are common and are best evaluated by CT.
5. An occult CSF leak, if not recognized, may result in significant morbidity. Suspected CSF leaks require neurosurgical consultation.
6. The best diagnostic modality for delineation of the extent of injuries is CT of the facial bones.

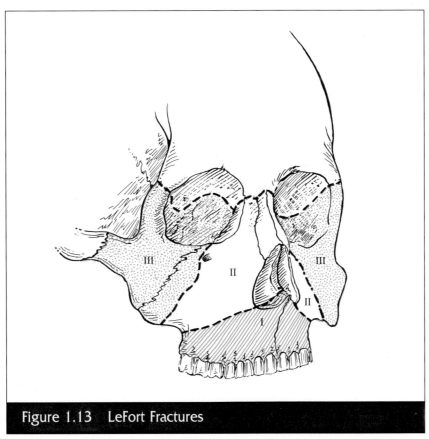

Figure 1.13   LeFort Fractures

Illustration of the fracture lines of LeFort I (alveolar), LeFort II (zygomatic maxillary complex), and LeFort III (cranial facial dysostosis) fractures.

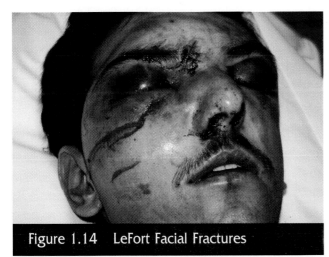

Figure 1.14   LeFort Facial Fractures

Clinical photograph of patient with blunt facial trauma. Note the ecchymosis and edema. This patient sustained a LeFort II/III fracture (a LeFort II fracture on one side and a LeFort III on the other), and associated intracranial hemorrhages. (Courtesy of Stephen Corbett, MD.)

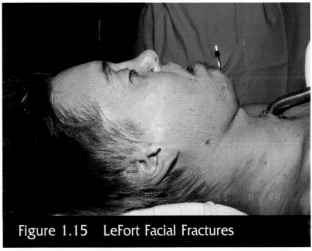

Figure 1.15   LeFort Facial Fractures

Clinical photograph of patient with blunt facial trauma. Patient demonstrates the classic "dish face" deformity (depressed midface) associated with bilateral LeFort III fractures. (Courtesy of Robert Schnarrs, MD.)

Associated Clinical Features

Blowout fractures occur when the globe sustains a direct blunt force. There are two mechanisms of injury. The first is a true blowout fracture where all energy is transmitted to the globe. The spherical globe is stronger than the thin orbital floor, and the force is transmitted to the thin orbital floor or medially through the ethmoid bones with the resultant fracture. The object causing the injury must be smaller than 5 to 6 cm, otherwise the globe is protected by the surrounding orbit. Fists or small balls are the typical causative agents. This mechanism of injury is more likely to cause entrapment and globe injury. The second mechanism of injury occurs when the energy from the blow is transmitted to the infraorbital rim causing a buckling of the orbital floor. Entrapment and globe injury is less likely with this mechanism of injury. Patients with blowout fractures have periorbital ecchymosis and lid edema (Figs. 1.16, 1.17), but may sustain eye injuries as well, including chemosis, subconjunctival hemorrhage, or infraorbital numbness from injury to the infraorbital nerve. Other eye injuries should be sought and ruled out with a careful physical examination and include corneal abrasion, hyphema, enophthalmos, proptosis, iridoplegia, dislocated lens, retinal tear, retinal detachment, and ruptured globe. If the inferior rectus muscle is extruded into the fracture, it may become entrapped, and upward gaze is limited with resultant diplopia (Figs. 1.18, 1.19). Due to the communication with the maxillary sinus, subcutaneous emphysema is common.

Differential Diagnosis

Orbital contusions present with similar physical findings. Orbital rim fractures are clinically similar to orbital blowout fractures. Other facial fractures (zygoma, tripod, LeFort) may involve the orbital floor, but involve more extensive injuries to the face outside of the orbit.

ED Treatment and Disposition

Plain radiography to include a Caldwell view (showing orbital rim and walls) and a Waters view (orbital floor and roof) demonstrates the fracture. Patients without eye injury or entrapment may be treated conservatively with ice and analgesics, and referred for follow-up in 2 to 3 days. Patients with blood in the maxillary sinus are usually treated with antibiotics. Strongly consider an ophthalmology consultation in patients with a true blowout fracture (all energy transmitted to the globe), since up to 30% of these patients sustain a globe injury. Patients with entrapment should receive a CT of the orbits and be referred on a same-day basis. Most specialists will observe fractures with entrapment for 10 to 14 days to allow for resolution of edema prior to operative repair.

Clinical Pearls

1. Enophthalmos, limited upward gaze, diplopia with upward gaze, or infraorbital anesthesia from entrapment or injury to the infraorbital nerve should heighten suspicion of a blowout fracture.
2. Compare the pupillary level on the affected side with the unaffected side, since it may be lower from prolapse of the orbital contents into the maxillary sinus. Subtle abnormalities may be appreciated as an asymmetric corneal light reflex (Hirschberg's reflex).
3. Subcutaneous emphysema on clinical examination, a soft-tissue teardrop along the roof of the maxillary sinus on plain film, or an air-fluid level in the maxillary sinus on plain film should also be interpreted as evidence of a blowout fracture.

4. Some patients present with unusual complaints, such as their eye swelling up after blowing their nose (from subcutaneous emphysema) or air bubbles emanating from the tear duct.

5. Carefully examine the eye for visual acuity, hyphema, or retinal detachment. Remember to assess the nose for a septal hematoma.

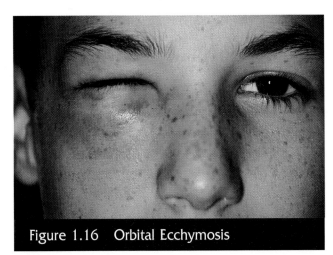

Figure 1.16   Orbital Ecchymosis

Sustained from blunt trauma to the globe, with some of the force directed to the inferior orbital rim. This patient presents with subtle signs only (ecchymosis and swelling with no entrapment or eye injury), yet has the classic signs on plain films (Figure 1.17). This patient demonstrates that orbital floor fractures can present with subtle physical findings. (Courtesy of Kevin J. Knoop, MD, MS.)

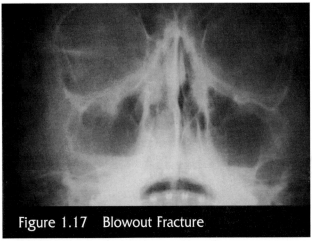

Figure 1.17   Blowout Fracture

Plain film demonstrating a fracture of the floor of the right orbit, with a teardrop sign due to extruded orbital contents. There is an associated air-fluid level in the maxillary sinus due to blood. Note the two lines seen at the inferior orbit: the infraorbital rim and inferior floor of the orbit. These are well visualized on the unaffected side, but disrupted on the affected side. (Courtesy of Kevin J. Knoop, MD, MS.)

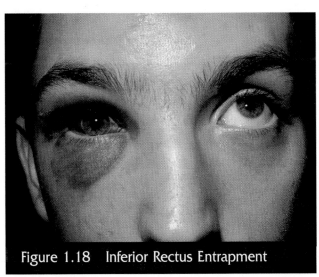

Figure 1.18   Inferior Rectus Entrapment

The inferior rectus muscle is entrapped within the blowout fracture. When the patient tries to look upward, the affected eye has limited upward gaze. The patient experiences diplopia with this maneuver. (Courtesy of Lawrence B. Stack, MD.)

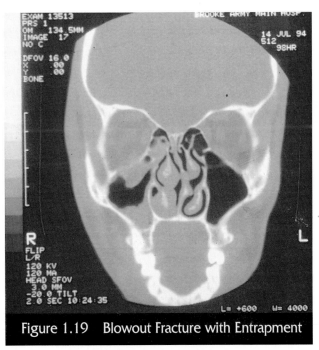

Figure 1.19   Blowout Fracture with Entrapment

CT of the patient demonstrating the entrapped muscle extruding into the maxillary sinus. (Courtesy of Lawrence B. Stack, MD.)

Associated Clinical Features

A history of blunt trauma, mandibular pain, and possible malocclusion is normally seen with mandibular fractures. A step-off in the dental line (Fig. 1.20) or ecchymosis or hematoma to the floor of the mouth are often present. Mandibular fractures may be open to the oral cavity as manifested by gum lacerations. Dental trauma may be associated. Other clinical features include inferior alveolar or mental nerve paresthesia, loose or missing teeth, dysphagia, trismus, or ecchymosis of the floor of the mouth (considered pathognomonic) (Fig. 1.21). Multiple mandibular fractures are present in more than 50% of cases because of the ring like structure of the mandible. Mandibular fractures are often classified as favorable or unfavorable, depending on the location and resultant displacement forces exerted by the associated musculature. Those fractures displaced by the masseter muscle are unfavorable (Fig. 1.22) and inevitably require fixation, whereas fractures that are not displaced by traction are favorable and in some cases will not require fixation. Injuries creating unstable mandibular fractures may create airway obstruction, because the support for the tongue is lost. Mandibular fractures are also classified based on the anatomic location of the fracture (Fig. 1.23).

Differential Diagnosis

Contusions have a similar presentation and can be differentiated only radiographically. Dislocation of the mandibular condyles may also result from blunt trauma and will always have associated malocclusion typified by an inability to close the mouth. Isolated dental trauma may have a similar presentation, and underlying mandibular fracture should be ruled out.

ED Disposition and Treatment

The best view for evaluating mandibular trauma is a dental panoramic view, which should be obtained if available. Plain films should include anteroposterior (AP), bilateral oblique, and a Townes view to evaluate the condyles. Nondisplaced fractures can be treated with analgesics, soft diet, and referral to oral surgery in 1 to 2 days. Displaced fractures, open fractures, and fractures with associated dental trauma need more urgent referral. All mandibular fractures should be treated with antibiotics effective against anaerobic oral flora (clindamycin, Amoxicillin clavalanate), and tetanus prophylaxis should be given if needed. The Barton's bandage has been suggested to immobilize the jaw in the ED.

Clinical Pearls

1. The presence of disfiguring facial injuries can be distracting. The primary consideration in the evaluation of the patient with facial fractures is the assessment and treatment of life-threatening injuries.
2. Any patient with trauma and malocclusion should be considered to have a mandibular fracture.
3. The most sensitive sign of a mandibular fracture is malocclusion. The jaw will deviate toward the side of a unilateral condyle fracture on maximal opening of the mouth. A nonfractured mandible should be able to hold a tongue blade between the molars tightly enough to break it off. There should be no pain when attempting to rotate the tongue blade between the molars.

4. Bilateral parasymphaseal fractures may cause acute airway obstruction in the supine patient. This is relieved by pulling the subluxed mandible and soft tissue forward and, in patients in whom the cervical spine has been cleared, by elevating the patient to a sitting position.

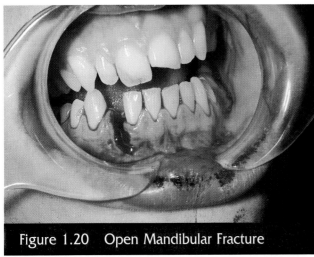

Figure 1.20   Open Mandibular Fracture

The open fracture line is evident clinically. There is slight misalignment of the teeth present. (Courtesy of Edward S. Amrhein, DDS.)

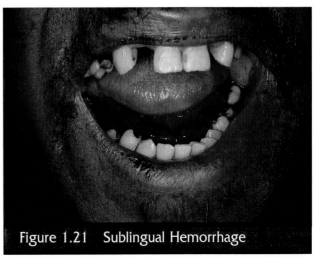

Figure 1.21   Sublingual Hemorrhage

Hemorrhage or ecchymosis in the sublingual area is pathognomonic for mandibular fracture. (Courtesy of Daniel L. Savitt, MD.)

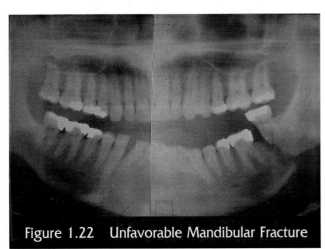

Figure 1.22   Unfavorable Mandibular Fracture

Dental panoramic view demonstrating a mandibular fracture with obvious misalignment due to the distracting forces of the masseter muscle. (Courtesy of Edward S. Amrhein, DDS.)

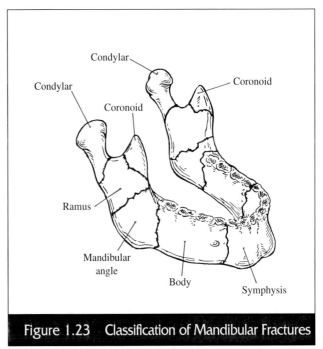

Figure 1.23   Classification of Mandibular Fractures

Classification based on anatomic location of the fracture.

Associated Clinical Features

Injuries to the external ear may be open or closed. Blunt external ear trauma may cause a hematoma (otohematoma) of the pinna (Fig. 1.24), which if untreated, may result in cartilage necrosis and chronic scarring or further cartilage formation and permanent deformity ("cauliflower ear") (Fig. 1.25). Open injuries include lacerations (with and without cartilage exposure) and avulsions (Fig. 1.26).

Differential Diagnosis

These injuries are normally self-evident. Pinna hematomas and contusions can sometimes be difficult to distinguish, but flocculence is the hallmark of the hematoma.

ED Treatment and Disposition

Pinna hematomas must undergo incision and drainage or large needle aspiration using sterile technique, followed by a pressure dressing to prevent reaccumulation of the hematoma. This procedure may need to be repeated several times, hence, after emergency department drainage, the patient is treated with antistaphylococcal antibiotics and referred to ENT or plastic surgery for follow-up in 24 h. Lacerations must be carefully examined for cartilage involvement, and if present, copious irrigation, closure, and postrepair oral antibiotics covering skin flora are indicated. Simple skin lacerations may be repaired primarily with nonabsorbable 6-0 sutures. The dressing after laceration repair is just as important as the primary repair. If a compression dressing is not placed, hematoma formation can occur. Complex lacerations or avulsions normally require ENT or plastic surgery referral.

Clinical Pearls

1. Pinna hematomas may take hours to develop, so give patients with blunt ear trauma careful discharge instructions, with a follow-up in 12 to 24 h to check for hematoma development.
2. Failure to adequately drain a hematoma, reaccumulation of the hematoma owing to a faulty pressure dressing, or inadequate follow-up increases the risk of infection of the pinna (perichondritis) or of a disfiguring cauliflower ear.
3. Copiously irrigate injuries with lacerated cartilage, which are usually able to be managed by primary closure of the overlying skin. Direct closure of the cartilage is rarely necessary and is indicated only for proper alignment, which helps lessen later distortion. Use a minimal number of absorbable 5-0 or 6-0 sutures through the perichondrium.
4. Lacerations to the lateral aspect of the pinna should be minimally debrided because of the lack of tissue at this site to cover the exposed cartilage.
5. In the case of an avulsion injury, the avulsed part should be cleansed, wrapped in saline-moistened gauze, placed in a sterile container, then placed on ice to await reimplantation by ENT.

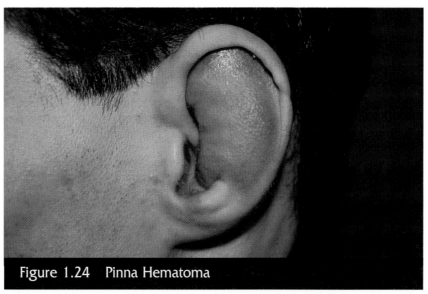

Figure 1.24   Pinna Hematoma

A hematoma has developed and is characterized by swelling, discoloration, ecchymosis, and flocculence. Immediate incision and drainage or aspiration is indicated, followed by an ear compression dressing. (Courtesy of C. Bruce MacDonald, MD.)

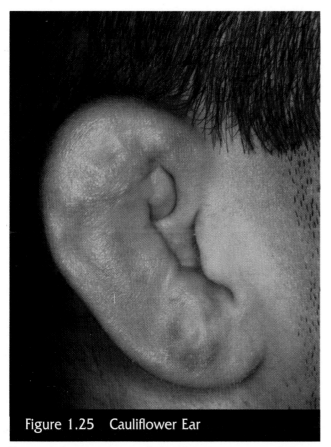

Figure 1.25   Cauliflower Ear

Repeated pinna trauma or undrained hematomas can result in cartilage necrosis and subsequent deforming scar formation. (Courtesy of Timothy D. McGuirk, DO.)

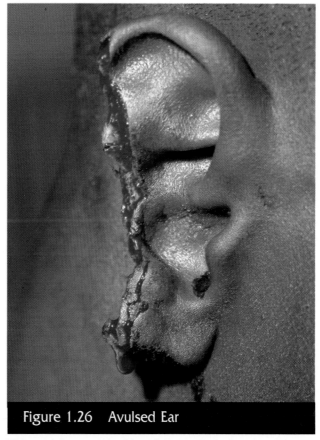

Figure 1.26   Avulsed Ear

This ear injury, sustained in a fight, resulted when the pinna was bitten off. Plastic repair is needed. Wrap the avulsed part in sterile gauze soaked with saline, and place in a sterile container on ice. (Courtesy of David W. Munter, MD.)

Associated Clinical Features

Blunt frontal area trauma may result in a depressed frontal sinus fracture. Often, there is an associated laceration (Fig. 1.27). Isolated frontal fractures (Fig. 1.28) normally do not have the associated features of massive blunt facial trauma such as seen in LeFort II and III fractures. Careful nasal speculum examination may reveal blood or CSF leak high in the nasal cavity. Posterior table involvement can lead to mucopyocoele or epidural empyema as late sequelae. Involvement of the posterior wall of the frontal sinus may occur and result in cranial injury or dural tear.

Differential Diagnosis

Simple lacerations or contusions of the frontal area may not involve fractures. Frontal fractures may be part of a complex of facial fractures such as seen in frontonasoethmoid fractures, but generally more extensive facial trauma is required.

ED Treatment and Disposition

Frontal sinus fractures revealed on plain films of the frontal bones, including a PA, lateral, and Waters view, may be quite subtle. The extent of the frontal injury, especially posterior table involvement, is best investigated with bone windows on CT (Fig. 1.29). Fractures involving only the anterior table of the frontal sinus can be treated conservatively with referral to ENT or plastic surgery in 1 to 2 days. Fractures involving the posterior table require urgent neurosurgical referral. Frontal sinus fractures are usually covered with high-dose antibiotics against both skin and sinus flora (second- or third-generation cephalosporins). ED management also includes control of epistaxis, application of ice packs, and analgesia.

Clinical Pearls

1. Explore every frontal laceration digitally before repair. Digital palpation is sensitive for identifying frontal fractures, although false positives from lacerations extending through the periosteum can occur.
2. Communication of irrigating solutions with the nose or mouth indicates a breach in the frontal sinus.
3. For serious injuries, a CT scan is mandatory to assess the posterior aspect of the sinus and for possible intracranial injury.

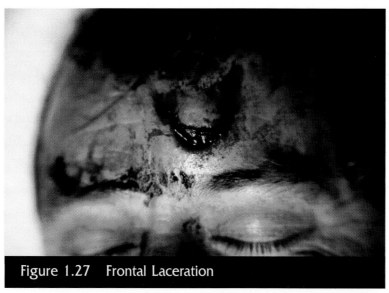

Figure 1.27   Frontal Laceration

Any laceration over the frontal sinuses should be explored to rule out a fracture.
This laceration was found to have an associated frontal fracture. (Courtesy of
David W. Munter, MD.)

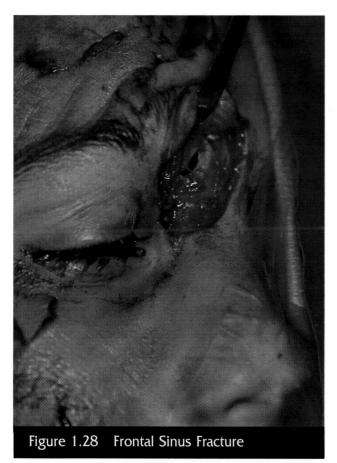

Figure 1.28   Frontal Sinus Fracture

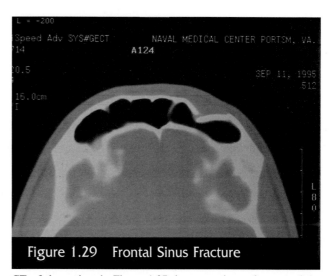

Figure 1.29   Frontal Sinus Fracture

CT of the patient in Figure 1.27 demonstrating a fracture of the
anterior table of the frontal sinus. (Courtesy of David W. Munter,
MD.)

Fracture defect seen at the base of a laceration over the frontal sinus.
(Courtesy of Jeffrey Kuhn, MD.)

Associated Clinical Features

Normally the result of blunt orbital trauma, the exophthalmos develops as a retrobulbar hematoma pushes the globe outward. Patients present with periorbital edema, ecchymosis (Fig. 1.30), a marked decrease in visual acuity, and an afferent pupillary defect in the involved eye. The exophthalmos, which may be obscured by periorbital edema, can be better appreciated from a superior view (Fig. 1.31). Visual acuity may be affected by the direct trauma to the eye, compression of the retinal artery, or more rarely, neuropraxia of the optic nerve.

Differential Diagnosis

Periorbital ecchymosis and edema can result from blunt trauma without a retrobulbar hematoma. Traumatic chemosis can present with exophthalmos. Visual impairment can result from retinal detachment, hyphema, globe rupture, or any number of nontraumatic conditions. Nontraumatic exophthalmos can be caused by cavernous sinus thrombosis, a complication of frontal sinusitis, or endocrine (thyrotoxicosis) disorders.

ED Treatment and Disposition

CT is the best modality to determine the presence and extent of a retrobulbar hematoma and associated facial or orbital fractures (Fig. 1.32). Referral to ENT and ophthalmology is indicated on an urgent basis. An emergent lateral canthotomy decompresses the orbit and can be performed in the ED. Emergency treatment can be sight-saving.

Clinical Pearls

1. The retrobulbar hematoma and resultant exophthalmos may not develop for hours. Give careful discharge instructions to any patient with periorbital trauma.
2. Perform a careful ophthalmic examination with visual acuity, since associated conditions such as hyphema or retinal detachment are common.
3. A subtle exophthalmos may be detected by looking down over the head of the patient and viewing the eye from the coronal plane.
4. Lateral canthotomy is indicated for emergent treatment of patients with traumatic exophthalmos who demonstrate profound ischemic signs and symptoms of an afferent pupillary defect and decreased vision.
5. An afferent pupillary defect in a patient with blunt trauma to the face or eye with normal visual acuity may be pharmacologically induced.

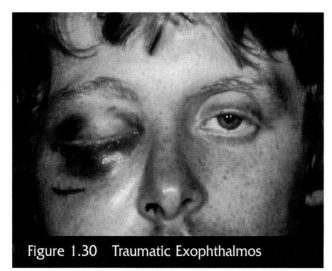

Figure 1.30   Traumatic Exophthalmos

Blunt trauma resulting in periorbital edema and ecchymosis, which obscures the exophthalmos in this patient. The exophthalmos is not obvious in the AP view and can therefore be initially unappreciated. Figure 1.31 shows the same patient viewed in the coronal plane from over the forehead. (Courtesy of Frank Birinyi, MD.)

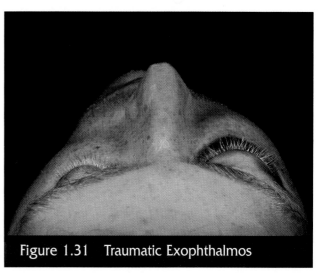

Figure 1.31   Traumatic Exophthalmos

Superior view demonstrating the right-sided exophthalmos. (Courtesy of Frank Birinyi, MD.)

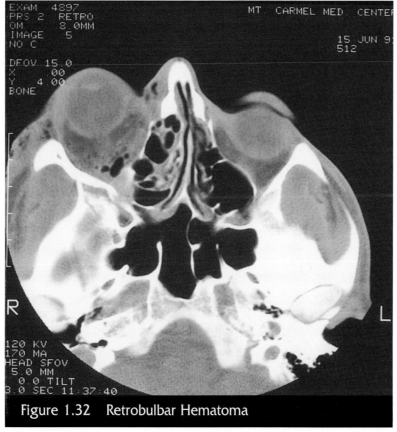

Figure 1.32   Retrobulbar Hematoma

CT of the patient in Figs. 1.30, 1.31 with right retrobulbar hematoma and traumatic exophthalmos. (Courtesy of Frank Birinyi, MD.)

EYE

CHAPTER 2

OPHTHALMOLOGIC CONDITIONS

Frank Birinyi
Thomas F. Mauger

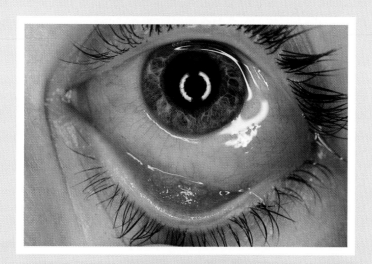

NEONATAL CONJUNCTIVITIS (OPHTHALMIA NEONATORUM)

Associated Clinical Features

Neonatal conjunctivitis is a newborn conjunctival infection acquired either during birth (during passage through the mother's cervix and vagina) or from cross infection in the neonatal period. Microbiologic etiologies include *Chlamydia trachomatis,* viruses (herpes simplex), and bacteria (*Neisseria gonorrhoeae, Staphylococcus aureus, Streptococcus pneumoniae,* groups A and B streptococci, *Haemophilus* species, *Pseudomonas aeruginosa,* and *Escherichia coli*). Of these, *S. aureus* is the most frequent, and *N. gonorrhoeae* is the most important. Clinical findings in neonatal conjunctivitis include drainage, conjunctival hyperemia, chemosis, and lid edema.

N. gonorrhoeae presents as a hyperacute bilateral conjunctivitis. Distinctive findings include a copious purulent drainage (Fig. 2.1) and preauricular adenopathy. The incubation period, like that for sexually transmitted *N. gonorrhoeae,* is 3 to 5 days. In chlamydial conjunctivitis the incubation period is 5 to 12 days. Distinctive clinical features of chlamydial conjunctivitis may include unilateral conjunctivitis and concomitant otitis media or pneumonia. Herpes simplex conjunctivitis generally begins 2 to 14 days after birth; fluorescein staining demonstrates epithelial dendrites.

Differential Diagnosis

Dacryocystitis, corneal abrasions, foreign body, and an obstructed nasolacrimal duct present with redness and tearing. Neonatal glaucoma may also be mistaken for conjunctivitis; findings include eye pain, photophobia, corneal haze, corneal enlargement, and excessive tearing.

ED Treatment and Disposition

With any form of neonatal conjunctivitis, smears and cultures are mandatory and therapy should begin immediately thereafter. Conjunctival (palpebral) scrapings for cultures and Gram's staining are more revealing than examination of the discharge itself. A neonate whose Gram's stain demonstrates gram-negative diplococci requires intravenous antibiotics (penicillin G, ceftriaxone, or cefotaxime) as well as topical penicillin. Treatment should also include frequent saline irrigation of the conjunctival cul-de-sac.

Chlamydial conjunctivitis is treated with oral erythromycin estolate. Neonatal bacterial conjunctivitis that is neither gonococcal nor chlamydial may be treated with antibiotic ointment (erthyromycin, tetracycline, gentamicin) and should be reevaluated in 24 h. In these cases, systemic therapy is needed only in the event of systemic disease. Herpes simplex conjunctivitis is treated with IV acyclovir and topical trifluorothymidine.

Evaluation of the newborn's parents should be undertaken in neonatal conjunctivitis due to gonococcus, chlamydia, or herpes simplex virus.

Clinical Pearls

1. The "rule of fives" is fairly accurate in predicting the most likely etiologic agent.

0 to 5 days	Gonococcus
5 days to 5 weeks	*Chlamydia*
5 weeks to 5 years	*Streptococcus* or *H. influenzae* species

2. The cornea should be examined for involvement. Corneal ulcers, perforation, permanent scarring, and blindness can quickly result from gonococcal eye infection in the neonate. It is one of the few urgent conjunctival infections.

3. A detailed maternal history may help with the diagnosis of neonatal conjunctivitis secondary to gonococcus, chlamydia, or herpes.

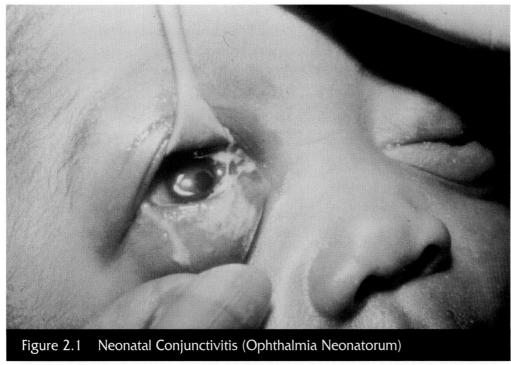

Figure 2.1   Neonatal Conjunctivitis (Ophthalmia Neonatorum)

Copious and purulent drainage in a newborn with neonatal gonococcal conjunctivitis. (Reprinted with permission of American Academy of Ophthalmology, *Eye Trauma and Emergencies: A Slide-Script Program.* San Francisco, 1985.)

Associated Clinical Features

Bacterial conjunctivitis is characterized by the acute onset of conjunctival injection and purulent drainage. *Staphylococcus aureus* is the most common cause in adults and children. Typically symptoms begin in one eye and spread to the other. Mucopurulent discharge (Fig. 2.2) results in sticking together of the eyelids on awakening. In some cases, lid edema and erythema, chemosis, and superficial punctate keratitis may develop.

The most severe form of acute purulent conjunctivitis is associated with *Neisseria gonorrhoeae*. Neisseriae are capable of invading an intact corneal epithelium, and infection can be seen at any age. Clinically symptoms are hyperacute in onset and include marked eyelid swelling along with tenderness, marked conjunctival hyperemia, pain, chemosis, and preauricular adenopathy. The discharge is prominent, thick, copious, and purulent. Corneal findings include a diffuse epithelial haze, epithelial defects, marginal infiltrates, and peripheral ulcerative keratitis that can rapidly progress to perforation.

Neonatal conjunctivitis is discussed separately.

Differential Diagnosis

Other etiologies of conjunctivitis (viral, allergic), as well as iritis, glaucoma, scleritis, and foreign body also present as a red eye.

ED Treatment and Disposition

Treatment involves local hygiene (warm moist compresses, frequent hand washing) and broad spectrum antibiotic drops (sulfacetamide, gentamicin). One drop every 3 h for 7 to 10 days is adequate and usually results in rapid resolution. If there is no response after 48 to 72 h, cultures and ophthalmologic consultation should be considered. Cultures should also be taken in cases of severe acute (hyperacute), persistent, refractory, or chronic conjunctivitis.

The treatment of gonococcal conjunctivitis is both systemic (ceftriaxone 1 g IM) and topical (penicillin G 100,000 U/mL every 2 h or bacitracin ophthalmic ointment 500 U/g every 2 h, tapering over 48 h to five times a day). Because of the frequent coexistence of chlamydia with gonococcal infections, patients should also receive treatment for *Chlamydia* (doxycycline 100 mg twice a day for 7 to 10 days in nonpregnant patients, azithromycin 1 g orally for pregnant patients). Patients with corneal involvement should be hospitalized to receive additional IV ceftriaxone (1 g every 12 h). Sexual partners should be advised and evaluated.

Clinical Pearls

1. Worsening symptoms during topical treatment with any antibiotic, especially Neosporin or a sulfonamide (e.g., Sodium Sulamyd), may represent a contact allergic reaction.
2. *N. gonorrhoeae* conjunctivitis must be considered in the sexually active adult with a purulent eye discharge.
3. Topical corticosteroids are contraindicated for conjunctivitis treatment because a herpetic cause would be greatly exacerbated.

4. In early or mild cases of bacterial conjunctivitis, symptoms may be limited to mild conjunctival infection without frankly purulent drainage evident to the physician. Thus, empiric antibiotic therapy is warranted in most cases of conjunctivitis.

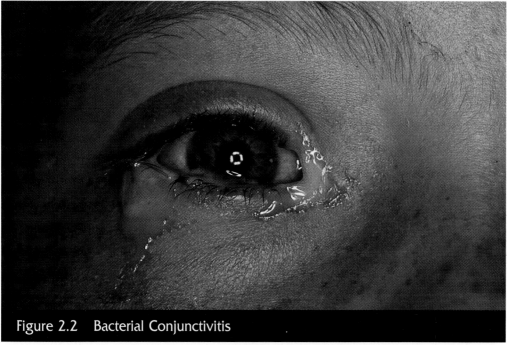

Figure 2.2   Bacterial Conjunctivitis

Mucopurulent discharge, conjunctival injection, and lid swelling, in a 10-year-old with *Haemophilus influenzae* conjunctivitis. (Courtesy of Frank Birinyi, MD.)

Associated Clinical Features

Viral conjunctivitis is a conjunctival infection caused most commonly by adenoviruses. Clinical features range in severity but usually are mild and typically include burning or irritation, conjunctival injection, lid edema, chemosis, and a thin, watery discharge. The infection usually begins in one eye; however, both eyes usually become involved because of autoinoculation (Fig. 2.3). The palpebral conjunctiva may demonstrate hyperemia and follicles. A punctate keratitis may appear several days after the onset of symptoms, followed several weeks later by subepithelial infiltrates. The visual acuity and pupillary reactivity are normal.

Pharyngoconjunctival fever, usually caused by adenovirus type 3, is highly infectious and should be considered if there is fever, upper respiratory tract infection (cold, flu, or sore throat), and preauricular adenopathy. It is seen predominantly in the young and institutionalized, with epidemics occurring in families, schools, and military camps.

Epidemic keratoconjunctivitis is discussed in the following section.

Differential Diagnosis

Similar symptoms are seen in allergic and bacterial conjunctivitis and other causes of a red eye (scleritis, glaucoma, iritis). Less common diagnoses include preseptal cellulitis and dacryoadenitis.

ED Treatment and Disposition

Many cases are self-limited and mild. Cool compresses are helpful. Meticulous hygiene (hand washing by the family and instrument cleaning by medical personnel) is necessary to prevent spread. Because the signs and symptoms of viral conjunctivitis are not always adequate in distinguishing it from bacterial conjunctivitis, antibacterial eyedrops are usually prescribed. Antivirals are ineffective against adenovirus. Symptoms may persist for several weeks, and follow-up is indicated if symptoms are not beginning to resolve in 4 to 7 days.

Clinical Pearls

1. Adenoviruses are the most common cause of acute conjunctivitis.
2. A complete eye examination is necessary to rule out other more serious causes of a red eye before the diagnosis of viral conjunctivitis is made.

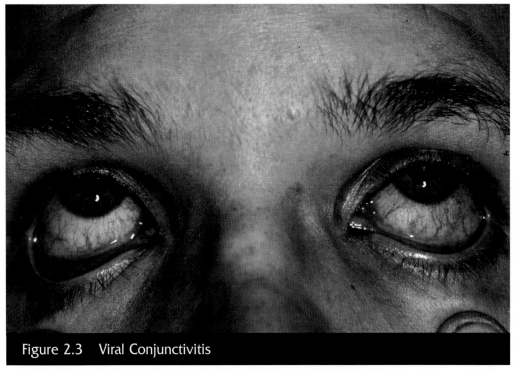

Figure 2.3   Viral Conjunctivitis

Note the classic asymmetric conjunctival injection. Symptoms first developed in the left eye, with symptoms spreading to the other eye a few days later. A thin, watery discharge is also seen. (Courtesy of Kevin J. Knoop, MD, MS.)

Associated Clinical Features

Epidemic keratoconjunctivitis (EKC) is a severe and highly contagious adenovirus infection involving the conjunctiva and cornea. Viral transmission usually occurs through direct or indirect contact with the ocular secretions of infected individuals. The incubation period after exposure is about 8 days. Initial symptoms include watery or mucopurulent discharge, foreign body sensation, and mild photophobia. Clinical findings include edema of the eyelids, chemosis, marked diffuse conjunctival hyperemia, subconjunctival hemorrhage, and a follicular and papillary conjunctival reaction (Fig. 2.4). Pseudomembranes overlying the palpebral conjunctiva and tender preauricular nodes may be present. A painful keratitis may develop (usually after 5 to 7 days) and initially appears as a fine punctate epithelial keratitis that stains with fluorescein (Figs. 2.5 and 2.6). These punctate lesions gradually coalesce to form coarse spots. Subepithelial infiltrates may develop centrally by the end of the second week. These lesions resolve and are replaced by small circular white subepithelial opacities (that do not stain with fluorescein) that may last months or even years. These are believed to result from host immune response rather than from active viral replication.

Symptoms usually begin unilaterally in young adults during the fall and winter months. Bilateral involvement may develop 4 to 5 days later, with less severe symptoms in the second eye, probably due to partial immune protection of the host. There are few to no systemic complaints. Thus in patients with systemic complaints and associated fever, upper respiratory tract infection, pharyngitis, otitis media, and diarrhea, the diagnosis is more likely to be pharyngoconjunctival fever (also caused by adenovirus).

Differential Diagnosis

Other viruses and causes of red eye (bacterial conjunctivitis, iritis, scleritis, glaucoma, herpetic infection) need to be considered.

ED Treatment and Disposition

Although EKC may be severe, the condition is self-limited and therapy is mainly palliative. Cool compresses, antipyretics, topical vasoconstrictors (Vasocon), and dark sunglasses provide symp-

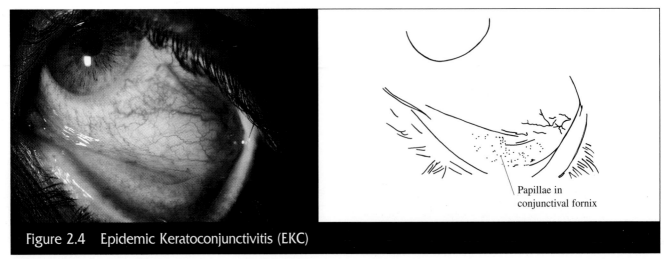

Papillae in
conjunctival fornix

Figure 2.4   Epidemic Keratoconjunctivitis (EKC)

Diffuse injection of the bulbar conjunctiva is seen in addition to a papillary reaction of the palpebral conjunctiva—a classic finding in EKC. (Courtesy of Katrina C. Santos.)

tomatic relief. Antibiotics and antivirals are ineffective. Topical broad spectrum antibiotic drops are usually prescribed, since it is difficult to distinguish viral causes from bacterial causes. In the presence of membrane formation, topical broad spectrum antibiotic ointments may be prescribed to lubricate and protect the cornea. The use of topical corticosteroids is controversial. They may have a role in those patients with marked symptoms (severe conjunctival pseudomembrane formation, severe foreign body sensation, reduced visual acuity secondary to epithelial or subepithelial keratitis). Although topical steroids do provide dramatic symptomatic relief, they have no beneficial therapeutic effect on the ultimate clinical outcome. Patients with EKC should limit their exposure to others for 2 weeks after the onset of the disease and use separate linens.

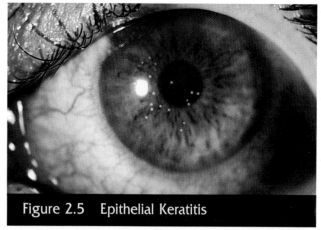

Figure 2.5   Epithelial Keratitis

This usually develops after 5 to 7 days and is seen as a fine punctate abrasion pattern over the cornea. (Courtesy of Katrina C. Santos.)

Clinical Pearls

1. A nonspecific adenovirus conjunctivitis will resolve in 10 to 14 days; a virulent adenovirus causing EKC will peak in 5 to 7 days, and may last 3 to 4 weeks.

2. Frequent hand washing and use of separate linens is advised for patients and family members to reduce exposure.

3. Pharyngoconjunctival fever should be considered if there is an associated fever, pharyngitis, and upper respiratory tract infection.

4. EKC may be nosocomially transmitted by tonometry (the footplate of the Schiøtz tonometer, the prism of the applanation tonometer), contaminated solutions (topical anesthetics), and the physician's fingers. Regular hand washing by the physician (and patient) and careful cleaning (using alcohol or Dakin's solution) and sterilization of instruments are therefore important. Adenovirus can be recovered for extended periods of time from these surfaces.

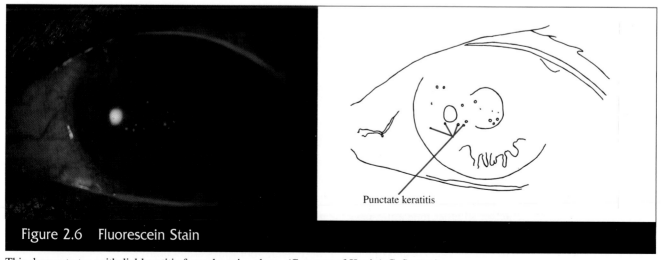

Punctate keratitis

Figure 2.6   Fluorescein Stain

This demonstrates epithelial keratitis from the prior photo. (Courtesy of Katrina C. Santos.)

Associated Clinical Features

Allergic conjunctivitis is a recurrent condition whereby airborne allergens (pollen) precipitate hypersensitivity reactions in the conjunctiva. The hallmark symptom of itching is due to a host of allergens including pollens (ragweed, grasses, trees, weeds), as well as animal dander, mold, or dust. Allergic conjunctivitis is usually transient and self-limited, and is seasonal if it is due to pollens. Associated clinical features include conjunctival injection and edema, burning, discharge (clear, white, or mucopurulent), and chemosis (swelling of the bulbar conjunctiva). Chemosis may be marked. Small to medium-sized papillae or follicles may be seen on the palpebral conjunctiva (Fig. 2.7). The eyelids may be red and swollen. There may be a personal or family history of atopy, eczema, asthma, and allergic rhinitis (hay fever).

Vernal conjunctivitis is an infrequent but serious form of allergic conjunctivitis that mainly affects young males (4 to 16 years of age) during the warm months or in tropical climates. In addition to the symptoms seen in allergic conjunctivitis (intense itching, drainage that is characteristically tenacious and ropy, and mild chemosis and conjunctival injection), a diffuse papillary hypertrophy develops with giant (cobblestone) papillae over the upper tarsal plate (Fig. 2.8). Corneal findings include a sterile ulcer (well delineated with an oval or shield shape and no surrounding haze or iritis), limbal follicles (infiltrates), Horner-Trantas' dots (superficial cellular and eosinophil infiltrates that straddle the limbus and appear as raised white dots), and superficial punctate keratopathy.

Differential Diagnosis

Other etiologies of a red eye (scleritis, iritis, glaucoma, bacterial conjunctivitis) should be considered.

ED Treatment and Disposition

The initial therapy of allergic conjunctivitis should be primarily aimed at the identification of the allergen and its elimination, if possible. The severity of the allergic condition is directly proportional to the level and duration of the allergen exposure. Limiting time outdoors (to avoid pollen-bearing wind), wearing goggles or glasses outdoors, or using air conditioners with appropriate filters should be suggested to decrease airborne allergen contact.

Cool compresses are recommended four times a day, as are topical tear substitutes 4 to 8 times a day. Topical antihistamines (e.g., Levcoabastine, four times a day) are helpful. Vasoconstrictor eyedrops are indicated for moderate or severe cases. Naphcon-A (1 to 2 drops every 3 to 4 h), now available over the counter, is frequently used and contains both an antihistamine (pheniramine) and a vasoconstrictor (naphazoline). Antibacterial eyedrops are prescribed if it is difficult to distinguish the etiology of the conjunctivitis. Elective ophthalmology follow-up is appropriate.

Lodoxamine 0.1%, a mast cell stabilizer similar to cromolyn, has been shown to be effective. Topical steroids may be prescribed after consultation with an ophthalmologist in those cases when all other modalities have been explored.

In vernal conjunctivitis, additional therapeutic agents include cromolyn sodium solution 4% (1 to 2 drops every 4 to 6 h) and aspirin (650 mg four times a day orally).

Clinical Pearls

1. Itching is the hallmark symptom of ocular allergy. Patients are usually the best source for identifying the allergen to which they are sensitive.
2. Topical corticosteroids may be used in severe cases but should not be prescribed by the ED physician without ophthalmology consultation. Complications of topical corticosteroid use include glaucoma, cataract formation, secondary infection, and corneal perforation.
3. Vernal conjunctivitis affects mainly children and adolescents and peaks in the warmer months.
4. Evert the upper lid to appreciate the large conjunctival papillae in vernal conjunctivitis. The cobblestone appearance is pathognomonic.

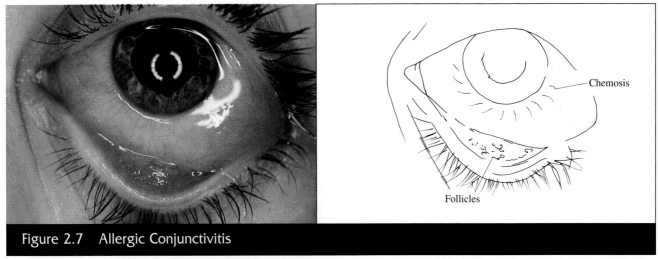

Figure 2.7   Allergic Conjunctivitis

Conjunctival injection, chemosis, and a follicular response in the inferior palpebral conjunctiva in this patient with allergic conjunctivitis secondary to cat fur. (Courtesy of Timothy D. McGuirk, DO.)

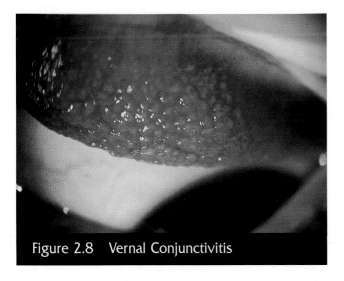

Figure 2.8   Vernal Conjunctivitis

The tarsal conjunctiva demonstrates giant papillae and a cobblestone appearance, pathognomonic for vernal conjunctivitis. (Courtesy of William Beck.)

Associated Clinical Features

A hordeolum is an acute infection and a localized abscess involving either the Meibomian glands, Zeis's glands, or Moll's glands. An internal hordeolum involves the Meibomian glands, and moderate swelling occurs. An external hordeolum (stye), involving glands of Zeis or Moll's glands, is smaller and more superficial (Fig. 2.9). A chalazion is a chronic granulomatous inflammation that develops as a foreign body reaction to sebum released into the surrounding tissue from the Meibomian glands. It may evolve from a hordeolum or may occur secondary to inspissation of sebum at the opening of the gland with subsequent gland rupture into the surrounding tissue. Chalazia are commonly seen in the ED (Fig. 2.10).

Common signs and symptoms include pain, focal swelling, erythema, and tenderness. If glands of Zeis are involved, the pathology is localized around the root of an eyelash. Focal inflammation around a chalazion may cause pointing of the lesion either anteriorly (toward the skin of the eyelid) or posteriorly (toward the tarsal conjunctiva) (Figs. 2.11 and 2.12). A chalazion may become sufficiently large as to press on the globe and cause astigmatism (corneal distortion that prevents focus). A chronic chalazion may appear as focal lid swelling without associated signs of inflammation.

There may be associated marginal blepharitis (a chronic low-grade inflammation of the lid margins with crusts around the lashes) or acne rosacea (a dermatologic condition with facial hyperemia, acneiform lesions, hypertrophy of sebaceous glands, and rhinophyma).

Differential Diagnosis

Sebaceous cell or squamous cell carcinoma should be suspected in older patients with recurrent or persistent lesions. Preseptal cellulitis should be considered if the entire lid is erythematous and edematous. Pyogenic granuloma has a similar appearance, but it has hypertrophic tissue, a vascular core, and bleeds easily. Dacryocystitis should be considered if the lesion involves the medial aspect of the lower lid.

ED Treatment and Disposition

The process may be self-limited, with spontaneous drainage and resolution within 5 to 7 days. Warm compresses (two to four times a day for 5 to 15 min) and topical broad spectrum antibiotic ointment (bacitracin or erythromycin, every 3 h, applied to the conjunctival sac) are almost always effective. Systemic antibiotics are unnecessary unless there is a significant cellulitis. If the mass persists beyond 3 or 4 weeks, or if the lesion is sufficiently large to distort vision, referral to the ophthalmologist should be made for incision and curettage or intralesional corticosteroid injection. Gentle scrubbing of the eyelids and lashes may be indicated if marginal blepharitis is noted.

Clinical Pearls

1. Excisional biopsy is indicated for recurrent chalazion to exclude malignancy.
2. *Staphylococcus aureus* is the most common bacterial pathogen.
3. Chalazia are often found in patients with marginal blepharitis, probably because the Meibomian gland orifices are blocked by the blepharitis infection.

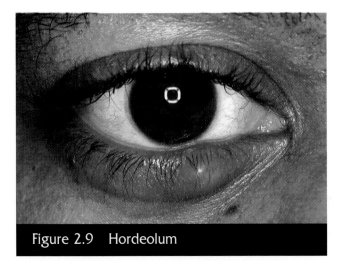

Figure 2.9 Hordeolum

Focal swelling and erythema at the lid margin are seen in this hordeolum. (Courtesy of Frank Birinyi, MD.)

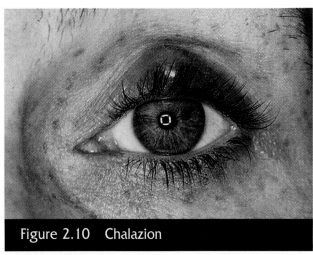

Figure 2.10 Chalazion

This chalazion shows nodular focal swelling and erythema. (Courtesy of Frank Birinyi, MD.)

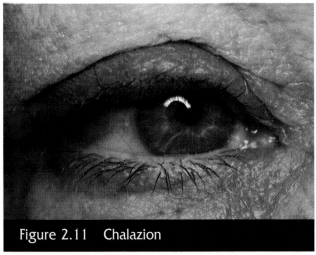

Figure 2.11 Chalazion

This chalazion is in an early stage. Lid swelling is evident with pointing of the chalazion to the inner tarsal conjunctiva. (Courtesy of Kevin J. Knoop, MD, MS.)

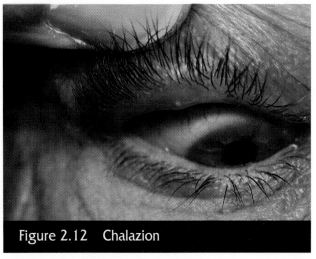

Figure 2.12 Chalazion

Pointing of the chalazion to the tarsal conjunctiva is more evident with slight lid eversion. (Courtesy of Kevin J. Knoop, MD, MS.)

Associated Clinical Features

Dacryocystitis, or inflammation of the lacrimal sac, is generally caused by a bacterial infection in the setting of an obstructed nasolacrimal duct. Hallmark findings are tearing (epiphora) and discharge. Acute dacryocystitis is associated with pain, swelling over the lacrimal sac (Fig. 2.13), and tenderness. Mucopurulent discharge may be expressed from the punctum when pressure is applied over the lacrimal sac. In adults, acute infection is due to *Staphylococcus aureus* or occasionally beta-hemolytic streptococci.

Dacryocystitis is usually seen in infants whose nasolacrimal passage remains closed (4 to 7% of newborns). In these cases, the duct normally opens spontaneously within the first month. Acute infection is uncommon in infants, but may develop secondary to *Haemophilus influenzae* and requires aggressive treatment to avoid orbital cellulitis. Organisms usually seen in chronic dacryocystitis include *Streptococcus pneumoniae* or, rarely, *Candida albicans.*

Dacryocystitis is uncommon in the intermediate age groups unless it follows chronic sinusitis, facial trauma, or (rarely) neoplasm.

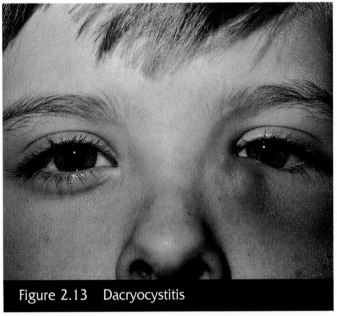

Figure 2.13   Dacryocystitis

Swelling and erythema over the medial lid and lacrimal sac developed in this 10-year-old patient with streptococcal pharyngitis. (Courtesy of Kevin J. Knoop, MD, MS.)

Differential Diagnosis

Chalazia, facial and orbital cellulitis, canaliculitis, canalicular stenosis, sinus tumors, ethmoid sinusitis, and mucoceles have similar features.

ED Treatment and Disposition

Acute dacryocystitis usually responds to oral antibiotics (amoxicillin-clavulanate), warm compresses, and gentle massage. Topical antibiotics may be used in chronic cases. Nonurgent ophthalmology or otolaryngology referral is required for definitive treatment—relief of the obstruction by dacryocystorhinostomy. In febrile and acutely ill cases of acute dacryocystitis, IV antibiotics (cefuroxime) are indicated.

In infants with chronic dacryocystitis, both topical and oral antibiotics may be used. Referral is indicated if signs do not regress by 6 to 9 months of age or if acute dacryocystitis develops.

Clinical Pearls

1. The swelling is localized to the extreme nasal aspect of the lower lid and is usually unilateral.
2. The diagnosis of acute dacryocystitis may be confirmed by pressure on the lacrimal sac and the expression of purulent material from the punctum. (The lacrimal sac and lacrimal fossa are situated in the inferior medial aspect of the orbit, not on the side of the nose.)
3. The incidence follows a bimodal distribution. Dacryocystitis usually occurs in infants or persons over 40 years of age.

Associated Clinical Features

Dacryoadenitis is an uncommon condition involving acute inflammation of the lacrimal gland. Symptoms are localized to the outer one-third of the upper eyelid and include swelling, conjunctival chemosis (Fig. 2.14), pain, erythema, tenderness, and tearing. Acute infections may demonstrate ipsilateral preauricular lymphadenopathy and fever. Associated organisms include bacteria (*Staphylococcus aureus, Neisseria gonorrhoeae,* streptococci) and viruses (mumps, Epstein-Barr, influenza, herpes zoster).

Differential Diagnosis

Chalazia, conjunctivitis, preseptal cellulitis, orbital cellulitis, and lacrimal gland tumor are other conditions to consider.

ED Treatment and Disposition

In the setting of acute bacterial infection, oral antibiotics (amoxicillin-clavulanate) are given for mild to moderate cases. In moderate to severe infections, IV antibiotics (ticarcillin-clavulanate) may be necessary. Viral dacryoadenitis (mumps) is treated with cool compresses and analgesics (acetaminophen). Nonemergent ophthalmology follow-up is appropriate. Outpatients should be instructed to return to the ED urgently for symptoms suggestive of orbital cellulitis (decreased ocular motility or proptosis).

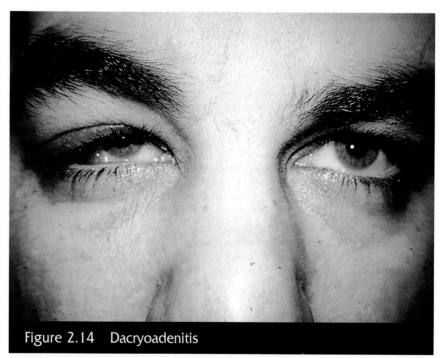

Figure 2.14   Dacryoadenitis

Unilateral localized swelling and chemosis are present laterally secondary to inflammation of the lacrimal gland. (Used with permission from American Academy of Ophthalmology: *External Disease and Cornea: A Multimedia Collection.* San Francisco, 1994.)

Clinical Pearls

1. The swelling is usually unilateral and localized over the lateral one-third of the upper lid and may impart an S-shaped curve to the lid margin.
2. Proptosis and limitation of ocular motion require an urgent CT scan and ophthalmology evaluation for orbital cellulitis.
3. Acute dacryoadenitis is most often seen in children as a complication of mumps, measles, or influenza. In adults, it is associated with gonorrhea, lacrimal gland trauma, or as a retrograde infection from bacterial conjunctivitis.
4. Chronic dacryoadenitis may be seen with lymphoma, leukemia, tuberculosis, and sarcoidosis.

Associated Clinical Features

A pinguecula (Latin, *pingueculus* meaning "fatty") is a degenerative lesion of the bulbar conjunctiva. It appears as a yellow-white amorphous subepithelial nodule adjacent to the limbus, usually nasally (Fig. 2.15). A pinguecula is usually asymptomatic. It may become episodically inflamed, gradually enlarge over time, or become a pterygium.

A pterygium is a benign proliferation of fibrovascular tissue within the bulbar conjunctiva that extends onto the peripheral cornea. Typically a pterygium assumes a triangular configuration with the apex of the lesion directed toward the pupil (Fig. 2.16). Growth occurs from this apex onto the limbal cornea. Pterygia are often preceded by pingueculae. Risk factors are exposure to ultraviolet light (sunlight), wind, and dust. Pterygia are more commonly bilateral and, like pingueculae, the nasal portion of the conjunctiva is more commonly involved than the temporal portion. Pterygia may be asymptomatic or become inflamed. They give rise to mild symptoms of irritation and foreign body sensation. Decreased visual acuity may develop if the visual axis is involved or the lesion induces astigmatism (irregular corneal curvature resulting in refractive error).

Differential Diagnosis

A pseudopterygium, a scar in the bulbar conjunctiva extending onto the cornea secondary to previous ocular inflammation (chemical burn, trauma, infection) may also have a similar appearance. Episcleritis, corneal ulcer, and conjunctival neoplasm should be considered in the differential diagnosis.

ED Treatment and Disposition

A patient with mild disease can be treated with artificial tears or a topical vasoconstrictor (naphazoline). In more severe cases, topical steroids may be prescribed after consultation. Nonemergent referral to an ophthalmologist is appropriate. Excision of a pinguecula (or pterygium) is indicated if the lesion interferes with contact lens wear, becomes chronically inflamed, or constitutes a cosmetic problem. Pterygia are excised if they cause persistent discomfort, encroach significantly on the cornea to involve the visual axis, or restrict extraocular muscle movement.

Clinical Pearls

1. Pterygia are a particular problem in sunny, hot, and dusty regions. Eye protection (goggles, sunglasses) helps to reduce the irritation.
2. Pterygia and pingueculae are usually found on the nasal conjunctiva, adjacent to the limbus. They are usually bilateral and always in the horizontal meridian.

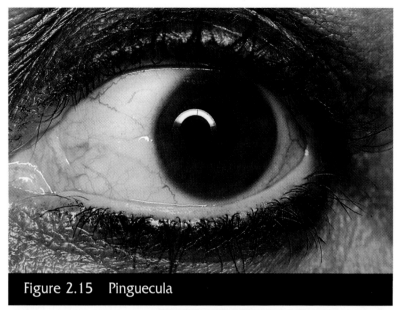

Figure 2.15   Pinguecula

A small area of yellowish "heaped up" conjunctival tissue is seen adjacent to the limbus on the nasal aspect. (Courtesy of Kevin J. Knoop, MD, MS.)

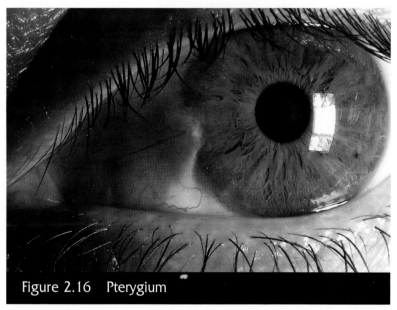

Figure 2.16   Pterygium

This pterygium appears as a raised vascular triangular area of bulbar conjunctiva that encroaches on the cornea. (Courtesy of the Department of Ophthalmology, Naval Medical Center, Portsmouth, VA.)

Associated Clinical Features

Scleritis is a destructive and serious inflammation involving the sclera, which is the tough, flexible white outer covering of the posterior portion of the eye. (Anteriorly the sclera is continuous with the cornea.) Pain, tearing, and photophobia are prominent features. The pain may radiate to the forehead, brow, or jaw. Ocular movement is usually painful.

Patients with scleritis have an intensely red eye with a violaceous or purple hue, secondary to engorgement of the deep vessels (Fig. 2.17). These vessels do not move when the overlying tissues are moved with a cotton-tipped applicator, nor do they blanch with topical phenylephrine 2.5%. Scleral edema is seen with slit-lamp biomicroscopy. Corneal involvement, iritis (with cells and flare in the anterior chamber), and decreased visual acuity frequently accompany scleritis.

The sclera is composed of collagen and elastic fibers, and therefore is subject to the connective tissue diseases (rheumatoid arthritis, systemic lupus erythematosus) that affect the body elsewhere. Granulomatous disorders (sarcoidosis, tuberculosis) have also been associated with scleritis.

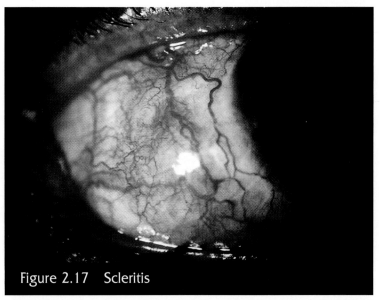

Figure 2.17   Scleritis

A prominent generalized vascular injection is present. These vessels do not move when the overlying conjunctiva is moved with a cotton-tipped applicator. (Courtesy of Thomas F. Mauger, MD.)

Differential Diagnosis

Other causes of a red eye (conjunctivitis, iritis, episcleritis, trauma, glaucoma) should be considered. Scleritis may be confused with an inflamed pinguecula, pterygium, foreign body, or tumor.

ED Treatment and Disposition

Urgent ophthalmology consultation and systemic therapy are required. Oral NSAIDs (indomethacin, ibuprofen) are recommended. Systemic steroids are added if oral NSAIDs are ineffective or for severe scleritis. Topical steroids are only occasionally effective. Immunosuppressive therapy (cyclophosphamide) is sometimes required, especially for progressive cases. Appropriate treatment of associated systemic autoimmune disease is also important.

Clinical Pearls

1. Scleritis, unlike episcleritis which may be self-limited, is destructive.
2. The eye is usually exquisitely tender, and patients frequently complain of severe pain. Episcleritis, on the other hand, is rarely associated with pain or significant tenderness.
3. Women are more commonly affected than men.

Associated Clinical Features

Episcleritis is focal inflammation and vasodilatation of the deep subconjunctival (episcleral) tissue. The episclera (Tenon's capsule) is a thin layer of vascular elastic tissue overlying the sclera that acts as a synovial membrane for smooth movement of the eye. Episcleral vessels are large, run in a radial direction, and can be seen beneath the conjunctiva.

Patients may complain of mild pain, foreign body sensation, mild tenderness, irritation, photophobia, and excessive lacrimation. The affected eye appears normal, except for a sector of episcleral and conjunctival hyperemia and edema. The condition is localized; is pink, purple, or bright red; and is pie-shaped with its apex toward the limbus (Fig. 2.18). Visual acuity is normal. There is no history of trauma or purulent discharge. Episodes may be recurrent.

Episcleritis is frequently an isolated condition, and the etiology is unknown. Episcleritis has been associated with gout, autoimmune conditions (systemic lupus erythematosus, rheumatoid arthritis, Sjögren's syndrome), and infectious disorders (coccidioidomycosis, syphilis, herpes zoster, tuberculosis).

Differential Diagnosis

Other considerations include conjunctivitis and other causes of a red eye, such as iritis, acute glaucoma, trauma, corneal ulcer, scleritis, pinguecula, and phlyctenule (similar to episcleritis except that a nodule is present in the center of the lesion).

ED Treatment and Disposition

For mild cases, the condition is self-limited and may spontaneously resolve after several weeks. Artificial tears and topical vasoconstrictors (naphazoline) may be used. Oral NSAIDs have been shown to be effective in those cases associated with rheumatoid arthritis or systemic lupus erythematosus. Topical steroids are only occasionally used. Urgent referral is indicated if scleritis is suspected.

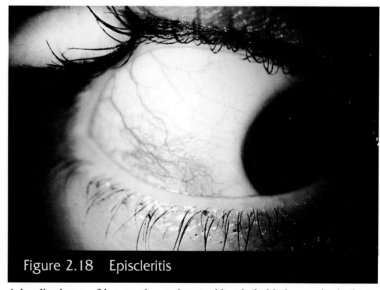

Figure 2.18   Episcleritis

A localized area of hyperemia consistent with episcleritis is seen in the lower lateral quadrant of the eye. (Courtesy of Thomas F. Mauger, MD.)

Clinical Pearls

1. Although other causes of a red eye demonstrate a generalized redness, episcleritis is easily recognizable because it is localized. Conjunctival vessels blanch with topical phenylephrine, clearly identifying the underlying episcleral injection.
2. Episcleritis is unilateral two-thirds of the time, and is seen in young and middle-aged adults. The sex incidence is equal.

Associated Clinical Features

Glaucoma refers to a heterogeneous group of disorders causing optic nerve damage, usually in association with elevated intraocular pressure (IOP). It is a major (and preventable) cause of blindness. In acute angle closure glaucoma (AACG), the elevated IOP is due to an obstruction to outflow of aqueous humor from the anterior chamber. Aqueous humor is initially produced by the ciliary body and first enters the posterior chamber. It then passes between the posterior surface of the iris and the lens to enter the anterior chamber. After circulating within the anterior chamber, the aqueous humor leaves through the trabecular meshwork of the anterior chamber angle to enter Schlemm's canal. In AACG the peripheral iris abuts this trabecular meshwork, and the angle is said to be closed. Aqueous outflow is blocked as a result. Normal IOP is 10 to 21 mmHg; it rises to between 50 and 100 mmHg in AACG.

Patients predisposed for AACG are typically not aware that they are at risk. They are usually hyperopic (farsighted). Anatomically these patients have congenitally narrow anterior chamber angles and, hence, are vulnerable to AACG, since the angle can be occluded more easily. In addition, these patients have a greater than normal area of contact between the posterior surface of the iris and the lens. This impedes the flow of aqueous from the posterior chamber to the anterior chamber through the pupil, and a pressure differential results between the posterior and anterior chambers, with increased pressure in the posterior chamber. This condition, known as relative pupillary block, produces a forward bowing of the peripheral iris (iris bombé), resulting in relative angle closure because of the contact between the peripheral iris and the trabecular meshwork. AACG may be precipitated by pupillary dilation, whereby the peripheral iris is further pushed against the trabecular meshwork, thereby closing the angle. This may occur, for example, with the use of sympathomimetics (over the counter cold preparations containing pseudoephedrine), the use of anticholinergics (antiemetics such as prochlorperazine, antipsychotics such as haloperidol, tricyclics such as amitriptyline), or in physiologic situations (low illumination, stress, fatigue). AACG may be inadvertently precipitated in the ED patient treated for corneal abrasion with a cycloplegic (cyclopentolate). Therefore the anterior chamber depth should always be evaluated in ED patients receiving cycloplegics.

AACG presents as an acutely inflamed eye. Eye pain or headache are prominent and can be described as a brow ache. Nausea and vomiting are common and may be in the presenting complaints. Other symptoms include blurred vision, rainbow-colored halos around lights, and photophobia. Clinical findings on examination include tearing, conjunctival infection with a perilimbal ("ciliary") flush (Fig. 2.19), a cloudy ("steamy") cornea (Fig. 2.20), a nonreactive and middilated pupil, mild anterior chamber inflammation, and increased intraocular pressure. Also, the anterior chamber is shallow; this is demonstrated by a penlight held laterally and directed nasally (Fig. 2.21). In an eye with a normal anterior chamber, the entire iris will be illuminated by the penlight. In an eye with a narrow angle or shallow anterior chamber, a shadow is cast on the nasal side of the iris secondary to the forward bowing of the iris. Alternatively, slit-lamp biomicroscopy may also be used to assess the anterior chamber depth. Funduscopic examination demonstrates optic cupping only if there is preexisting glaucoma.

Tonometers available in the ED for measurement of IOP include the air-puff noncontact tonometer, the Schiøtz tonometer, the Tono-Pen, and the applanation tonometer. Tactile tonometry, using the examiner's fingers to ballot the globe, can usually detect AACG in patients with markedly elevated IOP.

Differential Diagnosis

Similar conditions include temporal arteritis, acute iritis, ulcer, and other causes of a red eye (conjunctivitis, trauma, scleritis, keratitis, foreign body).

ED Treatment and Disposition

AACG is an ophthalmologic emergency, and treatment is directed at reducing the IOP. The IOP can be lowered by agents that decrease the production of aqueous humor or increase the outflow. Decreased production of aqueous is accomplished with the use of topical beta blockers (timolol solution, 0.5%, 1 to 2 drops every 10 to 15 min for three doses, then 1 drop every 12 h) and acetazolamide, a carbonic anhydrase inhibitor (500 mg IV every 12 h or 500 mg PO every 6 h). Aqueous outflow is increased by the use of topical miotics (pilocarpine 2%, 1 drop every 30 min until the pupil is constricted, then 1 drop every 6 h), which stimulate miosis to pull the peripheral iris taut from the trabecular meshwork. Hyperosmotic agents (mannitol 20%, 1 to 2 g/kg body weight IV over 30 to 60 min; isosorbide 45%, 1.5 g/kg body weight PO; glycerol 75%, 1 to 1.5 g/kg body weight PO) reduce the intraocular pressure. Topical steroids (prednisolone acetate 1%, 1 drop every 15 to 30 min for four doses, then hourly) are given. Typically, hyperosmotics and steroids are used in consultation with an ophthalmologist.

When the IOP is 50 mmHg or greater, topical miotics may be ineffective secondary to iris constrictor ischemia. In this situation corneal indentation may be used. Indentation of the cornea displaces the aqueous to the peripheral anterior chamber, temporarily opening the angle. This may successfully decrease the IOP and abort the attack; if the IOP has been longstanding, however, it more likely will be unsuccessful. Corneal indentation is performed with topical anesthetics and any smooth instrument such as the Goldmann applanation prism. The prism is held with the fingers and firm pressure applied for 30 s.

The definitive treatment of AACG is laser peripheral iridectomy, done usually after the IOP normalizes.

Clinical Pearls

1. The anterior chamber depth should always be evaluated in ED patients who are given cycloplegics, so that AACG is not iatrogenically precipitated.
2. In light of the associated severe headache and vomiting, patients with AACG may easily be misdiagnosed as having a migraine headache or a CNS catastrophe.
3. Treatment of nausea and vomiting with anticholinergics may worsen the problem.
4. The unaffected eye will also have a narrow anterior chamber and should be treated prophylactically (pilocarpine 0.5%). The presence of a shallow anterior chamber in only one eye casts doubt on the diagnosis of AACG, since AACG is the result of an anatomic configuration that is almost always bilateral.
5. Patients may be able to recall previous milder attacks.

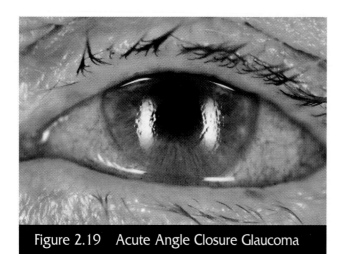

Figure 2.19   Acute Angle Closure Glaucoma

The cornea is edematous, manifested by the indistinctness of the iris markings and the irregular corneal light reflex. Conjunctival hyperemia is also present. (Courtesy of Kevin J. Knoop, MD, MS.)

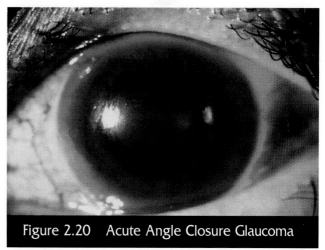

Figure 2.20   Acute Angle Closure Glaucoma

Note the cloudy or "steamy" appearance of the cornea and the mid-position pupil. Conjunctival hyperemia is not as evident. (Courtesy of Gary Tanner, MD.)

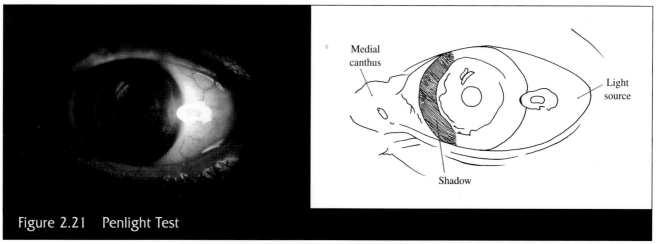

Figure 2.21   Penlight Test

A penlight, held laterally and directed nasally, projects a shadow on the nasal side of an iris with a shallow anterior chamber. This patient presented with acute angle closure glaucoma. (Courtesy of Alan B. Storrow, MD.)

Associated Clinical Features

The uvea is the middle coat of the eye and is composed of the iris, ciliary body, and choroid. Uveitis refers to inflammation within the uvea, and anterior uveitis localizes the inflammation to the anterior chamber, iris, ciliary body, and anterior vitreous.

In most cases of anterior uveitis, no definitive cause can be determined. A significant number, however, are associated with medically treatable systemic disease. These include inflammatory disorders (juvenile rheumatoid arthritis, rheumatoid arthritis, sarcoidosis, Behcet's disease, Sjögren's syndrome), HLA-B27-associated conditions (ankylosing spondylitis, Reiter's syndrome), and infectious processes (tuberculosis, toxoplasmosis, herpes simplex, herpes zoster, cytomegalovirus (CMV), syphilis, AIDS). Finally, lymphoma and Kawasaki's disease may also manifest as an anterior uveitis. Therefore aggressive attempts to determine the underlying cause of the uveitis is warranted.

Clinical features include conjunctival hyperemia, hyperemic perilimbal vessels ("ciliary flush") (Fig. 2.22), decreased visual acuity, photophobia, miosis, pupil irregularities (secondary to anterior or posterior synechiae formation), tearing, and pain. A hypopyon (a layer of white blood cells in the dependent portion of the anterior chamber) may be seen (Fig. 2.23). The slit-lamp examination may demonstrate cells and flare. The term *cells* refers to the finding of inflammatory cells seen in the anterior chamber, having the appearance of dust in a sunbeam (Fig. 2.24); *flare* is light scatter secondary to inflammatory cells and proteins circulating within the aqueous and anterior chamber, and has the appearance of a headlight in fog (Fig. 2.25). Other significant slit-lamp findings in anterior uveitis include keratic precipitates, which are agglutinated inflammatory cells adherent to the posterior corneal endothelium (Fig. 2.26). Keratic precipitates appear either as fine gray-white deposits or as large, flat confluent deposits with a greasy surface ("mutton fat"). The intraocular pressure (IOP) may be elevated secondary to inflammatory debris within the trabeculae obstructing outflow, or the IOP may be decreased secondary to decreased aqueous humor production by the inflamed ciliary body.

Differential Diagnosis

Other conditions presenting with a red eye include glaucoma, conjunctivitis (bacterial, viral, allergic), scleritis, episcleritis, keratitis, and corneal ulcer. A hypopyon can also be seen with severe corneal ulcerations and penetrating trauma to the anterior chamber.

ED Treatment and Disposition

In light of the association of anterior uveitis with systemic disease, the evaluation of a uveitis patient in the ED is a systemic evaluation, with history, general medical examination, and laboratory testing to elucidate a possible underlying etiology.

Treatment of the anterior uveitis itself is nonspecific. Topical cycloplegics (atropine) and corticosteroids are prescribed in conjunction with the ophthalmologist. Although nonspecific, this therapy greatly reduces the amount of scarring. Antibiotics are not usually prescribed or helpful unless there is a bacterial origin. Prompt ophthalmology follow-up is important if steroids are to be prescribed.

Clinical Pearls

1. A constricted (miotic) pupil with anterior chamber cells and flare are key diagnostic features of anterior uveitis.

2. When cells and flare are visualized in the anterior chamber using the slit-lamp, the cells appear as dust particles in a sunbeam, and the flare (the slit-lamp beam) appears as a car headlight cutting through fog.

3. The presence of anterior uveitis requires a search for associated systemic illness.

4. The Henkind test (shining light in the uninvolved eye resulting in pain in the involved eye) is not reliable in diagnosing anterior uveitis. On the other hand, pain with accommodation has been shown to be highly specific for anterior uveitis.

5. Topical analgesics do not significantly ameliorate the pain of anterior uveitis, unlike many of the common conditions seen in the ED (e.g. corneal abrasions).

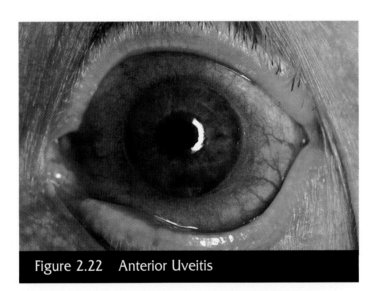

Figure 2.22   Anterior Uveitis

Marked conjunctival injection and perilimbal hyperemia ("ciliary flush") are seen in this patient with recurrent iritis. (Courtesy of Kevin J. Knoop, MD, MS.)

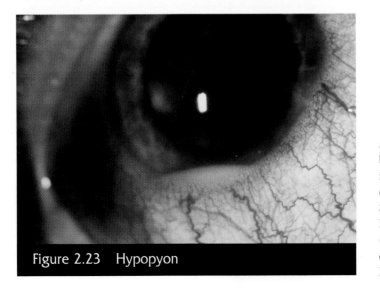

Figure 2.23   Hypopyon

A thin layering of white blood cells is present in the inferior anterior chamber. (Used with permission from Spalton DJ, Hitchings RA, Hunter PA (eds): *Atlas of Clinical Ophthalmology,* 2nd ed. Mosby-Wolfe Limited, London, UK, 1994.)

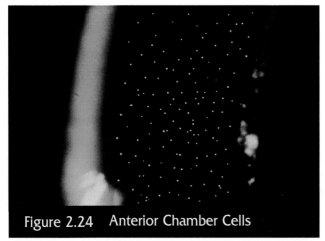

Figure 2.24   Anterior Chamber Cells

Cells in the anterior chamber are a sign of inflammation or bleeding and appear similar to particles of dust in a sunbeam. They are best seen with a narrow slit-lamp beam directed obliquely across the anterior chamber. (Used with permission from Spalton DJ, Hitchings RA, Hunter PA (eds): *Atlas of Clinical Ophthalmology,* 2nd ed. Mosby-Wolfe Limited, London, UK, 1994.)

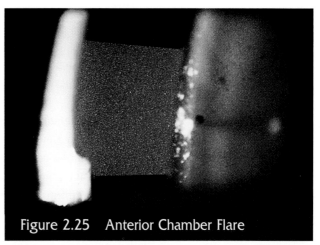

Figure 2.25   Anterior Chamber Flare

Flare in the anterior chamber represents an elevated concentration of plasma proteins from inflamed, leaking intraocular blood vessels. Flare seen in a slit-lamp beam appears similar to a car headlight cutting through the fog. (Used with permission from Spalton DJ, Hitchings RA, Hunter PA (eds): *Atlas of Clinical Ophthalmology,* 1st ed. Mosby-Wolfe Limited, London, UK, 1984.)

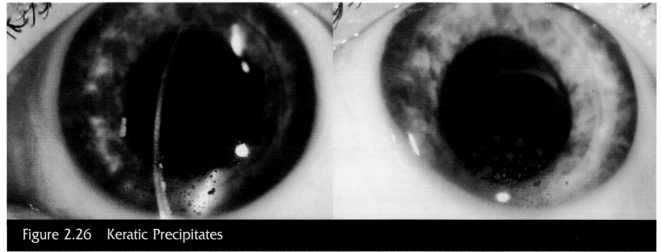

Figure 2.26   Keratic Precipitates

Deposits of cells on the *endothelial* layer of the cornea are seen in these photographs. (Used with permission from Spalton DJ, Hitchings RA, Hunter PA (eds): *Atlas of Clinical Ophthalmology,* 2nd ed. Mosby-Wolfe Limited, London, UK, 1994.)

Associated Clinical Features

Herpes zoster ophthalmicus develops secondary to activation of latent varicella zoster virus within the trigeminal ganglion. Neuronal spread of the virus through the ophthalmic division of the trigeminal nerve results in crops of grouped vesicles in a dermatomal distribution (Fig. 2.27).

Herpes zoster keratitis is a common ophthalmic complication of herpes zoster ophthalmicus infection, although almost any ophthalmic abnormality in both anterior and posterior segments may be seen with herpes zoster ophthalmicus. Conjunctivitis, keratitis, and iritis are common. Common corneal lesions include a punctate epithelial keratitis (fine or coarse superficial defects), anterior stromal infiltrates, neurotrophic keratitis, and dendriform (pseudodendritic) keratitis. Pseudodendrites form from mucous deposition, are usually peripherally located, and stain only moderately with fluorescein. They may be differentiated from the dendrites of herpes simplex infection in that the pseudodendrites lack the rounded terminal bulbs at the end of the branches, and are broader and more plaquelike; when they are wiped from the cornea, an intact epithelium remains, unlike the epithelial defect seen with herpes simplex.

Corneal anesthesia or hypoesthesia is a frequent complication of herpes zoster keratitis. The majority, however, recover normal sensitivity within 2 to 3 months. With neurotrophic keratitis, however, corneal anesthesia is permanent.

Differential Diagnosis

Herpes simplex keratitis may similarly present with rash, red eye, and dendriform keratitis. Ocular complications of herpes zoster ophthalmicus may follow the rash by many months to years; they have a highly variable presentation that mimics almost any disease in the anterior pole of the eye.

ED Treatment and Disposition

Mild punctate epithelial keratitis and dendriform keratitis are self-limited and clear within a few days. For moderate or severe disease, however, debridement, warm compresses, lubricants (artificial tears), and topical broad spectrum antibiotics (to prevent secondary infection) may be recommended. Oral famciclovir (500 mg three times a day for 7 days) or acyclovir (800 mg five times a day for 10 days), if given within 72 h of onset, may ameliorate the course of the disease and the keratitis. (The effect on post-herpetic neuralgia is controversial.) Topical antivirals are generally not useful for herpes zoster. However, in those cases in which the diagnosis is not secure, it is probably advisable to add topical antivirals (trifluridine, 1%, 1 drop q 2 hrs. while awake) to assure coverage of herpes simplex. Cycloplegics (cyclopentolate) are used if an iritis is present. An ophthalmology consult is necessary.

The use of systemic steroids has been shown to reduce the incidence and severity of keratitis. Its effect on post-herpetic neuralgia is unclear. The use of oral steroids must be weighed against the risks, including systemic dissemination of the varicella zoster virus. Topical steroids have been shown to be effective in those cases with stromal infiltrates, since the infiltrates probably represent an immune response to soluble viral antigen.

Nonnarcotic and narcotic analgesics may be prescribed.

Clinical Pearls

1. A careful eye examination with corneal staining should be performed in patients with herpes zoster ophthalmicus to rule out corneal involvement.

2. Patients with skin lesions on the nose (Hutchinson's sign) are at higher risk for ocular involvement with herpes zoster since the sensory innervation to both the eye and the side of the tip of the nose is supplied by the nasociliary branch of the first division of the fifth cranial nerve. However, the eye may be involved without nasal involvement.

3. Corneal hypoesthesia and the appearance of dendrites with fluorescein staining are seen in both herpes zoster ophthalmicus and herpes simplex keratitis.

4. The severity of the cutaneous disease does not necessarily correlate with the severity of the ocular disease.

5. The prognosis is good and recurrences, unlike herpes simplex keratitis, are rare.

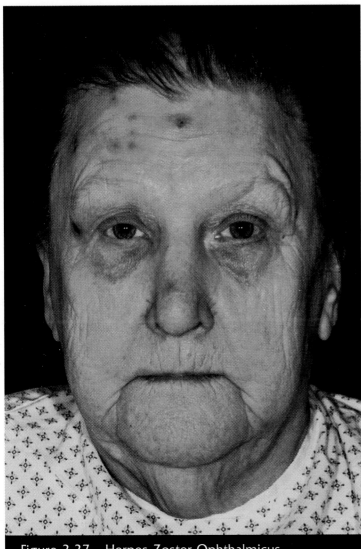

Figure 2.27 Herpes Zoster Ophthalmicus

A healing, vesicular rash in the distribution of the ophthalmic division (V1) of the trigeminal nerve is present in this 72-year-old diabetic patient. The presence of the lesion on the tip of the nose (Hutchinson's sign) increases the risk of ocular involvement. (Courtesy of Frank Birinyi, MD.)

Associated Clinical Features

Herpes simplex keratitis is a corneal infection by the herpes simplex virus (HSV). In general HSV keratitis is accompanied by pain, irritation, foreign body sensation, redness, photophobia, tearing, and occasionally decreased visual acuity. In cases of HSV with corneal anesthesia, symptoms may be minimal.

As in herpes infections elsewhere in the body, ocular HSV infection may be primary or recurrent. In primary infection, usually seen in children up to the age of 15, HSV presents as a unilateral blepharitis (with vesicles on an erythematous base, frequently at a mucocutaneous border), conjunctivitis (with follicles, papillae, and purulent discharge), or keratoconjunctivitis. Epithelial disease is usually punctate; dendritic ulcers are only rarely seen in primary disease. A palpable and tender preauricular node may be felt.

In recurrent disease, keratoconjunctivitis (Fig. 2.28), blepharitis, or iritis is seen, and the cornea is more likely to be involved (Fig. 2.29). With fluorescein staining, the cornea itself may manifest a keratitis that is classically dendritic (Fig. 2.30). HSV dendrites most commonly occur in the center of the cornea, and their branches have characteristic terminal bulbs at the end of each branch. Other patterns of fluorescein staining include a superficial punctate keratitis (particularly early in the course), stellate keratitis, and a geographic ulcer. Geographic ulcers are often the result of the use of topical steroids on dendritic lesions. Faint subepithelial infiltrates and edema can also be seen corresponding in shape to the original epithelial lesion. Corneal sensitivity in the area of the dendrite or geographic ulceration is characteristically reduced or anesthetic, whereas uninvolved areas may show normal or reduced sensation. Recurrences may be triggered by immunosuppression, fever, ultraviolet light exposure, trauma, systemic illness, stress, or menstruation. Herpetic corneal lesions occasionally scar, and a permanently decreased visual acuity can result if the ulcer involves the central cornea. With repeated and protracted episodes of HSV keratitis, ulcerations persist; in some patients, melting and perforation of the corneal stroma ensue.

Differential Diagnosis

Other causes of red eye (scleritis, iritis, glaucoma, conjunctivitis) should be considered. A similar fluorescein appearance may be seen with herpes zoster virus, recurrent corneal erosions, or a healing corneal abrasion.

ED Treatment and Disposition

Ophthalmology consultation is required. Oral acyclovir is given and is more beneficial if given early in the course. Primary herpetic ocular disease is often self-limited and relatively benign; acyclovir and antivirals (e.g., trifluridine) may be given. In primary or recurrent HSV infections, treatment of ulcerations includes debridement, topical antiviral agents (e.g., trifluridine), and topical broad spectrum antibiotics. Cycloplegics (e.g., homatropine) are used if iritis is present.

In case of refractory or advanced herpetic stromal keratitis (believed to be an immune-mediated hypersensitivity reaction to the fixed herpes antigen within the stroma), topical steroids, in addition to antivirals and cycloplegics, may be prescribed by the ophthalmologist.

Clinical Pearls

1. HSV is the most common cause of corneal ulceration and the most common infectious cause of corneal blindness in the Western hemisphere.

2. HSV dendrites, when stained with fluorescein, appear as branching lesions with club-shaped or beadlike extensions called terminal bulbs at the end of each branch. In primary HSV disease, however, dendritic ulcers are rare.

3. Other patterns of fluorescein staining in HSV infection include a superficial punctate keratitis. This is seen particularly in primary disease and early in the course of recurrent disease.

4. Recurrent HSV eye infections occur in about one-third of cases within 2 years of the first attack. Identification of a trigger mechanism may aid in control.

5. With recurrent attacks, corneal pain may be diminished owing to increasing corneal hypoesthesia.

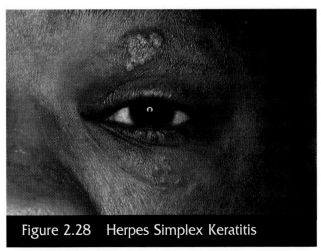

Figure 2.28   Herpes Simplex Keratitis

This 23-year-old has a history of ocular herpes infections since childhood. Grouped vesicles on an erythematous base with mild lid swelling are seen. The conjunctiva is mildly hyperemic. (Secondary impetigo may be present.) (Courtesy of Frank Birinyi, MD.)

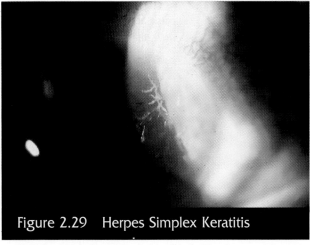

Figure 2.29   Herpes Simplex Keratitis

A slit-lamp view of unstained dendritic lesions is seen. (Courtesy of Lawrence B. Stack, MD.)

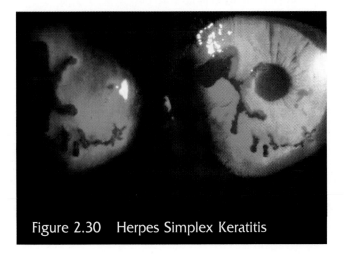

Figure 2.30   Herpes Simplex Keratitis

Fluorescein (*left*) and rose Bengal (*right*) stains demonstrate characteristic dendritic patterns. Whereas fluorescein staining is used to detect epithelial defects, rose Bengal staining additionally demonstrates degenerating or dead epithelial cells and is particularly good for demonstrating the club-shaped terminal bulbs at the end of each branch. (Used with permission from American Academy of Ophthalmology: *External Disease and Cornea: A Multimedia Collection,* San Francisco, 1994.)

Associated Clinical Features

A corneal ulcer is an inflammatory and ulcerative condition involving the cornea. Similar terms include infectious keratitis, bacterial keratitis, and ulcerative keratitis. Common etiologies include bacteria (*Staphylococcus, Streptococcus, Pseudomonas*) and viruses (herpes simplex). Keratitis secondary to herpes simplex is discussed separately. Corneal ulcers are commonly associated with extended wear soft contact lenses, whereby a minor corneal abrasion permits bacteria to penetrate the cornea. Infections secondary to fungi (*Aspergillus, Candida*) and protozoa (*Acanthamoeba*) are rare. However fungal infection should be suspected in cases of ocular trauma involving vegetable matter (a tree branch), chronic corneal disease (herpes keratitis), or cases involving steroid use. Contaminated contact lens solutions may contain bacteria or *Acanthamoeba*.

Symptoms associated with corneal ulcer include pain, photophobia, decreased vision, discharge, and a foreign body sensation. The ulcer appears as a corneal stromal infiltrate associated with conjunctival hyperemia (Fig. 2.31), a miotic pupil, chemosis, lid edema, and lid erythema. Slit-lamp biomicroscopy demonstrates an epithelial defect with fluorescein uptake. Findings in the anterior chamber include cells (inflammatory cells that appear as dust in a sunbeam) and flare (light scatter seen secondary to cells and proteins), keratic precipitates (inflammatory cells that have coalesced and adhered to the cornea), and hypopyon (a layer of white blood cells in the inferior or dependent portion of the anterior chamber).

Differential Diagnosis

Other possibilities include a sterile ulcer, residual corneal foreign body, rust ring, and sterile corneal infiltrate (secondary to an immune reaction to contact lens, solution, or *Staphylococcus*). Other causes of a red eye (conjunctivitis, glaucoma, scleritis) should also be considered.

ED Treatment and Disposition

Corneal ulcers should be treated as an ophthalmologic emergency and assumed to be bacterial until proved otherwise. An emergent ophthalmology consult is indicated, and stains and cultures should be obtained as expeditiously as possible before antibiotic treatment has commenced. Intensive topical treatment is the most effective route to treat corneal infections. Topical fluoroquinolone antibiotics (ciprofloxacin) may be given hourly. Fortified (concentrated) cefazolin and gentamicin may be used in combination, every 30 to 60 min. Subconjunctival injections of antibiotics (every 12 to 24 h) are used in very severe cases. Systemic antibiotics are not usually used except in cases in which the organism may have extended to the sclera (*Pseudomonas*) or if there is a high risk of concurrent systemic disease (*Neisseria, Haemophilus*). Cycloplegics are usually recommended for the accompanying iritis. Epithelial debridement may be beneficial. Steroids and an eye patch are contraindicated in the initial management. A contact lens wearer must discontinue contact lens wear.

Clinical Pearls

1. A bacterial corneal infection must be treated as an ophthalmologic emergency.
2. Corneal injury, including recent contact lens procedures, is a risk factor for the development of a corneal ulcer.

3. *Pseudomonas aeruginosa* is capable of destroying the cornea within 6 to 12 h. It should be suspected by its aggressive course, thick yellow-green or blue-green mucopurulent tenacious exudate, and ground-glass edema surrounding the ulcer.

4. *Acanthamoeba,* a ubiquitous protozoa, should be suspected in contact lens wearers with contaminated lens solutions or who swim wearing their contact lens. These patients characteristically have pain out of proportion to their clinical findings.

5. Infectious ulcers tend to develop centrally, away from the vascular supply (and immune system) of the limbus. A hypopyon is usually sterile, except in fungal ulcers.

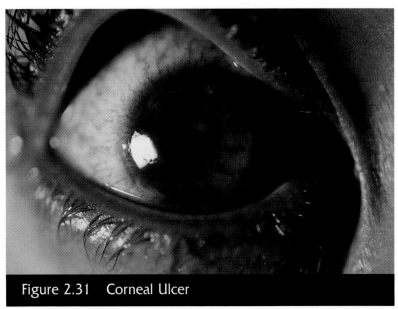

Figure 2.31   Corneal Ulcer

A circular corneal infiltrate is seen at 12 o'clock; conjunctival hyperemia is present. (A rectangular flash reflection is seen at 9 o'clock.) A mild limbal flush is noted superiorly. (Courtesy of Lawrence B. Stack, MD.)

Associated Clinical Features

Anisocoria is unequal pupil size. In room lighting the normal diameter of pupils is 3 to 5 mm. Pupil size is larger in childhood and smaller with age. Anisocoria of 1 to 2 mm may be a normal finding and is found in 5 to 20% of normal individuals. With normal (physiologic) anisocoria, the pupil size disparity is the same in light as in dark. In addition the pupils react normally to light and accommodation, are perfectly round, and no ptosis is present.

Differential Diagnosis

Associated redness, pain, or neurologic symptoms (ptosis, limited eye movements, abnormal re-activity) suggest that the anisocoria is secondary to underlying pathology. The most serious causes of anisocoria are neurogenic. In the setting of trauma, severe headache, or following in-tracranial surgery, anisocoria and a third-nerve palsy with ptosis and extraocular muscle palsies are early signs of an aneurysm or an expanding supratentorial mass with tentorial herniation.

In pathologic anisocoria, it may be difficult to ascertain which is the abnormal pupil. In this situation, pupil sizes in light and dark should be compared. Anisocoria that is greater in the dark suggests that the smaller pupil is abnormal; anisocoria that is greater in the light suggests that the larger is the abnormal pupil. Anisocoria with an abnormal small pupil may be secondary to Horner's syndrome, a long-standing Adie's pupil, iritis, or eyedrops (pilocarpine). Horner's syn-drome causes ptosis and pupil miosis secondary to interruption of sympathetic fibers to the pupil. An Adie's pupil is initially dilated, but may become smaller than the unaffected pupil over time; etiologies of an Adie's pupil include orbit trauma, infection, zoster, diabetes, autonomic neu-ropathies, and Guillain-Barré syndrome. Anisocoria with an abnormal large pupil may be seen with an early Adie's pupil, ocular trauma (with iris sphincter damage) (Fig. 2.32), eyedrops (at-ropine, phenylephrine), or inadvertent contamination from a scopolamine patch.

ED Treatment and Disposition

The evaluation of anisocoria in the ED is dependent on the clinical presentation. A patient with the acute onset of anisocoria with an altered mental status or severe headache should be aggres-sively evaluated and treated as a neurosurgical emergency. A patient with long-standing aniso-coria, on the other hand, may be discharged to follow-up with an ophthalmologist.

Pilocarpine may be helpful to the ED physician to differentiate nontraumatic causes of aniso-coria where one pupil is abnormally dilated, for example, Adie's pupil, third-nerve palsy, or phar-macologic dilation. With low concentrations of pilocarpine (0.125%), an Adie's pupil will con-strict significantly more than the unaffected pupil. With higher concentrations (1%), constriction occurs in those patients with third-nerve palsy but not with pharmacologic dilation.

Clinical Pearls

1. Compare pupil sizes in light and dark. In physiologic or normal anisocoria, the pupil size disparity is the same in light as in dark. Anisocoria that is greater in the dark suggests that the smaller pupil is abnormal; anisocoria greater in the light suggests that the larger pupil is abnormal.

2. An old photograph or driver's license viewed with an ophthalmoscope may be helpful to document the prior existence of anisocoria.

3. Some brands of eye makeup contain belladonna alkaloids, which can cause mydriasis.

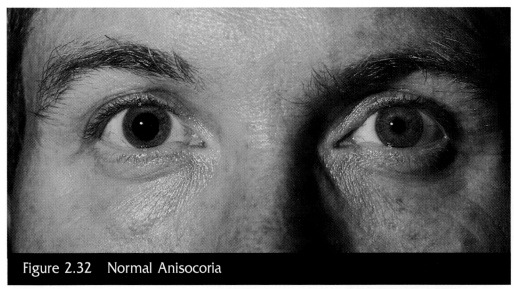

Figure 2.32 Normal Anisocoria

Marked chronic anisocoria secondary to prior trauma. (Courtesy of Kevin J. Knoop, MD, MS.)

Associated Clinical Features

Horner's syndrome consists of loss of innervation to the dilator pupillae muscle and the superior tarsal (Müller's) muscle, secondary to a lesion of the sympathetic pathway. Clinical features include unilateral miosis, 1 to 2 mm unilateral ptosis (Fig. 2.33), and anhidrosis on the ipsilateral face and neck. Slight elevation of the lower lid and conjunctival injection may also be noted on the affected side. Light and near reactions are intact. Patients themselves may be asymptomatic.

Associated clinical findings are secondary to the neurologic lesion and its location. The causes of Horner's syndrome may involve first-order neurons (stroke or tumor in the brain stem), second-order neurons (spinal cord trauma or tumor, syringomyelia; cervical chain involvement by a Pancoast tumor, cervical rib, or tumor), or third-order neurons (internal carotid artery dissection or aneurysm, herpes zoster virus).

Horner's syndrome is often idiopathic.

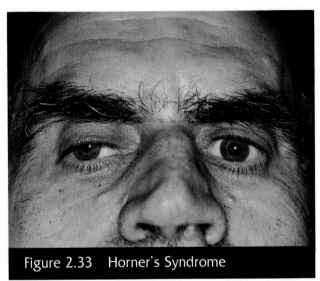

Figure 2.33 Horner's Syndrome

Unilateral miosis and ptosis are seen in this patient with Horner's syndrome and sarcoma metastatic to the spine. (Courtesy of Frank Birinyi, MD.)

Differential Diagnosis

Ptosis is seen in third-nerve palsies (berry aneurysm). Miosis may be due to eyedrops (pilocarpine), iritis, an Argyll Robertson pupil (a syphilitic pupil that accommodates but does not react), and long-standing Adie's pupil. An Adie's pupil is initially dilated (with minimal or no reaction to light), but may become smaller than the unaffected pupil over time. It is seen secondary to orbit trauma, infection, zoster, diabetes, autonomic neuropathies, and Guillain-Barré syndrome.

Pupillary inequality may be due to physiologic anisocoria.

ED Treatment and Disposition

ED treatment is directed toward diagnosing the underlying lesion. A Horner's syndrome of new onset probably requires an extensive workup and admission to the hospital. A chronic Horner's is more likely to be benign.

Clinical Pearls

1. A true Horner's pupil does not dilate in response to cocaine as does the normal pupil.
2. An old photograph or driver's license viewed with an ophthalmoscope may be helpful for comparison.

Associated Clinical Features

A Marcus Gunn pupil is indicative of a defect in the anterior visual pathway (retina, optic nerve, chiasm). It is best appreciated by the swinging flashlight test which discloses differences in afferent stimuli between the two eyes (Fig. 2.34). To perform this, a flashlight is directed onto one pupil and then the other. The critical observation to be made when evaluating the pupillary response is the initial response of the pupils when stimulated with light. The normal pupillary response to bright light is an initial constriction followed by a small amount of dilation. Normally the brief interval required to move the light from one eye to the other permits the pupils to begin to dilate. Under normal circumstances, when the light reaches the second eye, both pupils then initially constrict. In the abnormal situation, however, should the pupils instead dilate, the second pupil is said to have an afferent pupillary defect (APD) (Fig. 2.35). This positive finding indicates asymmetric function of the anterior visual pathway, that is, the eye with an APD perceives less light.

The swinging flashlight test is a useful screening technique and one of the most important assessments to make on the patient who complains of decreased vision. The test helps to differentiate whether the decreased vision is due to a media problem (cataract) or is due to optic nerve dysfunction. Although sensitive, the swinging flashlight test is not specific. Pathology may be anywhere anterior to the optic chiasm. Although a large retinal lesion may produce an APD, a positive finding almost always indicates a lesion in the optic nerve on the affected side.

In patients with an APD, associated findings might include decreased visual acuity and decreased visual fields. Funduscopic findings occasionally demonstrate the basis for the APD. These include a central retinal vein or artery occlusion, optic nerve pallor, optic nerve cupping, or severe vitreal hemorrhage.

An APD in the absence of gross ocular disease indicates a neurologic lesion in the anterior visual pathway. A Marcus Gunn pupil is best seen in conditions involving the optic nerve such as ischemic optic neuropathy, optic neuritis (including that seen with multiple sclerosis), retrobulbar optic neuritis, tumor, and glaucoma. Other conditions associated with an APD include central retinal artery or vein occlusion and a lesion of the optic chiasm or tract. Mild APD may be seen with vitreous hemorrhage, macular degeneration, retinal detachment, or other retinal disease. Small opacities do not produce an APD.

Differential Diagnosis

An Adie's pupil, seen predominately in young women, is unilaterally dilated. The reaction to light, both direct and consensual, is diminished or absent. An Argyll Robertson pupil (seen in neurosyphilis) is usually bilateral and miotic, and does not respond to light stimulation, but it does accommodate.

ED Treatment and Disposition

The finding of a Marcus Gunn pupil is nonspecific. A neurologic evaluation (history, physical examination, and CT scan) is important to assess for treatable conditions. In the absence of gross ocular or neurologic disease, a clinically stable patient may be discharged from the ED with ophthalmology follow-up.

Clinical Pearls

1. Ocular opacities such as a cataract do not result in a Marcus Gunn pupil. A dense vitreous hemorrhage, however, is capable of producing a mild defect.

2. Dim room illumination may be helpful when performing the swinging flashlight test. The patient should focus on an object 15 ft away to avoid the pupil constriction normally seen with accommodation.

3. The normal pupil response to bright light is an initial constriction followed by a small amount of dilation. In performing the swinging flashlight test, it is important to assess the initial reaction seen. In the Marcus Gunn pupil, this initial reaction is dilation.

4. In the swinging flashlight test, *both* pupils will dilate when the flashlight moves from the normal eye to the affected eye, since pupil size is centrally mediated (midbrain).

5. If the affected eye is additionally damaged or paralyzed, an APD can still be assessed by observing the response of the normal pupil with light shined alternatively in each eye. That is, the swinging flashlight test is performed as before, but the physician maintains attention on the normal eye. As the light shines in the affected eye, the *normal* eye dilates due to the consensual response of the affected eye, which perceives less light than the normal eye.

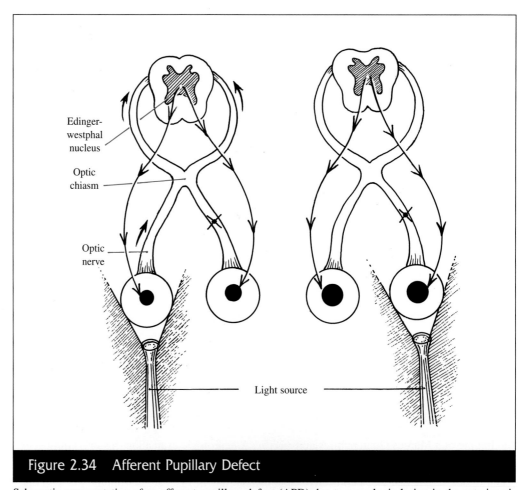

Figure 2.34   Afferent Pupillary Defect

Schematic representation of an afferent pupillary defect (APD) due to neurologic lesion in the anterior visual pathway.

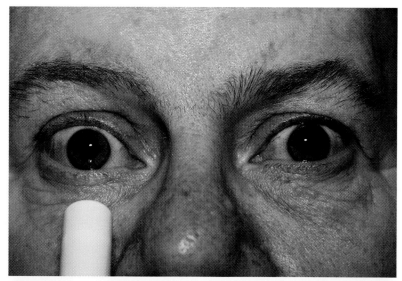

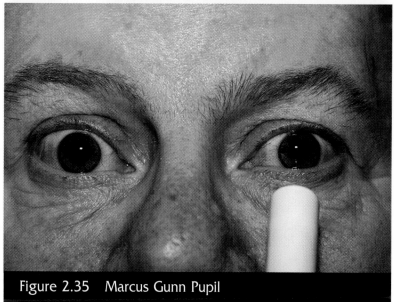

Figure 2.35   Marcus Gunn Pupil

These photographs demonstrate an afferent pupillary defect of the left pupil. When the light shines in the affected left eye, the pupils are less constricted compared with when the light shines in the right eye. Thus, when swinging the light from the right pupil to the left, the pupils appear to dilate. The anisocoria here is subtle. (Courtesy of Frank Birinyi, MD.)

Associated Clinical Features

The third cranial nerve controls the pupillary constrictor muscle, all extraocular muscles (except the lateral rectus and superior oblique muscles), and the levator palpebrae muscle. Loss of third-nerve function therefore results in a dilated and unreactive pupil, limited extraocular movements, and ptosis (Fig. 2.36).

The most important causes of an isolated third-nerve palsy are uncal herniation and aneurysm. A third-nerve palsy is in fact the most common sign of a berry aneurysm of the posterior communicating artery at its junction with the internal carotid artery. Parasympathetic fibers that control pupil constriction lie on the surface of the oculomotor nerve. The nerve runs alongside the posterior communicating artery, and therefore these fibers are particularly susceptible to compressive lesions. In uncal herniation, enlarging lesions in the middle fossa or temporal lobe commonly push the medial edge of the uncus toward the midline and over the edge of the tentorium, compressing the underlying third nerve.

A third-nerve palsy may be congenital, traumatic (subdural or epidural hematoma), or nontraumatic. Nontraumatic etiologies in addition to aneurysm include cerebral vascular accident (including Weber's syndrome, with oculomotor palsy and contralateral hemiplegia), cavernous sinus disease, brain tumor or leukemia, zoster, syphilis, and migraine. Third-nerve palsies may occur in children as a complication of meningitis and viral syndromes.

An isolated third-nerve palsy is a common sign of diabetic or hypertensive microvascular disease. In this situation, the palsy rarely affects the pupil ("pupil sparing"). This sparing is the result of the superficial pupillary fibers of the oculomotor nerve having a dual blood supply, with blood vessels supplied from both the core of the nerve as well as the sheath.

Associated clinical findings seen with a third-nerve palsy include headache, loss of accommodation, and exotropia (the affected pupil faces laterally, secondary to the unopposed action of the lateral rectus). Diplopia is not usually a complaint because of significant ptosis.

Differential Diagnosis

Unilateral pupil dilation is also seen with minor eye trauma, eyedrops (atropine), inadvertent contamination from a scopolamine patch, and an Adie's pupil (a dilated and minimally or nonreactive pupil, seen unilaterally and most often in young women). Myasthenia gravis, thyroid disease, temporal arteritis, and orbital inflammatory pseudotumor also have similar features. Ptosis may also be seen in Horner's syndrome.

ED Treatment and Disposition

The etiology of a third-nerve palsy must be delineated to determine appropriate treatment. A patient with a third-nerve palsy or unilateral dilating pupil with concomitant altered mental status must be treated as a neurosurgical emergency and requires immediate evaluation for an aneurysm or uncal herniation. Once signs of uncal herniation appear, deterioration may proceed rapidly and patients may deteriorate from full consciousness to deep coma in a few hours. In the setting of head trauma and increased intracranial pressure, measures to reduce the intracranial pressure include elevation of the head of the bed, hyperventilation, mannitol, and burr holes.

Patients with third-nerve palsies with pupil involvement should be hospitalized. Patients with vasculopathic risk factors and pupil-sparing third-nerve palsies may be discharged from the ED following their evaluation provided close follow-up is arranged.

Clinical Pearls

1. Uncal herniation and a berry aneurysm may have as their first sign a unilateral dilating pupil. Patients with the abrupt onset of headache and third-nerve palsy require immediate neurosurgical evaluation.
2. The most common cause of an isolated third-nerve palsy is a berry aneurysm of the posterior communicating artery.
3. In patients with third-nerve palsies whose pupil is unaffected (pupil sparing), the etiology is usually hypertensive or diabetic vascular disease.

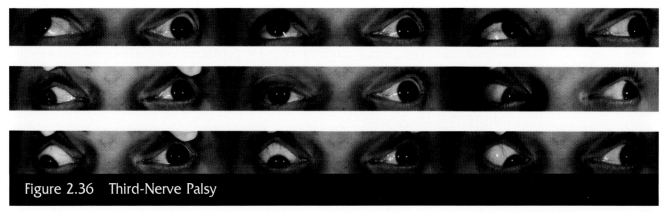

Figure 2.36   Third-Nerve Palsy

This composite shows the classic defects of a third cranial nerve palsy in all fields of gaze. The pupil is dilated. Conjugate eye movement is present in only one position, when the affected eye gazes laterally to the affected side (intact lateral rectus). When gaze is directly ahead, exotropia is seen, secondary to the unopposed lateral rectus muscle of the affected side. (Courtesy of Frank Birinyi, MD.)

Associated Clinical Features

The sixth cranial nerve (abducens nerve) innervates the lateral rectus muscle and is the most common single muscle palsy. Paralysis produces loss of abduction (Fig. 2.37) and horizontal diplopia. The diplopia is accentuated with gaze toward the affected side. Patients tend to turn their face toward the affected eye to limit their diplopia. Other eye movements are normal; the lid and pupil are not affected.

The nerve may be infarcted by microvascular changes secondary to diabetes, hypertension, migraine, or arteriosclerosis. The abducens nucleus may be involved in a cerebrovascular accident, in which case other brain stem findings are usually present. Other causes of abducens palsy include intracranial tumor, head trauma, cavernous sinus lesions (meningioma, metastasis, thrombosis, invasive nasopharyngeal carcinoma, aneurysm, carotid-cavernous fistula), infection (meningitis, Lyme disease, viruses), increased intracranial pressure, Arnold-Chiari malformation, arteriovenous malformation, giant cell arteritis, multiple sclerosis, and sarcoidosis. In children, a sixth-nerve palsy may follow a viral infection or may be acquired during birth with injury to the muscle or nerve.

An isolated sixth-nerve palsy is not usually due to an aneurysm. When associated with lesions in the cavernous sinus, cranial nerves III, IV, and V (ophthalmic and maxillary divisions) are also affected.

Differential Diagnosis

Thyroid eye disease, orbital inflammatory pseudotumor, myasthenia gravis, Duane's syndrome (congenital absence of the sixth nerve), Parinaud's syndrome (dorsal midbrain syndrome), and medial rectus entrapment (by an ethmoid fracture) have similar findings.

ED Treatment and Disposition

There is no treatment for the palsy itself except for patching the affected eye if diplopia is bothersome. ED care is directed toward determining and treating, if necessary, the underlying etiology. The aggressiveness of the workup is guided by the presence or absence of concomitant systemic disease (diabetes) and other clinical signs (other cranial nerve palsies). Commonly no underlying pathology is found.

Clinical Pearls

1. Isolated sixth-nerve palsy is usually not secondary to an aneurysm.
2. Compression of the sixth nerve can occur in cavernous sinus disorders, but associated findings usually include involvement of cranial nerves III, IV, and V (ophthalmic and maxillary divisions).

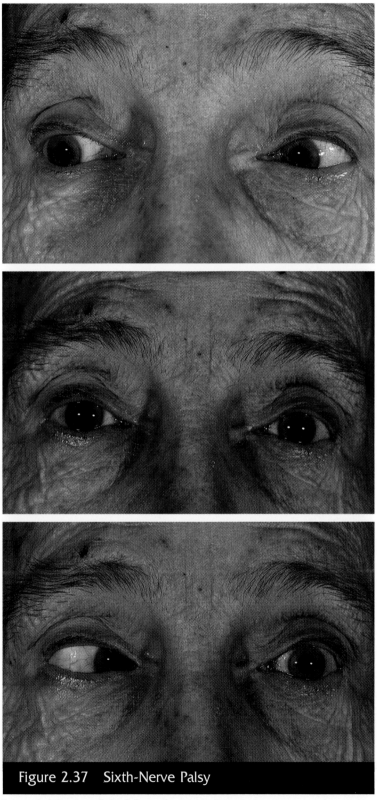

Figure 2.37   Sixth-Nerve Palsy

Loss of abduction of the left eye is seen in lateral gaze demonstrating an iso-lated sixth-nerve palsy. (Courtesy of Frank Birinyi, MD.)

EYE

CHAPTER 3

FUNDUSCOPIC FINDINGS

David Effron
Beverly C. Forcier
Richard E. Wyszynski

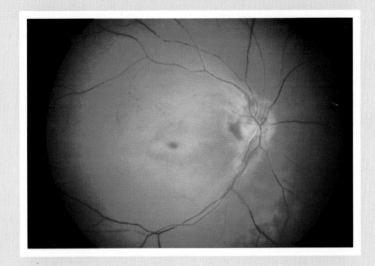

Associated Clinical Features

Disk

The disk is pale pink, approximately 1.5 mm in diameter, with sharp, flat margins (Fig. 3.1). The physiologic cup is located within the disk and usually measures less than six-tenths the disk diameter. The cups should be approximately equal in both eyes.

Vessels

The central retinal artery and central retinal vein travel within the optic nerve, branching near the surface into the inferior and superior branches of arterioles and venules, respectively. Normally the walls of the vessels are not visible; the column of blood within the walls is visualized. The venules are seen as branching, dark red lines. The arterioles are seen as bright red branching lines, approximately two-thirds or three-fourths the diameter of the venules.

Macula

An area of the retina located temporal to the disk; it is void of capillaries. The fovea is an area of depression, approximately 1.5 mm in diameter (similar to the optic disk) in the center of the macula. The foveola is a tiny pit located in the center of the fovea. These areas correspond to central vision.

Background

The background fundus is red; there is some variation in the color, depending on the amount of individual pigmentation and the visibility of the choroidal vessels beneath the retina.

Clinical Pearls

1. Fundal examination should be an integral part of any eye examination.
2. The cup/disk ratio is slightly larger in the African-American population.
3. The normal fundus should be void of any hemorrhages, exudates, or tortuous vasculature.

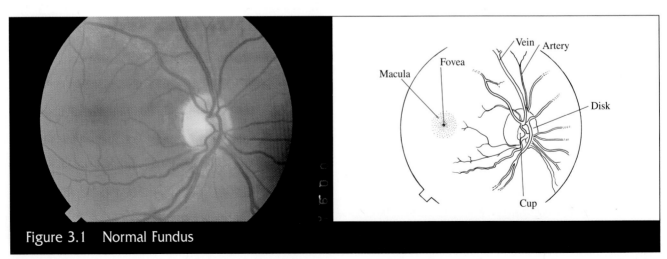

Figure 3.1   Normal Fundus

The disk has sharp margins and is normal color with a small central cup. Arterioles and venules have normal color, sheen, and course. Background is normal color. The macula is enclosed by arching temporal vessels. The fovea is located by a central pit. (Courtesy of Beverly C. Forcier, MD.)

Associated Clinical Features

Age-related macular degeneration, the leading cause of blindness in the elderly, increases in incidence with each decade over 50. Degeneration of the macula may be evidenced by accumulation of either drusen (small, discrete, round, punctate nodules), or soft drusen (larger, pale yellow or gray without discrete margins that may be confluent) (Fig. 3.2A and B). Most patients with drusen have good vision, although there may be decreased visual acuity and distortion of vision. There may be associated pigmentary changes and atrophy of the retina. Vision may slowly deteriorate if atrophy occurs.

Patients with early or late degenerative changes of their macula are at risk of developing subretinal neovascularization (SRNV), which is associated with distortion of vision, blind spots, and decreased visual acuity. Macular appearance may show dirty gray lesions, hemorrhage, retinal elevation, and exudation (Fig. 3.3).

Differential Diagnosis

Hereditary macular degenerations, other acquired macular disorders, including toxicities, and retinal exudation may present similarly.

Hemorrhages and exudates can present from vascular disease, ocular disorders such as inflammations or infections, tumors, trauma, and hereditary disorders.

ED Treatment and Disposition

Patients with drusen need ophthalmologic evaluation every 6 to 12 months, or sooner if visual distortion or decreasing visual acuity develops. If a patient complains of deterioration of visual acuity or image distortion, prompt ophthalmic evaluation is warranted, probably including fluorescein angiography. If SRNV is present, laser treatment may be indicated.

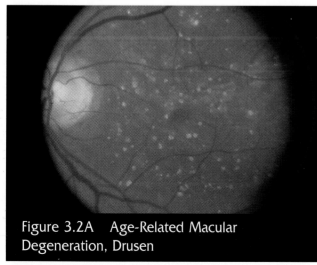

Figure 3.2A Age-Related Macular Degeneration, Drusen

Typical macular drusen and retinal pigment epithelial (RPE) atrophy (scalloped pigment loss) in age-related macular degeneration. (Courtesy of Richard E. Wyszynski, MD.)

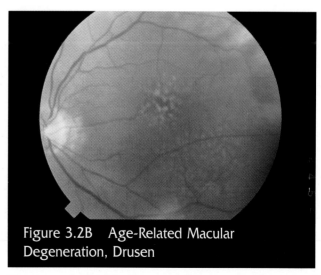

Figure 3.2B Age-Related Macular Degeneration, Drusen

Drusen are clustered in the center of the macula. (Courtesy of Richard E. Wyszynski, MD.)

Clinical Pearls

1. Age-related macular degeneration is the leading cause of blindness in the United States in patients older than 65 years of age.
2. Patient may have normal peripheral vision.
3. Untreated SRNV can lead to visual loss within a few days.
4. Patients frequently complain of distortion with SRNV.

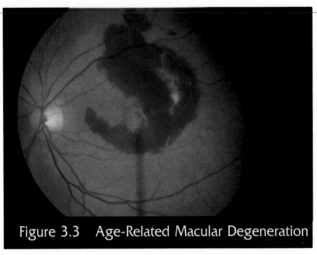

Figure 3.3   Age-Related Macular Degeneration

Hemorrhage seen beneath the retina in association with subretinal neovascularization. (Courtesy of Richard E. Wyszynski, MD.)

Associated Clinical Features

Hard exudates (Figure 3.4A) are refractile, yellowish deposits with sharp margins composed of fat-laden macrophages and serum lipids. Occasionally the lipid deposits form a partial or complete ring (called a circinate ring) around the leaking area of pathology. If the lipid leakage is located near the fovea, a spoke, or star-type distribution of the hard exudates is seen.

Cotton wool spots, or soft "exudates," are actually microinfarctions of the retinal nerve-fiber layer, and appear white with soft or fuzzy edges (Fig. 3.4B).

Inflammatory exudates are secondary to retinal or chorioretinal inflammation.

Differential Diagnosis

Hard exudation and cotton wool spots are associated with vascular diseases such as diabetes mellitus, hypertension, and collagen vascular diseases, but can be seen with papilledema and other ocular conditions. Inflammatory exudates are seen in patients with such diseases as sarcoidosis and toxoplasmosis.

ED Treatment and Disposition

Routine referral for ophthalmologic and medical workup is appropriate.

Clinical Pearls

1. Hard exudates which are intraretinal may easily be confused with drusen that occur near Bruch's membrane, which separates the retina from the choroid.

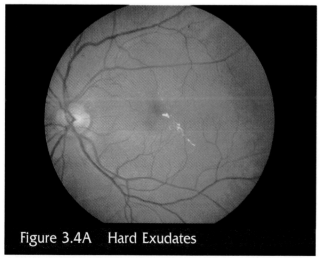

Figure 3.4A   Hard Exudates

Linear collection of yellow lipid deposits with sharp margins in macula. (Courtesy of Beverly C. Forcier, MD.)

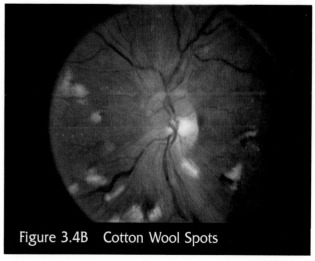

Figure 3.4B   Cotton Wool Spots

White lesions with fuzzy margins, seen here approximately one-fifth to one-fourth disk diameter in size. Orientation of cotton wool spots generally follows the curvilinear arrangement of the nerve fiber layer. Intraretinal hemorrhages and intraretinal vascular abnormalities are also present. (Courtesy of Richard E. Wyszynski, MD.)

Associated Clinical Features

Roth's spots are retinal hemorrhages with a white or yellow center (Fig. 3.5). They are seen in patients with a host of diseases such as anemia, leukemia, multiple myeloma, diabetes mellitus, collagen vascular disease, other vascular disease, intracranial hemorrhage in infants, septic retinitis, and lung carcinoma.

Differential Diagnosis

Flamed-shaped or splinter hemorrhages, or dot-blot hemorrhages may resemble Roth's spots.

ED Treatment and Disposition

Routine referral for general medical evaluation is appropriate.

Clinical Pearls

1. Roth's spots are not pathognomonic for any particular disease process and can represent a variety of clinical conditions.
2. These lesions represent red blood cells surrounding inflammatory cells.

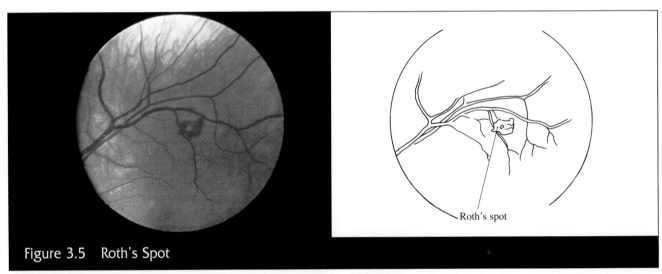

Figure 3.5 Roth's Spot

Retinal hemorrhage with pale center. (Courtesy of William E. Cappaert, MD.)

Associated Clinical Features

Plaques, if present, are often found at arteriolar bifurcations (Fig. 3.6). Patients may have signs and symptoms of vascular disease including a "source" of emboli such as carotid bruits or stenosis, aortic stenosis, aneurysms, or atrial fibrillation. Amaurosis fugax, a transient loss of vision, which is often described as a curtain of darkness obscuring vision with restoration of sight within a few minutes, may be present in the history.

Differential Diagnosis

Cholesterol emboli (Hollenhorst plaques) associated with generalized atherosclerosis often from carotid atheroma are bright, highly refractile plaques; platelet emboli (carotid artery or cardiac thrombus) are white and very difficult to visualize; and calcific emboli (cardiac valvular disease) are irregular and white or dull gray and much less refractile.

ED Treatment and Disposition

Referral for routine general medical evaluation is appropriate unless the patient presents with signs or symptoms consistent with showering of emboli, transient ischemic attack, or cerebrovascular accident, in which case referral for admission is indicated.

Clinical Pearls

1. Retinal emboli may produce a loss of vision, either transient or permanent in nature.
2. Arteriolar occlusion may occur either in a central or peripheral branch location.

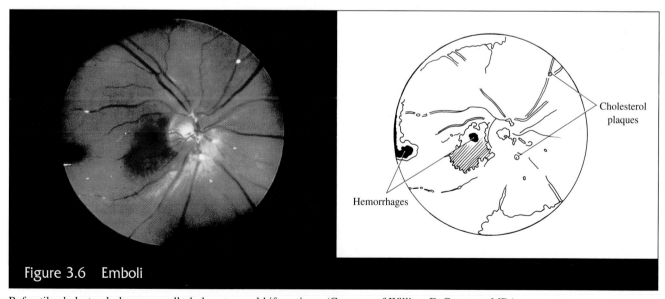

Figure 3.6   Emboli

Refractile cholesterol plaques usually lodge at vessel bifurcations. (Courtesy of William E. Cappaert, MD.)

Associated Clinical Features

The typical patient experiences a sudden, painless monocular loss of vision, either segmental or complete. Visual acuity may range from finger counting or light perception to complete blindness. Fundal findings include these: most of the fundus is pale due to retinal edema; the fovea does not have the edema, and thus appears as a cherry red spot; the retinal arterioles are narrow and irregular; the retinal venules have a "boxcar" appearance (Fig. 3.7).

Differential Diagnosis

Arteriosclerosis, arterial hypertension, carotid artery disease, diabetes mellitus, and valvular heart disease are the most common systemic disorders associated with CRAO. Other associated disorders include vascular disorders, trauma, and coagulopathies. Temporal arteritis may present with similar visual complaints.

ED Treatment and Disposition

Attempts to restore retinal blood flow may be beneficial if performed in a very narrow time window after the acute event. This may be accomplished by (1) decreasing intraocular pressure with topical beta-blocker eyedrops or intravenous acetazolamide; (2) ocular massage, applied with cyclic pressure on the globe for 10 s, followed by release, then repeated. Urgent consultation with an ophthalmologist if the CRAO is less than a few hours old is indicated to determine if more aggressive acute therapy (paracentesis) is warranted. However, such aggressive treatment rarely alters the poor prognosis. Medical evaluation and treatment of associated findings may be warranted.

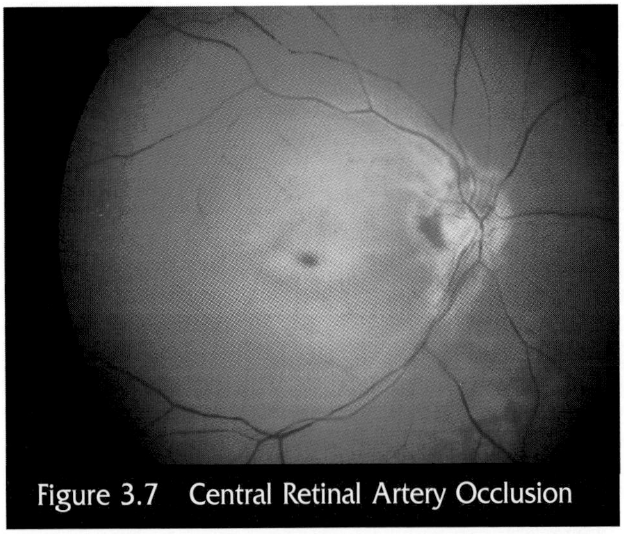

Figure 3.7   Central Retinal Artery Occlusion

The retinal pallor due to retinal edema is well demonstrated contrasting with the "cherry red spot" of the nonedematous fovea. Note the vascular narrowing and the "boxcar" appearance of the venules. (Courtesy of Richard E. Wyszynski, MD.)

Clinical Pearls

1. History should focus on how long ago the episode occurred. If the loss of vision occurred recently, then the patient should be triaged and examined quickly so as to consult an ophthalmologist within the treatment window.
2. Sudden painless monocular vision loss is typical.
3. CRAO may be associated with temporal arteritis. This diagnosis should be strongly considered in all patients presenting with signs and symptoms of CRAO who are older than 55 years.

Associated Clinical Features

Patients are usually older individuals and complain of sudden, painless visual loss in one eye. The vision loss is usually not as severe as CRAO and may vary from normal to hand motion. Funduscopy in a classic, ischemic CRVO shows a "blood and thunder" fundus: hemorrhages (including flame, dot or blot, preretinal, and vitreous) and dilation and tortuosity of the venous system. The arterial system often shows narrowing. The disk margin may be blurred. Cotton wool spots and edema may be seen (Fig. 3.8).

Differential Diagnosis

Retinal detachment, papilledema, and central retinal artery occlusion can have a similar appearance.

ED Treatment and Disposition

Treatment is rarely effective in preventing or reversing the damage done by the occlusion and is directed toward systemic evaluation to identify and treat contributing factors, hopefully decreasing the chance of contralateral CRVO. Ophthalmologic evaluation is necessary to confirm the diagnosis, estimate the amount of ischemia, and follow the patient so as to minimize sequelae of possible complications such as neovascularization and neovascular glaucoma.

Clinical Pearls

1. Sudden painless visual loss in one eye should be evaluated promptly to determine its etiology.
2. Look for the classic "blood and thunder" funduscopic findings.
3. Consider the differential diagnosis of acute *painful* (glaucoma, retrobulbar neuritis) versus *painless* vision loss (central retinal artery occlusion, anterior ischemic optic neuropathy, retinal detachment, subretinal neovascularization, and vitreous hemorrhage).

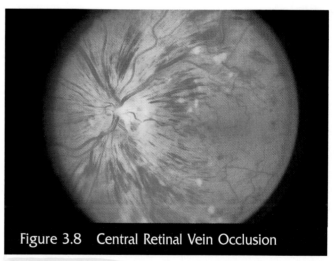

Figure 3.8   Central Retinal Vein Occlusion

The amount of hemorrhage is the most striking feature in this photograph. Also note the blurred disk margin, the dilation and tortuosity of the venules, and the cotton wool spots. Retinal edema is suggested by blurring of the retinal details. (Courtesy of Department of Ophthamology, Naval Medical Center, Portsmouth, VA.)

Associated Clinical Features

Fundus changes that may be seen with hypertension include generalized and focal narrowing of arterioles, generalized arteriolar sclerosis (copper or silver wiring), arteriovenous crossing changes, hemorrhages (usually flame-shaped), retinal edema and exudation, cotton wool spots, microaneurysms, and disk edema (Fig. 3.9).

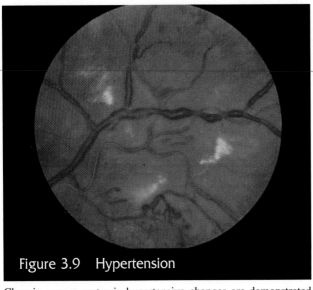

Figure 3.9 Hypertension

Chronic, severe systemic hypertensive changes are demonstrated by hard exudates, increased vessel light reflexes, and sausage-shaped veins. (Courtesy of Richard E. Wyszynski, MD.)

Differential Diagnosis

Diabetic retinopathy, many hemopoietic and vascular diseases, traumas, localized ocular pathology, papilledema should all be considered.

ED Treatment and Disposition

Medical treatment of hypertension.

Clinical Pearls

1. Hypertensive arteriolar findings may be reversible if organic changes have not occurred in the vessel walls.
2. Always consider hypertensive retinopathy in the differential diagnosis of papilledema.

Associated Clinical Features

The early ocular manifestations of diabetes mellitus are referred to as background diabetic retinopathy (BDR). Fundus findings include flame or splinter hemorrhages (located in superficial nerve fiber layer) or dot and blot hemorrhages (located deeper in the retina), hard exudates, retinal edema, and microaneurysms (Fig. 3.10A and B). If these signs are located in the macula, the patient's visual acuity may be decreased or at risk of becoming compromised, requiring laser treatment. Preproliferative diabetic retinopathy can show BDR changes plus cotton wool spots, intraretinal microvascular abnormalities, and venous beading. Proliferative diabetic retinopathy is demonstrated by neovascularization at the disk (NVD) or elsewhere (NVE) (Fig. 3.10C). These require laser therapy owing to risk of severe visual loss from sequelae: vitreous hemorrhage, tractional retinal detachment, severe glaucoma.

Differential Diagnosis

Many vascular and hemopoietic diseases, such as collagen vascular disease, sickle cell trait, hypertension, hypotension, anemia, leukemia, inflammatory and infectious states, and ocular conditions can be associated with some of or all the above signs.

ED Treatment and Disposition

Routine ophthalmologic referral for laser or surgical treatment is indicated.

Clinical Pearls

1. Periodic ophthalmologic evaluations are recommended.
2. Microaneurysms typically appear 10 years after the initial onset of diabetes, although they may appear earlier in patients with juvenile diabetes.

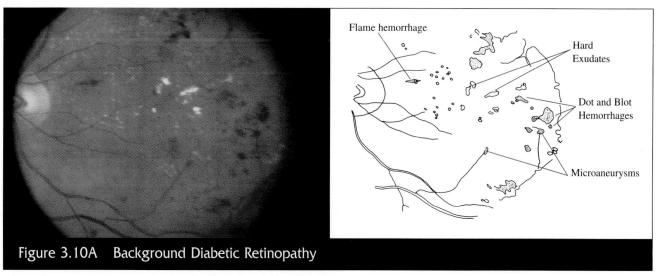

Figure 3.10A   Background Diabetic Retinopathy

Hard exudates, dot hemorrhages, blot hemorrhages, flame hemorrhages, and microaneurysms are present. Because these changes are located within the macula, this is classified as diabetic maculopathy. (Courtesy of Richard E. Wyszynski, MD.)

3. Control of blood sugar alone does not prevent the development of vasculopathy.
4. Blurred vision can also occur from acute increases in serum glucose, causing lens swelling and a refractive shift even in the absence of retinopathy.

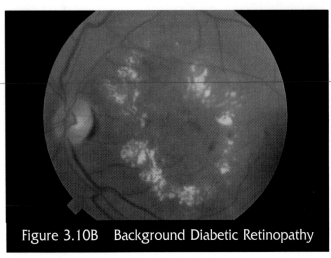

Figure 3.10B   Background Diabetic Retinopathy

An example of diabetic maculopathy with a typical circinate lipid ring. (Courtesy of Richard E. Wyszynski, MD.)

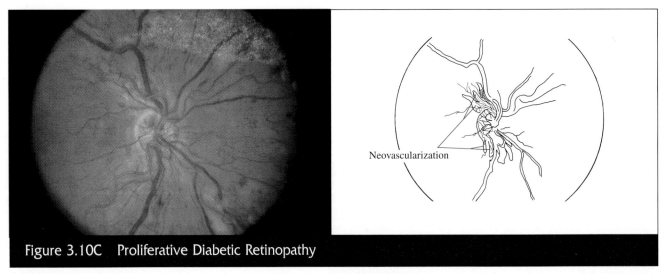

Neovascularization

Figure 3.10C   Proliferative Diabetic Retinopathy

In addition to the signs seen in background and preproliferative diabetic retinopathy, neovascularization is seen here coming off the disk. (Courtesy of Richard E. Wyszynski, MD.)

Associated Clinical Features

Patients may complain of sudden loss or deterioration of vision in the affected eye, although bilateral hemorrhage can occur. The red reflex is diminished or absent, and the retina is obscured because of the bleeding. Large sheets or three-dimensional collections of red to red-black blood may be detected (Fig. 3.11A and B).

Differential Diagnosis

Multiple underlying etiologies include proliferative diabetic retinopathy, retinal or vitreous detachments, hematologic diseases, trauma (ocular, or shaken baby syndrome), subarachnoid hemorrhage, collagen vascular disease, infections, macular degeneration, and tumors.

ED Treatment and Disposition

Refer to an ophthalmologist and an appropriate physician for associated conditions. Ophthalmic observation, photocoagulation, and surgery are all part of the therapeutic regimen. Bedrest may help to increase visualization.

Clinical Pearl

1. The patient's vision may improve somewhat after a period of sitting or standing as the blood layers out.

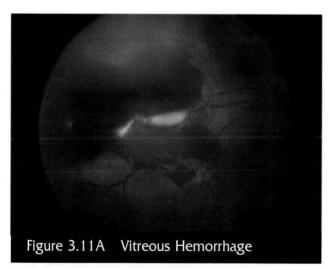

Figure 3.11A Vitreous Hemorrhage

Large amount of vitreous hemorrhage associated with metallic intraocular foreign body. The large quantity of blood obscures visualization of retinal details. (Courtesy of Richard E. Wyszynski, MD.)

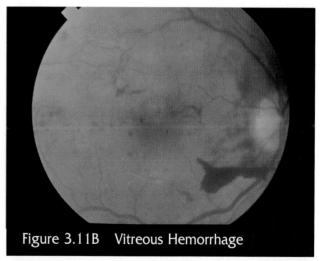

Figure 3.11B Vitreous Hemorrhage

Smaller amount of vitreous hemorrhage is more easily photographed. Gravitational effect on the vitreous blood creates appearance of flat meniscus (keel-shaped blood) in this patient with vitreous hemorrhage associated with proliferative diabetic retinopathy. (Courtesy of Richard E. Wyszynski, MD.)

Associated Clinical Features

Patients often complain of monocular, decreased visual function and may describe a shadow or curtain descending over their eye. Other complaints include cloudy or smoky vision, floaters, or flashes of light. Central visual acuity is diminished with macular involvement. Fundal examination may reveal a billowing or tentlike elevation of retina compared with adjacent areas. The elevated retina often appears gray. Retinal holes and tears may be seen, but often the holes, tears, and retinal detachment cannot be seen without indirect ophthalmoscopy (Fig. 3.12A and B).

Differential Diagnosis

Retinal detachments due to retinal tears or holes can be associated with trauma, previous ocular surgery, nearsightedness, family history of retinal detachment, and Marfan's disease. Retinal detachments due to traction on the retina by an intraocular process can be due to systemic influences in the eye, such as diabetes mellitus or sickle cell trait. Occasionally retinal detachments are due to tumors or exudative processes that elevate the retina. Symptoms of "light flashes" may occur with vitreous changes in the absence of retinal pathology. Patients may note flashes of light occurring only in a darkened environment because of the mechanical stimulation of the retina from the extraocular muscles, usually in a nearsighted individual.

ED Treatment and Disposition

Urgent ophthalmologic evaluation and treatment is warranted.

Clinical Pearls

1. Often patients have had sensation of flashes of light that occur in a certain area of a visual field in one eye corresponding to the pathologic pulling on the corresponding retina.
2. Visual loss may be gradual or sudden.

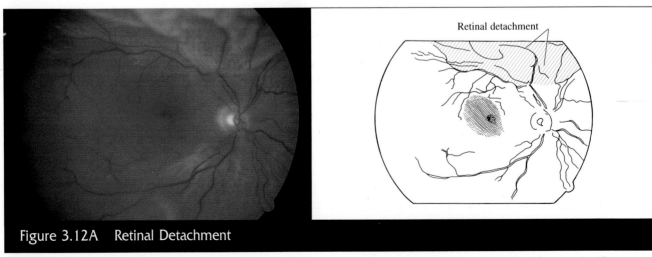

Figure 3.12A   Retinal Detachment

Red, flat, well-focused macula is contrasted with the pale, undulating, out-of-focus elevated retina surrounding the macula. (Courtesy of Richard E. Wyszynski, MD.)

Associated Clinical Features

Patient may complain of the gradual onset of the following visual sensations: floaters, scintillating scotoma (quivering blind spots), decreased peripheral visual field, and metamorphopsia (wavy distortion of vision). CMV infiltrates appear as focal, small, white lesions in the retina that look like cotton wool spots. CMV is a necrotizing virus that is spread hematogenously so that damage is concentrated in the retina adjacent to the major vessels and the optic disk. Often hemorrhage is involved with significant retinal necrosis (dirty white with a granular appearance), giving the "pizza pie" or "cheese and ketchup" appearance (Fig. 3.13). Optic nerve involvement and retinal detachments can be present.

Differential Diagnosis

The differential includes other infections such as toxoplasmosis, other herpesviruses, syphilis, and occasionally other opportunistic infections.

ED Treatment and Disposition

Reversal, if possible, of immunosuppression. Ganciclovir and foscarnet have been used with some effectiveness.

Clinical Pearls

1. HIV retinopathy consists of scattered retinal hemorrhages and scattered, multiple cotton wool spots that resolve over time, whereas CMV lesions will typically progress.
2. Although exposure to the CMV virus is widespread, the virus rarely produces a clinically recognized disease in nonimmunosuppressed individuals.

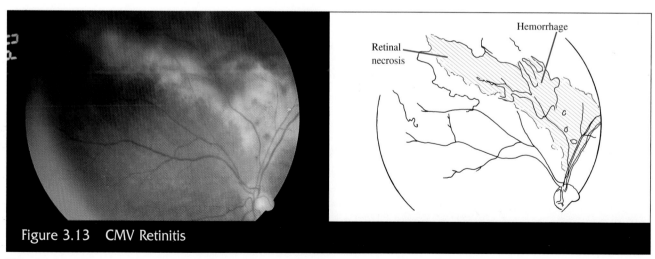

Figure 3.13   CMV Retinitis

"Pizza pie" or "cheese and ketchup" appearance is demonstrated by hemorrhages and the dirty, white, granular-appearing retinal necrosis adjacent to major vessels. (Courtesy of Richard E. Wyszynski, MD.)

Associated Clinical Features

Papilledema refers to swelling of the optic nerve head, usually in association with elevated intracranial pressure. The optic disks are hyperemic with blurred disk margins; the venules are dilated and tortuous. The optic cup may be obscured by the swollen disk. There may be flame hemorrhages and infarctions (white indistinct cotton wool spots) in the nerve fiber layer and edema in the surrounding retina (Fig. 3.14).

Differential Diagnosis

Ocular inflammation (e.g., papillitis), tumors or trauma, central retinal artery or vein occlusion, optic nerve drusen, and marked hyperopia may present with similar findings.

ED Treatment and Disposition

Expeditious ophthalmologic and medical evaluation is warranted.

Clinical Pearls

1. The top of a swollen disk and the surrounding unaffected retina will not both be in focus on the same setting on direct ophthalmoscopy.
2. Papilledema is a bilateral process, though it may be slightly asymmetric. A unilateral swollen disk suggests a localized ocular or orbital process.
3. Vision is usually normal acutely, though the patient may complain of transient visual changes. The blind spot is usually enlarged.
4. Diplopia from a cranial nerve VI palsy can be associated with increased intracranial pressure and papilledema.

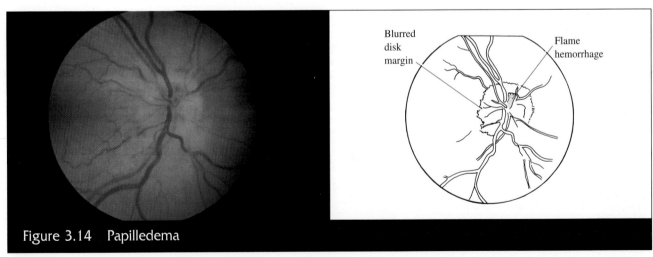

Figure 3.14 Papilledema

Disk is hyperemic and swollen with loss of sharp margins. The venules are dilated and tortuous. The cup is obscured. A small flame hemorrhage is seen at 12 to 1 o'clock on the disk margin. (Courtesy of Department of Ophthalmology, Naval Medical Center, Portsmouth, VA.)

Associated Clinical Features

Most cases of optic neuritis are retrobulbar and have no changes in the fundus, or optic disk, during the acute episode. With time, variable optic disk pallor may be present (Fig. 3.15A and B). Typical retrobulbar optic neuritis presents with sudden or rapidly progressing monocular vision loss in patients younger than 50 years. There is a central visual field defect that may extend to the blind spot. There is pain on movement of the globe. The pupillary light response is diminished in the affected eye. Over time the vision improves partially or completely, and there may be minimal or severe optic atrophy that develops. Papillitis, inflammation of the intraocular portion of the optic nerve, will have disk swelling with a few flame hemorrhages and possible cells in the vitreous.

Differential Diagnosis

Optic neuritis must be differentiated from papilledema (bilateral disk swelling, typically with no acute visual loss with the exception of transient visual changes), ischemic neuropathy (pale, swollen disk in older individual with sudden monocular vision loss), tumors, metabolic or endocrine disorders, or ocular conditions. Most cases of optic neuritis have unknown etiology. Some known causes of optic neuritis include demyelinating disease, infections (including viral, syphilis, tuberculosis, sarcoidosis), or inflammations from contiguous structures (sinuses, meninges, orbit).

ED Treatment and Disposition

Treatment is controversial, and often none is recommended. Oral steroids may worsen prognosis in certain cases. Intravenous steroids may be considered after consultation with an ophthalmologist.

Clinical Pearls

1. Monocular vision loss with pain on palpation of the globe or with eye movement are clinical clues to the diagnosis.
2. Sudden or rapidly progressing central vision loss is characteristic.
3. Most cases of acute optic neuritis are retrobulbar. Thus ophthalmoscopy shows a normal fundus.

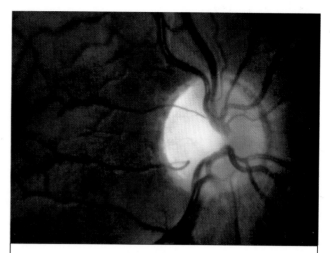

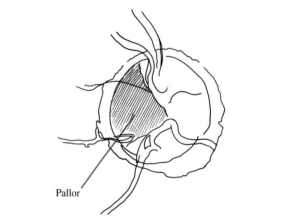

Pallor

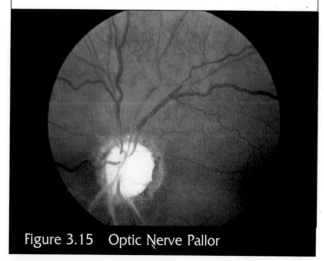

Figure 3.15 Optic Nerve Pallor

Optic nerve pallor, either segmental (*top*) or generalized (*bottom*) are nonspecific changes that may be associated with a previous episode of optic neuritis or other insults to the optic nerve. (Courtesy of Richard E. Wyszynski, MD.)

Associated Clinical Features

Anterior ischemic optic neuropathy presents with sudden visual field loss (often altitudinal) usually involving fixation, in an older individual. The loss is usually stable after onset, with no improvement, and only occasionally, progressive over several days to weeks. Pale disk swelling is present involving a sector or the full disk, with accompanying flame hemorrhages (Fig. 3.16).

Differential Diagnosis

The common, nonarteritic causes of AION (probably arteriosclerosis) need to be differentiated from arteritic, such as giant cell arteritis. The latter, if untreated, will involve the other eye in 75% of cases, often in a few days to weeks. These elderly individuals often have weight loss, masseter claudication, weakness, myalgias, elevated sedimentation rate, and painful scalp, temples, or forehead.

ED Treatment and Disposition

Routine ophthalmologic and medical evaluation is appropriate.

Clinical Pearls

1. Consider AION in an elderly patient with sudden, usually painless visual field loss.
2. Rule out giant cell arteritis. These patients tend to be older (age >55) and may have associated CRAO or cranial nerve palsies (III, IV, or VI) with diplopia.

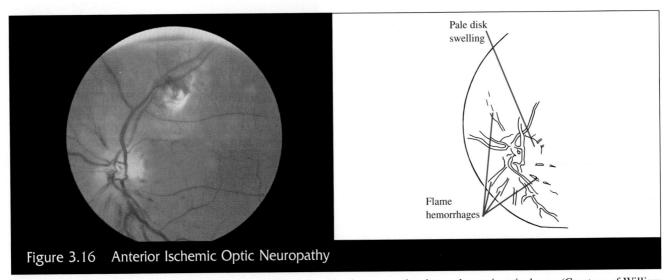

Figure 3.16   Anterior Ischemic Optic Neuropathy

Pale disk swelling and flame hemorrhages are present. This patient also has an unrelated toxoplasmosis retinal scar. (Courtesy of William E. Cappaert, MD.)

Associated Clinical Features

Narrow or closed angle glaucoma results from a physical appositional impedence of aqueous humor outflow. Symptoms range from complaints of colored halos around lights and blurred vision to severe pain (may be described as a headache or brow ache) associated with nausea and vomiting. Intraocular pressures are markedly elevated. Perilimbal vessels are injected, the pupil mid-dilated and poorly reactive to light, and the cornea may be hazy and edematous (see also Chapt. 2 for external ocular images).

Two-thirds of glaucoma patients have open angle glaucoma due to an abnormality of primary tissues responsible for the outflow of fluid out of the eye. Often they are asymptomatic. They may have a family history of glaucoma. Funduscopy may show asymmetric cupping of the optic nerves (Fig. 3.17). The optic nerve may show notching, local thinning of tissue, or disk hemorrhage. Optic cups enlarge, especially vertically, with progressive damage. Tissue loss is associated with visual field abnormalities, usually in arcuate patterns. The intraocular pressure often, but not always, is greater than 21.

Differential Diagnosis

Acute Glaucoma

Painful visual loss (retrobulbar optic neuritis, iritis, endophthalmitis), referred pain from nonophthalmic source.

Chronic Glaucoma

Normal variants, ocular conditions like disk drusen or optic neuropathy.

ED Treatment and Disposition

Acute Narrow Angle Glaucoma

Emergent ophthalmologic consultation and administration of medications to decrease IOP (intraocular pressure). Beta-blocker drops (timolol), carbonic anhydrase inhibitors (acetazolamide), cholinergic stimulating drops (pilocarpine), hyperosmotic agents (osmoglyn), and alpha-adrenergic agonists (apraclonidine) may be employed prior to laser or surgical iridotomy (see also Chapt. 2).

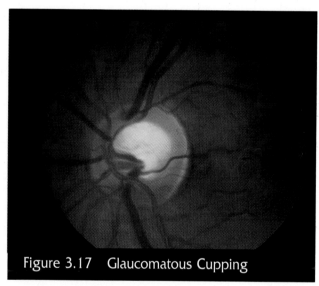

Figure 3.17   Glaucomatous Cupping

The cup is not central; it is elongated toward the rim supero temporally. (Courtesy of Department of Ophthalmology, Naval Medical Center, Portsmouth, VA.)

Open Angle Glaucoma

Long-term ophthalmic evaluation and treatment with medications and laser or surgery.

Clinical Pearls

1. A high index of suspicion must be maintained since associated complaints such as nausea, vomiting, and headache may obscure the diagnosis.

2. Open angle glaucoma usually causes no symptoms other than gradual loss of vision.
3. Congenital glaucoma is rare. However, because of prognosis if diagnosis is delayed, consider congenital glaucoma in infants and children with any of the following: tearing, photophobia, enlarged eyes, cloudy corneas.
4. Asymmetric cupping, enlarged cups, and elevated intraocular pressure are hallmarks of open angle glaucoma.

SUBHYALOID HEMORRHAGE IN SUB-ARACHNOID HEMORRHAGE (SAH)

Associated Clinical Features

Subhyaloid hemorrhage appears as extravasated blood beneath the retinal layer (Fig. 3.18). These are often described as "boat-shaped" hemorrhages to distinguish them from the "flame-shaped" hemorrhages on the superficial retina. They may occur as a result of blunt trauma, but are perhaps best known as a marker for subarachnoid hemorrhage. In SAH, the hemorrhages appear as a "puff" of blood emanating from the central disk.

Differential Diagnosis

SAH, shaken-baby syndrome, hypertensive retinopathy, and retinal hemorrhage should all be considered and aggressively evaluated.

ED Treatment and Disposition

No specific treatment is required for subhyaloid hemorrhage. Treatment is dependent on the underlying etiology. Appropriate specialty referral should be made in all cases.

Clinical Pearl

1. A funduscopic examination looking for subhyaloid hemorrhage should be included in all patients with severe headache, unresponsive pediatric patients, or those with altered mental status.

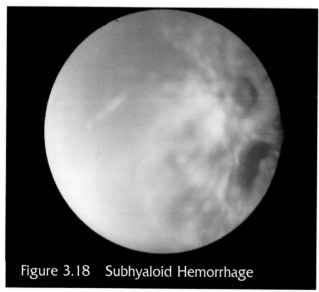

Figure 3.18 Subhyaloid Hemorrhage

Subhyaloid hemorrhage seen on funduscopic examination in a patient with subarachnoid hemorrhage. (Courtesy of Dallas E. Peak, MD.)

EYE

CHAPTER 4

OPHTHALMIC TRAUMA

Dallas E. Peak
Carey D. Chisholm
Kevin J. Knoop

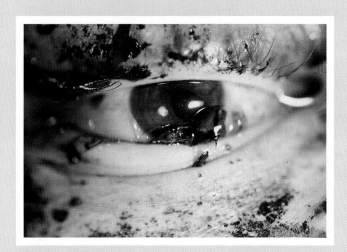

Associated Clinical Features

Corneal abrasions are heralded by the acute onset of eye discomfort accompanied by tearing and a foreign body sensation. Conjunctival injection may also be noted. If the area of abrasion is large or central, visual acuity may be affected. Large abrasions or delays in seeking care may be accompanied by photophobia and headache from ciliary muscle spasm. Associated findings or complications include traumatic iritis, hypopyon, or a corneal ulcer (described in Chap. 2). Examination before and after instillation of fluorescein, preferably with a slit lamp, usually reveals the defect (Figs. 4.1 and 4.2). Fluorescein pools and stains the area where corneal epithelium has been denuded.

Differential Diagnosis

Corneal foreign body, conjunctivitis, conjunctival foreign body, and corneal ulcer can present with similar complaints.

ED Treatment and Disposition

Instillation of topical anesthetic drops permits a better examination and relieves pain. A short-acting cycloplegic (e.g., cyclopentolate 0.5%, homatropine 5%) may reduce ciliary spasm and pain and should be considered in patients with larger abrasions or in those who complain of headache or photophobia. Topical antibiotic drops or ointment, preferably broad spectrum such as gentamicin, sulfacetamide, or erythromycin are used to prevent secondary bacterial infection. A soft double-layer patch may also be applied. Neither topical antibiotics nor patching have been scientifically validated, and routine use of these practices has recently been called into question. Follow-up is required for any patient who is still symptomatic after 12 h.

Clinical Pearls

1. Only sterile fluorescein strips should be used since the corneal epithelium, the primary barrier to infection, has been potentially disrupted.
2. Mucus may simulate the fluorescein uptake but its position changes with blinking.
3. Multiple linear corneal abrasions, the "ice-rink sign," may result from a foreign body adherent to the conjunctiva under the lid (Fig. 4.3). The lid should always be everted to rule out a retained foreign body.
4. A high index of suspicion of a perforating injury should be maintained for any abrasion which occurs as a result of grinding or striking metal on metal.
5. Fluorescein streaming away from an "abrasion" (Seidel's test) may be an indication of a corneal perforation.

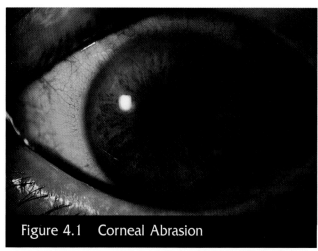

Figure 4.1   Corneal Abrasion

Seen under magnification from the slit lamp, corneal abrasion can sometimes be appreciated without fluorescein staining. This abrasion is seen without using the cobalt blue light. (Courtesy of Harold Rivera.)

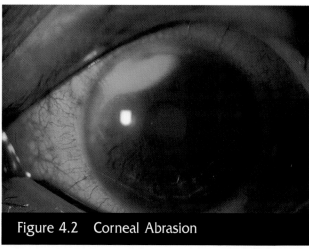

Figure 4.2   Corneal Abrasion

The same abrasion as Fig. 4.1 is seen under magnification from the slit lamp with fluorescein stain using the cobalt blue light. (Courtesy of Harold Rivera.)

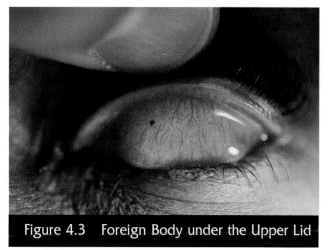

Figure 4.3   Foreign Body under the Upper Lid

Lid eversion is an essential part of the eye examination. (Courtesy of Kevin J. Knoop, MD, MS.)

Associated Clinical Features

Patients typically give a history of something in the eye or complain of foreign body sensation. If the foreign body overlies the cornea, the patient's vision may be affected. There may be tearing, conjunctival injection, and ciliary flush (Fig. 4.4). If several hours have elapsed since the occurrence of the injury, there may be headache and photophobia in addition to the above signs and symptoms.

Differential Diagnosis

The most important consideration in the differential is the possibility of a penetrating injury to the globe. A meticulous history about the mechanism of injury (grinding or metal on metal) must be elicited. Conjunctival foreign body, corneal abrasion, penetrating injury to the globe, intraocular foreign body, conjunctivitis, iritis, and glaucoma should also be considered.

ED Treatment and Disposition

If superficial, removal of the foreign body with a moist cotton-tipped applicator may be attempted; if unsuccessful, an eye spud, or small (25 gauge) needle may be used. After removal, if a residual corneal abrasion is present, instill an antibiotic solution or ointment. A "short-acting" cycloplegic (e.g., cyclopentolate 0.5%) should be considered in patients with complaints of headache or photophobia. Metallic foreign bodies are often accompanied by a "rust ring" discoloration of the surrounding corneal epithelium (Fig. 4.5). Removal of the rust ring can be attempted, either with a needle or preferably with a small burr drill device available commercially. Alternatively, the patient may be referred to an ophthalmologist the following day.

Clinical Pearls

1. Treatment of a suspected penetrating injury to the globe includes immediate referral, eye rest, protective patching (Fig. 4.6), and elevating the head of the bed.
2. If history of ocular penetration is present, a diligent search for foreign body with either plain x-rays or CT scan is indicated (Fig. 4.7).
3. Be sure to evert the upper lid and search carefully for foreign body. A foreign body adherent to the upper lid abrades the cornea producing the "ice-rink" sign, caused from multiple linear abrasions.
4. If a rust ring is present from a metallic foreign body, its removal can be attempted, or the patient may await ophthalmology follow-up in 24 h.
5. Multiple small corneal foreign bodies (e.g., glass or sand) may be removed by irrigating with normal saline or tap water. The instillation of a topical anesthetic facilitates the irrigation process.

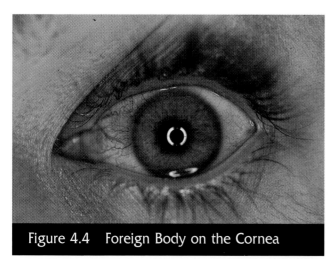

Figure 4.4   Foreign Body on the Cornea

A foreign body is lodged at 10 o'clock on the cornea. Note the localized ciliary flush in the surrounding conjunctiva at the limbus. (Courtesy of Kevin J. Knoop, MD, MS.)

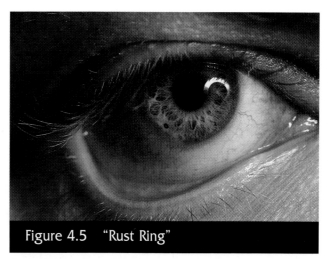

Figure 4.5   "Rust Ring"

A rust ring has formed from a foreign body (likely metallic) in this patient. A burr drill can be used for attempted removal, which if unsuccessful, can be reattempted in 24 h. (Courtesy of Kevin J. Knoop, MD, MS.)

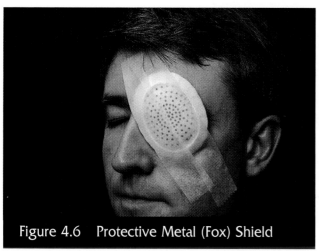

Figure 4.6   Protective Metal (Fox) Shield

A protective shield is used in the setting of a suspected or confirmed perforating injury. A patch may be fashioned from a cup if needed. (Courtesy of Kevin J. Knoop, MD, MS.)

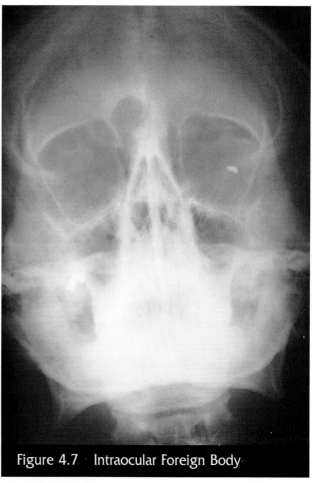

Figure 4.7   Intraocular Foreign Body

A metallic foreign body is seen on a plain radiograph and with comparison with a lateral film indicates the presence of an intraocular foreign body. (Courtesy of Department of Ophthalmology, Naval Medical Center, Portsmouth, VA.)

Associated Clinical Features

Eyelid lacerations should always prompt a thorough search for associated injury to the globe, penetration of the orbit, or involvement of surrounding structures (e.g., lacrimal glands, ducts, puncta) (Fig. 4.8). Depending on the mechanism of injury, a careful exclusion of foreign body may be indicated.

Differential Diagnosis

Laceration of the levator palpebrae musculature or tendinous attachments, laceration of the canthal ligamentous support, division of the lacrimal duct or puncta, and penetration of the periorbital septum should all be considered.

ED Treatment and Disposition

Eyelid lacerations involving superficial skin can be repaired with 6-0 nonabsorbable interrupted sutures which should remain in place for 3 days. Lacerations through an anatomic structure called the gray line (see Fig. 4.8), situated on the palpebral edge, require diligent reapproximation and should be referred. Other injuries that require specialty consultation for repair include:

Lacerations through the lid margins: these require exact realignment to avoid entropion or extropion.

Deep lacerations through the upper lid that divide the levator palpebrae muscles or their tendinous attachments: these must be repaired with fine, absorbable suture to avoid ptosis.

Lacrimal duct injuries: these are repaired by stenting of the duct, otherwise excessive spilling of tears (epiphora) will result.

Medial canthal ligaments: these must be repaired to avoid drooping of the lids.

The most important objectives are to rule out injury to the globe and to search diligently for foreign bodies.

Clinical Pearls

1. Lacerations of the medial one-third of the lid (Fig. 4.9) should always raise suspicion for injury to the lacrimal ducts or puncta as well as the medial canthal ligament.
2. A small amount of adipose tissue seen within a laceration is a sign that perforation of the orbital septum has occurred (since there is no subcutaneous fat in the lids themselves).
3. Injuries involving the orbital septum carry a higher than normal risk of globe injury and intraorbital foreign body, and carry a higher risk for orbital cellulitis. A CT scan and specialty consultation should be considered.
4. Any injury to the lids involving tissue loss or avulsion should be referred for specialty consultation.

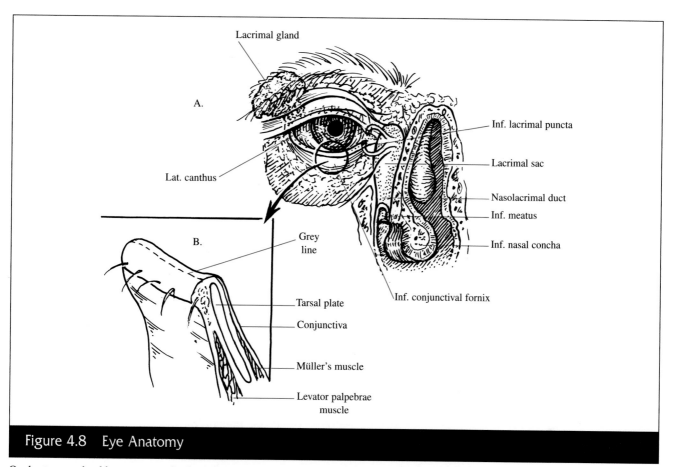

Figure 4.8 Eye Anatomy

Ocular trauma should prompt examination of surrounding anatomic structures for associated injuries.

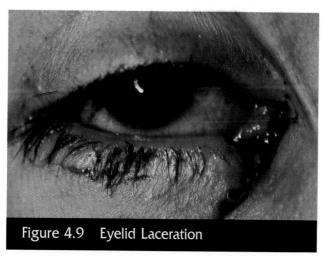

Figure 4.9 Eyelid Laceration

This laceration involving the medial third of the lid clearly violates the canalicular structures. The patient was struck by a person wearing a ring. (Courtesy of Kevin J. Knoop, MD, MS.)

Associated Clinical Features

Injury to the anterior chamber that disrupts the vasculature supporting the iris or ciliary body results in a hyphema. The blood tends to layer and because of gravity forms a meniscus (Fig. 4.10). Symptoms can include pain, photophobia, and possibly blurred vision secondary to obstructing blood cells. Nausea and vomiting may signal a rise in intraocular pressure (glaucoma) caused by blockage of the trabecular meshwork by blood cells or clot.

Differential Diagnosis

Hypopyon (pus within the anterior chamber), vitreous hemorrhage, iridodialysis, penetrating injury to the globe, and intraocular foreign body should be considered.

ED Treatment and Disposition

Prevention of further hemorrhage is the first goal. The patient should be kept at rest in the supine position with the head elevated slightly. A hard eye shield should be used to prevent further trauma from manipulation. Oral or parenteral pain medication and sedatives are appropriate, but avoid agents with antiplatelet activity (e.g., NSAIDs). Antiemetics should be used if the patient has nausea. Further treatment is at the discretion of specialty consultants, but may include topical and oral steroids, antifibrinolytics such as aminocaproic acid, or surgery. Intraocular pressure should be measured in all patients unless there is a suspicion of penetrating injury to the globe. If elevated, intraocular pressure should be treated with appropriate agents including topical beta blockers, pilocarpine, and if needed, osmotic agents (mannitol, sorbitol) and acetazolamide. The need for admission for small hyphemas is variable, since some centers admit all, whereas others individualize treatment. Ophthalmologic consultation is warranted to determine local practices.

Clinical Pearls

1. The patient should be told specifically not to read or watch television as these activities result in greater than usual ocular activity.
2. Depending on the severity of the initial hyphema, re-bleeding may occur in 10 to 25% of patients, commonly in 2 to 5 days as the original clot retracts and loosens.
3. Blood which is not absorbed from the anterior chamber may infiltrate and stain the cornea leaving a brown discoloration.
4. An "eightball" or total hyphema occurs when blood fills the entire anterior chamber. These require surgical evacuation.
5. Patients with sickle cell and other hemoglobinopathies are at risk for sickling of blood inside the anterior chamber (Fig. 4.11). This can cause a rise in intraocular pressure from physical obstruction of the trabecular meshwork.

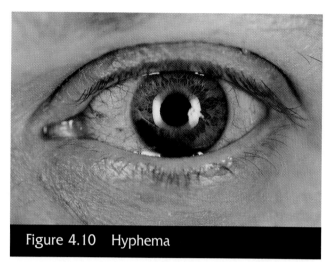

Figure 4.10   Hyphema

This hyphema has almost completely layered while the patient's head was tilted. Note the hazy greenish area at 6 o'clock in contrast to the remainder of the blue iris. This represents blood circulating in the anterior chamber that has not yet layered. (Courtesy of Kevin J. Knoop, MD, MS.)

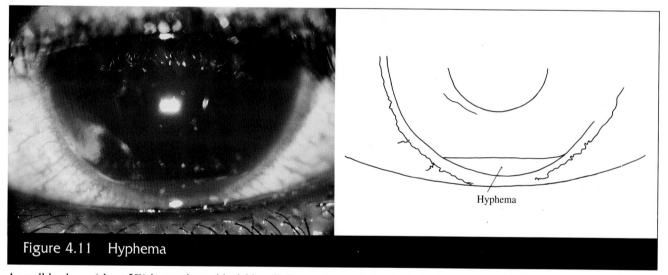

Figure 4.11   Hyphema

A small hyphema (about 5%) in a patient with sickle cell disease that needed to be drained. (Courtesy of Dallas E. Peak, MD.)

Associated Clinical Features

Traumatic iridodialysis is the result of an injury, typically blunt trauma, which pulls the iris away from the ciliary body. The resulting deformity appears as a lens-shaped defect at the outer margin of the iris (Fig. 4.12). Patients may present complaining of a "second pupil." As the iris pulls away from the ciliary body, a small amount of bleeding may result. Look closely for associated traumatic hyphema.

Differential Diagnosis

Traumatic hyphema, penetrating injury to the globe, scleral rupture, intraocular foreign body, and lens dislocation causing billowing of the iris should all be considered.

ED Treatment and Disposition

A remote traumatic iridodialysis requires no specific treatment in the emergency department. Recent history of ocular trauma should prompt a diligent slit-lamp examination for associated hyphema or lens discoloration. If hyphema is present, it should be treated as discussed (see "Hyphema"). Pure cases of iridodialysis may be referred for specialty consultation to exclude other injuries, or if the defect is large enough to result in monocular diplopia, surgical repair may be necessary.

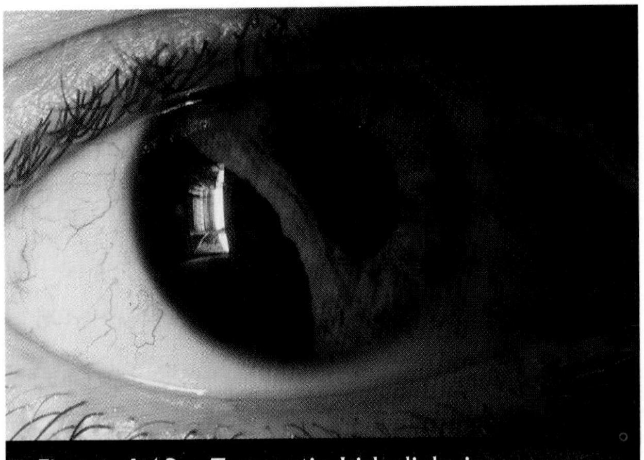

Figure 4.12   Traumatic Iridodialysis

The iris has pulled away from the ciliary body as a result of blunt trauma. (Courtesy of Department of Ophthalmology, Naval Medical Center, Portsmouth, VA.)

Clinical Pearls

1. The examination should carefully exclude posterior chamber pathology and hyphema.
2. A careful review of the history to exclude penetrating trauma should be made. If the history is unclear, CT scan may be used to exclude the presence of intraocular foreign body.
3. A careful examination includes searching for associated lens dislocation.

Associated Clinical Features

Lens dislocation may result from sudden blow to the globe with resultant stretching of the zonule fibers which hold the lens in place (Fig. 4.13). The patient may experience symptoms of monocular diplopia or gross blurring of images, depending on severity. The edge of the subluxed lens may be visible when the pupil is dilated (Fig. 4.14). If all the zonule fibers tear and the lens is dislocated, it may lodge in the anterior chamber or the vitreous.

Differential Diagnosis

Marfan's syndrome, tertiary syphilis, and homocystinuria may be present and should be considered in patients presenting with lens dislocation.

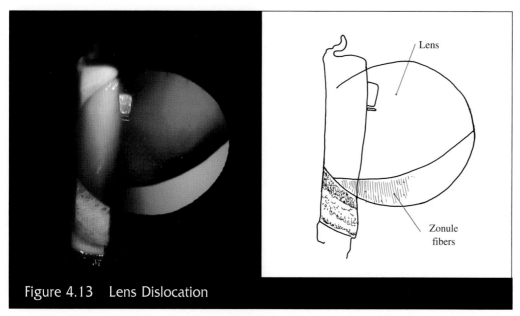

Figure 4.13   Lens Dislocation

Lens dislocation revealed during slit lamp examination. Note the zonule fibers which normally hold the lens in place. (Courtesy of Department of Ophthalmology, Naval Medical Center, Portsmouth, VA.)

ED Treatment and Disposition

Almost all require surgery if the lens is totally dislocated; partial subluxations may only require a change in refraction.

Clinical Pearls

1. Patients may experience lens dislocation with seemingly trivial trauma if they have an underlying coloboma of the lens (see Fig. 4.19), Marfan's syndrome, homocystinuria, or syphilis.
2. Iridodonesis is a trembling movement of the iris noted after rapid eye movements and is a sign of occult posterior lens dislocation.

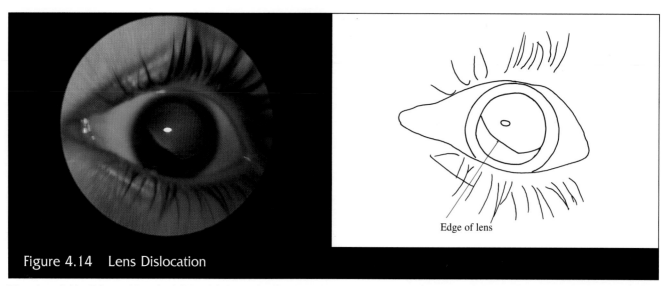

Figure 4.14   Lens Dislocation

The edge of this dislocated lens is visible with the pupil dilated as an altered red reflex. (Courtesy of Department of Ophthalmology, Naval Medical Center, Portsmouth, VA.)

Associated Clinical Features

Open globe injuries resulting from penetrating trauma can be subtle and easily overlooked. All are serious injuries. Signs to look for are loss of anterior chamber depth caused from leakage of aqueous humor, a teardrop-shaped pupil, or prolapse of choroid through the wound (Fig. 4.15).

Differential Diagnosis

Iridodialysis, corneal foreign body, and scleral rupture may have similar presentations.

ED Treatment and Disposition

All open globe injuries require specialty consultation. A Fox (metal) eye shield should be placed over the affected eye. No attempts to examine, measure pressures, or manipulate the eye should be made. Intravenous antibiotics to cover gram-positive organisms are appropriate. Sedation and aggressive pain management are crucial and should be used liberally to prevent or decrease expulsion of intraocular contents due to crying, activity, or vomiting. Antiemetics should be given if nausea is present. Tetanus immunization should be updated.

Clinical Pearls

1. When a large foreign body such as a pencil or nail protrudes from the globe, resist the temptation to remove it. Such objects should be left in place until definitive treatment in the operating room.
2. Control of pain, activity, and nausea may be sight-saving and require proactive use of appropriate medications.
3. Use of lid hooks, retractors (Fig. 4.16), or even retractors fashioned from paper clips (Fig. 4.17) is preferred to open the eyelids of trauma victims with blepharospasm or massive swelling. Attempts to do this with fingers can inadvertently increase the pressure on the globe.
4. Penetrating globe injuries are a relative contraindication to the sole use of depolarizing neuromuscular blockade (e.g., succinylcholine). Pretreatment with a small dose of nondepolarizing agent should be done to abolish the fasciculations and resultant increased intraocular pressure.

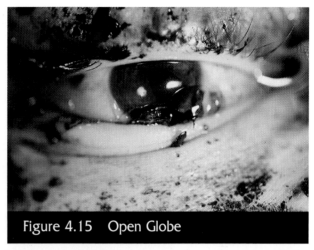

Figure 4.15   Open Globe

This injury is not subtle; extruded ocular contents (vitreous) can be seen; a teardrop pupil is also present. (Courtesy of Alan B. Storrow, MD.)

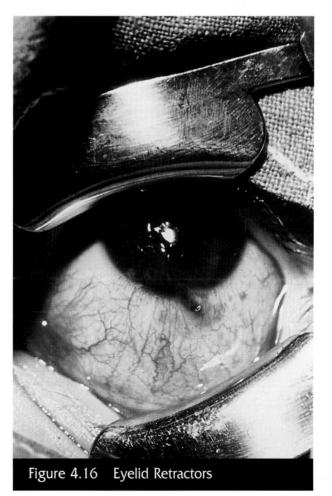

Figure 4.16   Eyelid Retractors

Retractors are used to gain exposure without applying pressure to the globe. (Courtesy of Dallas E. Peak, MD.)

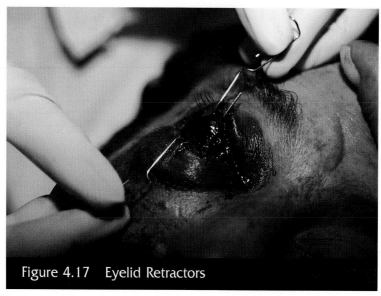

Figure 4.17   Eyelid Retractors

Retractors fashioned with paper clips can be used safely when standard retractors are not available. (Courtesy of Kevin J. Knoop, MD, MS.)

Associated Clinical Features

A forceful blow to the eye may result in a scleral rupture. The diagnosis is obvious when orbital contents are seen spilling from the globe itself. The diagnosis may be more occult in situations where only a tiny rent in the sclera has occurred. When rupture occurs at the limbus, a small amount of iris may herniate, resulting in an irregularly shaped pupil called a teardrop pupil (Fig. 4.18). A teardrop pupil may also be the result of a penetrating foreign body. Mechanism is the key to distinguishing these two causes. Another associated finding is bloody chemosis of the bulbar conjunctiva over the area of scleral rupture. This may be distinguished from a simple subconjunctival hematoma by bulging of the conjunctiva.

Differential Diagnosis

Subconjunctival hematoma, nontraumatic bloody chemosis, corneal-scleral laceration, intraocular foreign body, iridodialysis, and traumatic lens dislocation may have a similar presentation. A coloboma of the iris (Fig. 4.19) may appear similar to a teardrop pupil.

ED Treatment and Disposition

Urgent specialty consultation and operative management are mandatory. The eye should be protected by a Fox metal eye shield, and all further examination and manipulation of the eye should be discouraged to prevent prolapse or worsening prolapse of choriouveal structures. Tetanus status should be addressed. IV antibiotics to cover suspected organisms are appropriate. Adequate sedation and use of parenteral analgesics is encouraged. Antiemetics should be given proactively since vomiting may result in further prolapse of intraocular contents. CT scanning should be considered if the presence of a foreign body is suspected.

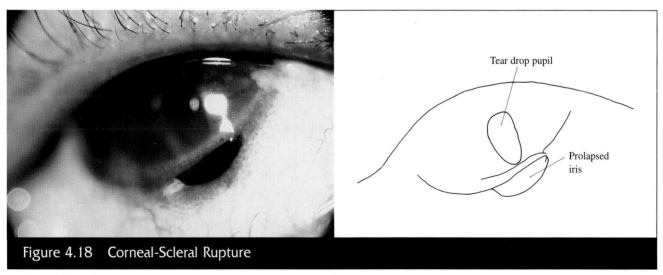

Figure 4.18   Corneal-Scleral Rupture

A teardrop pupil is present with a small amount of iris herniating from a rupture at the limbus. These injuries may initially go unnoticed. (Courtesy of Dallas E. Peak, MD.)

Clinical Pearls

1. The eyeball may appear deflated, or the anterior chamber excessively deep. Intraocular pressure will likely be decreased, but measurement should be avoided since this may worsen herniation of intraocular contents.

2. Rupture usually occurs where the sclera is the thinnest, at the point of attachment of extraocular muscles and at the limbus.

3. Bloody chemosis from scleral rupture is distinguished from subconjunctival hematoma by bulging of the conjunctiva. A subconjunctival hematoma is flat in appearance (see Fig. 4.20).

4. A teardrop pupil may be easily overlooked in the triage process or in the setting of multiple traumatic injuries.

5. Seidel's test (instillation of fluorescein and observing for fluorescein streaming away from the injury) may be used to diagnose subtle perforation.

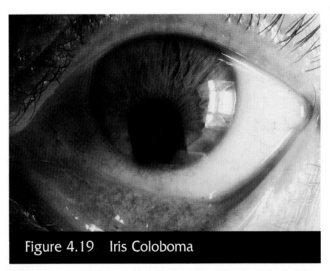

Figure 4.19   Iris Coloboma

Iris coloboma is a congenital finding resulting from incomplete closure of the fetal ocular cleft. It appears as a teardrop pupil and may be confused as a sign of scleral rupture. (Courtesy of Department of Ophthalmology, Naval Medical Center, Portsmouth, VA.)

Associated Clinical Features

A subconjunctival hemorrhage or hematoma occurs with often trivial events such as a cough, sneeze, or valsalva. The patient may present with some degree of duress secondary to the appearance of the bloody eye. The blood which is usually bright red and appears flat (Fig. 4.20). It is limited to the bulbar conjunctiva and stops abruptly at the limbus. This appearance is important to differentiate from bloody chemosis, which can occur with scleral rupture. Aside from appearance, this condition does not cause the patient any pain or diminution in visual acuity.

Differential Diagnosis

Scleral rupture, nontraumatic bloody chemosis (Fig. 4.21), conjunctivitis, iritis, corneal-scleral laceration, severe hypertension, and coagulopathy may have a similar appearance or presentation.

ED Treatment and Disposition

No treatment is required. The patient should be told to expect the blood to be resorbed in 2 to 3 weeks.

Clinical Pearls

1. Subconjunctival hematoma may be differentiated from bloody chemosis by the flat appearance of the conjunctival membranes.
2. A subconjunctival hematoma involving the extreme lateral globe after blunt trauma is very suspicious for zygomatic arch fracture.
3. Patients with nontraumatic bloody chemosis should be evaluated for an underlying metabolic (coagulopathy) or structural (cavernous sinus thrombosis) disorder.

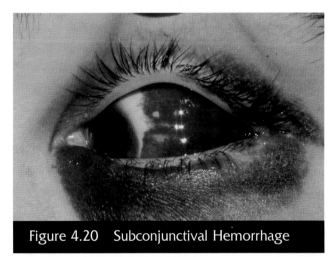

Figure 4.20   Subconjunctival Hemorrhage

Subconjunctival hemorrhage in a patient with blunt trauma. The flat appearance of the hemorrhage indicates its benign nature. (Courtesy of Dallas E. Peak, MD.)

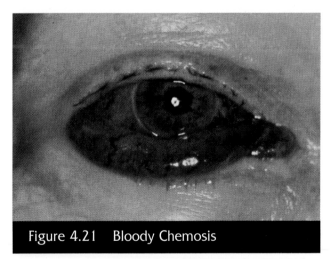

Figure 4.21   Bloody Chemosis

"Bloody chemosis was confused with" "subconjunctival hemorrhage" in this patient with no history of trauma and positive cranial nerve palsies. Cavernous sinus thrombosis was diagnosed. (Courtesy of Eric Einfalt, MD.)

Associated Clinical Features

Any trauma to the eye which disrupts the normal architecture of the lens may result in development of a traumatic cataract, a lens opacity (Fig. 4.22). The mechanism behind cataract formation involves fluid infiltration into the normally avascular and acellular lens stroma. The lens may be observed to swell with fluid and become cloudy and opacified. The time course is usually weeks to months following the original insult. Cataracts that are large enough may be observed by the naked eye. Those that are within the central visual field may cause blurring of vision or distortion of light around objects (e.g., halos).

Differential Diagnosis

Lens dislocation, intraocular foreign body, hypopyon, corneal abrasion, and hyphema can present with similar complaints. History and physical examination are helpful in discriminating most of these conditions from traumatic cataract.

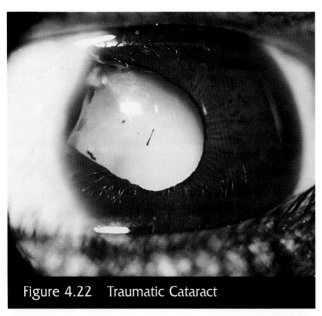

Figure 4.22 Traumatic Cataract

This traumatic cataract is seen as a large lens opacity overlying the visual axis. A traumatic iridodialysis is also present. (Courtesy of Dallas E. Peak, MD.)

ED Treatment and Disposition

No specific treatment is rendered in the emergency department for cases of delayed traumatic cataract. Routine ophthalmologic referral is indicated for most cases.

Clinical Pearls

1. Traumatic cataracts are a frequent sequela of lightning injury. All lightning strike victims should be warned of this possibility.
2. Cataracts may also occur as a result of electric current injury to the vicinity of the cranial vault.
3. Cataracts can be easily examined using the +10 diopter setting on an ophthalmoscope, or in more detail with a slit lamp.
4. Leukocoria results from a dense cataract, which causes loss of the red reflex.
5. If a cataract develops sufficient size and "swells" the lens, the trabecular meshwork may become blocked producing glaucoma.

EAR, NOSE, and THROAT

CHAPTER 5

EAR, NOSE, AND THROAT CONDITIONS

Edward C. Jauch
Alexander T. Trott
Kevin J. Knoop

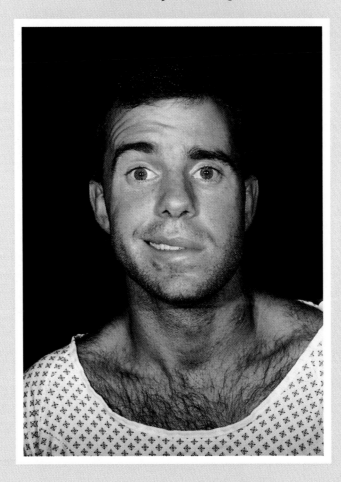

Associated Clinical Features

Children between the ages of 6 months and 2 years are at highest risk of developing otitis media (OM). Males, North American Eskimos, non-breast-fed infants, and children with craniofacial anomalies have the highest incidence of OM. Additionally, children who contract their first episode prior to their first birthday, have a sibling with a history of recurrent OM, are in day care, or have parents who smoke, are at increased risk of recurrent OM.

In its most basic form, OM is defined as an acute inflammation and effusion of the middle ear. Otoscopy of the middle ear should focus on color, position, translucency, and mobility. Compared with the tympanic membrane of a normal ear (Fig. 5.1), acute OM causes the tympanic membrane to appear dull, erythematous or injected, bulging, or less mobile (Figs. 5.2 and 5.3). The light reflex, normal tympanic membrane landmarks, and malleus become obscured.

There are many classifications, and hence presentations, of OM based on symptom duration and clinical presentation. Regardless of classification, the common pathogenesis of OM is eustachian tube dysfunction, allowing retention of secretions (serous otitis) (Figs. 5.4 and 5.5) and seeding of bacteria.

OM is caused by a wide variety of pathogens, including viral, bacterial, and fungal. The most common bacterial isolates are *Streptococcus pneumoniae, Haemophilus influenzae, Moraxella catarrhalis,* and *Streptococcus pyogenes.* Approximately 20% of middle ear effusion aspirations are sterile. The prevalence of β-lactamase–producing strains of *H. influenzae* and *M. catarrhalis* is variable but increasing.

Patient presentation and complaints vary with age. Infants with OM have vague, nonspecific symptoms such as irritability, lethargy, and decreased oral intake. Young children can be irritable, often febrile, and frequently pull at their ears, but they may also be completely asymptomatic. Older children and adults note ear pain, decreased auditory acuity, and occasionally, otorrhea.

Differential Diagnosis

Myringitis, otitis externa, tympanic membrane perforations, and herpes zoster can mimic otitis media. Less common causes of ear pain include temporomandibular joint disorders, odontogenic infections, and sinusitis. Tympanic membrane erythema can be caused by crying children in an otherwise healthy ear.

ED Treatment and Disposition

Although most cases of OM spontaneously resolve, most patients are treated with antibiotics and analgesics. Steroids, decongestants, and antihistamines do not alter the course in OM but may improve upper respiratory tract symptoms. Rarely, myringotomy may be needed for pain relief.

Antibiotic selection is widely variable. Amoxicillin is a suitable first choice for an acute OM. Alternatives for initial therapy include trimethoprim-sulfamethoxazole, erythromycin ethyl succinate with sulfisoxazole, and second-generation cephalosporins. If the patient continues to have symptoms 48 to 72 h after beginning antibiotics, amoxicillin with clavulanate, cefixime, or the newer macrolides may provide broader coverage.

Patients should be instructed to follow up in 10 to 14 days or return if symptoms persist or worsen after 48 h. Patients who have significant hearing loss, failed two complete courses of outpatient antibiotics during a single event, have chronic OM with or without acute exacerbations, or failed prophylactic antibiotics warrant referral to an otolaryngologist for further evaluation and possible tympanostomy tubes (Fig. 5.6).

Clinical Pearls

1. In children, recurrent OM is often due to food allergies.
2. Only 4% of children under 2 years old with OM develop temperatures greater than 104°F. Children with temperatures higher than 104°F or with signs of systemic toxicity should be closely evaluated for other causes of the illness before attributing the fever to OM.

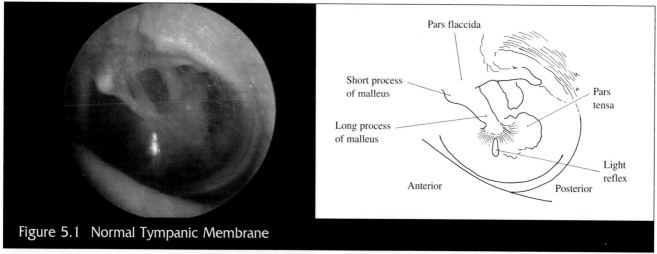

Figure 5.1   Normal Tympanic Membrane

Normal tympanic membrane anatomy and landmarks. (Courtesy of Richard A. Chole, MD, PhD.)

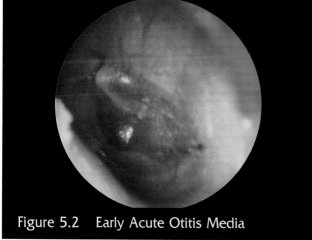

Figure 5.2   Early Acute Otitis Media

A mildly erythematous tympanic membrane is seen with a small purulent effusion in the middle ear. (Courtesy of C. Bruce MacDonald, MD.)

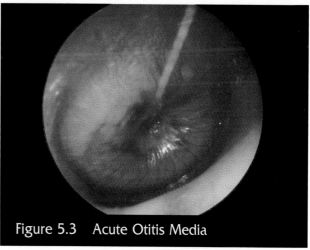

Figure 5.3   Acute Otitis Media

The middle ear is filled with purulent material behind an erythematous, bulging tympanic membrane. (Courtesy of Richard A. Chole, MD, PhD.)

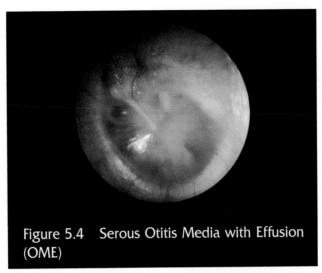

Figure 5.4   Serous Otitis Media with Effusion (OME)

Serous OME is commonly seen after acute otitis media, but is also common without this history. Any process that leads to obstruction of a eustachian tube will cause a middle ear effusion. A clear, amber-colored effusion with a single air-fluid level is seen in the middle ear behind a normal tympanic membrane. (Courtesy of C. Bruce MacDonald, MD.)

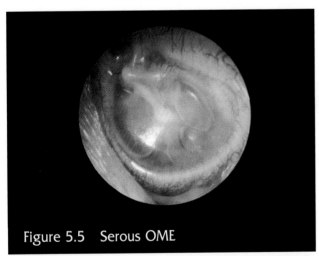

Figure 5.5   Serous OME

A clear, amber-colored effusion with multiple air-fluid levels is seen in the middle ear behind a normal tympanic membrane. (Courtesy of C. Bruce MacDonald, MD.)

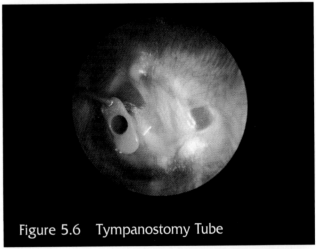

Figure 5.6   Tympanostomy Tube

Typical appearance of a tympanostomy tube in the tympanic membrane. These tubes will migrate to the periphery and eventually drop out. Occassionally, they will be found in the external ear canal. (Courtesy of C. Bruce MacDonald, MD.)

Associated Clinical Features

Bullous myringitis is a direct inflammation and infection of the tympanic membrane (TM) secondary to a viral or bacterial agent. Fluid-filled vesicles or bullae on an infected tympanic membrane are the hallmark of bullous myringitis (Fig. 5.7). Frequently, a concomitant otitis media with effusion is noted. Common bacterial agents are *Mycoplasma pneumoniae, Streptococcus pneumoniae,* and *Haemophilus influenzae.*

The onset of bullous myringitis is preceded by an upper respiratory tract infection and is heralded by sudden onset of ear pain, serosanguinous canal drainage, and frequently some degree of hearing loss. Otoscopy reveals bullae on either the inner or outer surface of the TM, often filled with red bloody fluid. Patients presenting with fever, hearing loss, and purulent drainage are more likely to have other concomitant infections such as otitis media and otitis externa.

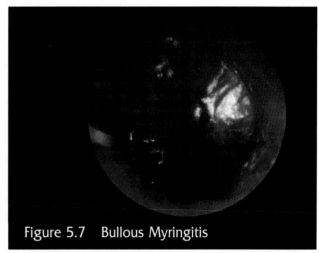

Figure 5.7   Bullous Myringitis

Several bullae, which may be blood- or fluid-filled, are seen distorting the surface of the tympanic membrane. (Courtesy of Richard A. Chole, MD, PhD.)

Differential Diagnosis

Barotrauma is usually associated with swimming, diving, or airplane travel. Herpes zoster oticus produces facial nerve palsy and facial pain. Otitis externa causes external auditory canal edema and drainage, whereas otitis media distorts the TM but rarely causes bullae.

ED Treatment and Disposition

Differentiation between viral and bacterial etiologies for tympanic membrane bullae is difficult but, fortunately, seldom necessary. Although most episodes spontaneously resolve, many physicians prescribe antibiotics, such as trimethoprim-sulfamethoxazole or a macrolide. Topical or systemic analgesics and oral decongestants may provide symptomatic relief. Referral is not necessary in most cases, unless bullae rupture is required for pain relief.

Clinical Pearl

1. Facial nerve paralysis associated with clear fluid-filled TM vesicles is characteristic of herpes zoster oticus.

Associated Clinical Features

Contrary to the origin suggested by their name, cholesteatomas are epidermoid inclusion cysts: collections of desquamating stratified squamous epithelium found in the middle ear or mastoid air cells. Congenital cholesteatomas are most frequently found in children and young adults. Acquired cholesteatomas originate from perforations of the tympanic membrane, usually marginally or in the pars flaccida, allowing migration of external auditory canal stratified squamous epithelium into the middle ear.

Cholesteatomas can be locally destructive of the middle ear ossicles and tympanic membrane and, through the production of collagenases, erode into the temporal bone, inner ear structures, mastoid sinus, or posterior fossa dura. Delays in treatment can lead to permanent conductive hearing loss or infectious complications.

Patients present with progressive hearing loss, foul-smelling ear drainage, and, in advanced stages, pain, headache, dizziness, facial paralysis, fever, or vertigo. Many cholesteatomas have an insidious progression without associated pain or symptoms. Cholesteatomas are seen on otoscopy as either a retraction pocket containing white debris or a yellow crust on the tympanic membrane with or without a perforation (Fig. 5.8). Middle ear cholesteatomas appear as a pearly white or yellow middle ear mass behind the tympanic membrane producing a focal bulge, in contrast to a more diffuse displacement of the tympanic membrane seen in otitis media. Radiographs and CT scans may reveal bony destruction.

Osteomas (sometimes called exostoses) are benign tumors of the external auditory canal (EAC) found in the deep meatus. Osteomas are associated with patients with recurrent cold water exposures, such as swimmers and divers. Osteomas are seen on otoscopy as single or multiple round shiny swellings of the bony external auditory canal (Fig. 5.9). A cerumen impaction or an otitis externa may obscure the examination.

Differential Diagnosis

Wax particles and external auditory canal (EAC) foreign bodies may resemble cholesteatomas on otoscopy. Furuncles are painful to palpation, whereas otitis externa and otitis media have EAC drainage and middle ear effusions, respectively.

ED Treatment and Disposition

Early diagnosis of a cholesteatomas is essential for proper referral. Water avoidance, topical and sometimes systemic antibiotics are important. Small cholesteatomas found in retraction pockets can be excised and a tympanostomy tube placed to equilibrate middle ear pressures. More extensive cholesteatomas may require surgical excision, tympanoplasty, and radical mastoidectomy. Osteomas require no medical or surgical management unless they become symptomatic.

Clinical Pearls

1. Persistent pain associated with headache, facial motor weakness, nystagmus, or vertigo suggests inner ear or intracranial involvement.
2. Polyps found on the tympanic membrane can indicate the presence of a cholesteatoma and require further evaluation to exclude its presence.

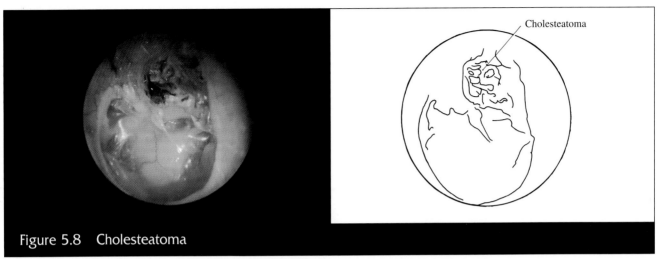

Figure 5.8   Cholesteatoma

A cholesteatoma is seen in this ear. Primary acquired cholesteatomas are thought to arise from gradual invagination of the pars flaccida, usually secondary to trauma. Note the yellow epithelial debris from the cholesteatoma in the area of the pars flaccida. Often there is an effusion and debris, which can distort the anatomy on otoscopy. (Courtesy of C. Bruce MacDonald, MD.)

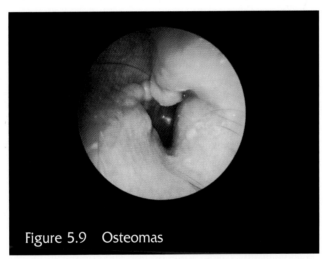

Figure 5.9   Osteomas

Multiple osteomas almost occlude the external auditory canal. The tympanic membrane can be seen in the center, past the osteomas. These are often seen in patients who are cold water swimmers. (Courtesy of C. Bruce MacDonald, MD.)

Associated Clinical Features

Acute tympanic membrane (TM) perforations are often the result of direct penetrating trauma, water or air pressure changes (barotrauma, blast injuries), chronic otitis media, corrosives, thermal injuries (electricity, lightning, heated objects), and iatrogenic causes (foreign body removal, tympanostomy tubes). TM perforations are occasionally complicated by damage to the ossicular chain, producing a more complete conductive hearing loss, temporal bone injuries, and cranial nerve damage.

Patients complain of sudden onset of ear pain, vertigo, tinnitus, and altered hearing after a specific event. Patients with posterior perforations present with a more profound deafness than those with anterior perforation sites. Physical examination of the TM reveals a slit-shaped tear or larger perforation with an irregular border. An acute perforation can have blood on the perforation margin and blood or clot in the canal (Fig. 5.10). The margins are smooth in subacute or chronic perforations (Fig. 5.11).

Differential Diagnosis

Congenital malformations, chronic perforations, residual perforations from tympanostomy tubes, and retraction pockets have more regular borders and no bleeding or TM erythema.

ED Treatment and Disposition

Treatment of acute tympanic membrane perforations is tailored to the mechanism. All easily removable foreign bodies should be extracted. Corrosive exposures require face, eye, and ear decontamination. Antibiotics and irrigation do not improve the rate or completeness of healing unless the injury is associated with otitis media. Systemic antibiotics should be used for perforations associated with otitis media, penetrating injury, and possibly water sport injuries (see "Otitis Media"). Topical steroids impede perforation closure.

Patients are instructed to avoid getting water in the ear while the perforation is healing and to return for symptoms of infection. All TM perforations should be referred to an otolaryngologist for follow-up and possible myringoplasty evaluation. Even though nearly 80% of all TM perforations spontaneously heal, some do not, and complications can develop.

Clinical Pearls

1. Cortisporin eardrops of any formulation have been shown to retard spontaneous healing and should be avoided.
2. Traumatic TM perforation associated with cranial nerve deficits or persistent vertigo requires immediate ENT consultation for possible temporal bone fractures and more extensive injuries.

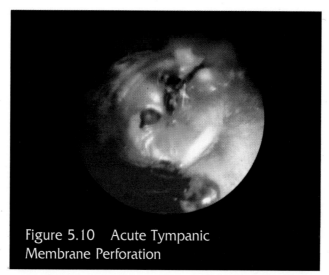

Figure 5.10   Acute Tympanic
Membrane Perforation

Acute tympanic membrane perforation with erythema of the canal
and tympanic membrane. Note the sharp edges of the perforation.
(Courtesy of Robin T. Cotton, MD.)

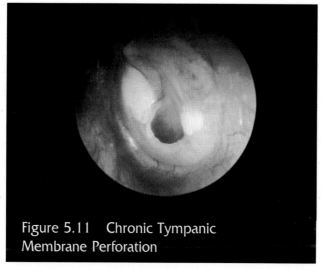

Figure 5.11   Chronic Tympanic
Membrane Perforation

Note absence of blood and erythema on the tympanic membrane
and the smooth perforation margins. (Courtesy of C. Bruce
MacDonald, MD.)

Associated Clinical Features

Otitis externa (OE) or "swimmer's ear," is an inflammation and infection (bacterial or fungal) of the auricle and external auditory canal (EAC). Typical symptoms include otalgia, pruritus, otorrhea, and hearing loss. Physical examination reveals EAC hyperemia and edema, (Fig. 5.12), otorrhea, malodorous discharge, occlusion from debris and swelling, pain with auricle manipulation, and periauricular lymphadenopathy.

Several factors predispose the EAC to infection: increased humidity and heat, water immersion, foreign bodies, trauma, hearing aids, and cerumen impaction. Bacterial otitis externa is primarily an infection due to *Pseudomonas* species or *Staphylococcus aureus.* Diabetics are particularly prone to infections by *Pseudomonas. Candida albicans,* and less commonly *Aspergillus niger* (Fig. 5.13).

Differential Diagnosis

Cholesteatomas and foreign bodies can produce a secondary OE. Periauricular cellulitis, herpes zoster oticus (Fig. 5.14), and malignant otitis externa have auricular and facial involvement. EAC dermatitis, eczema, and furuncles rarely produce EAC drainage.

ED Treatment and Disposition

Saline irrigation and suctioning is recommended to thoroughly evaluate the EAC. Topical antibiotic *suspensions* (containing polymyxin, neomycin, and hydrocortisone) with ear wicks are effective. Topical *solutions* are not pH-balanced and thus are irritating and may cause inflammation in the middle ear if a perforation is present. Systemic antibiotics are not indicated unless extension into the periauricular tissues is noted. Patients should avoid swimming and prevent water from entering the ear while bathing. Dry heat aids in resolution, and analgesics provide symptomatic relief. Follow-up should be arranged in 10 days for routine cases.

Clinical Pearls

1. Resistent cases may have an allergic component. These typically present with a dry, scaly EAC and are recurrent and chronic in nature.
2. Drying the EAC after water exposure with a 50:50 mixture of isopropyl alcohol and water, or acetic acid (white vinegar) minimizes recurrence. If the TM is possibly perforated, isopropyl alcohol should be avoided.
3. Often the symptoms are out of proportion to the visible findings, necessitating narcotic analgesia.

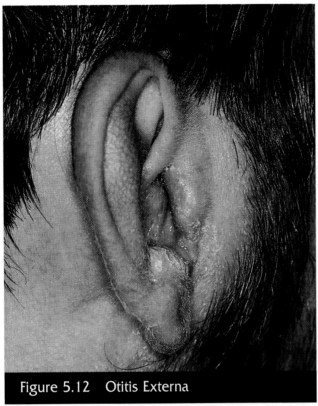

Figure 5.12   Otitis Externa

A discharge is seen coming from the external auditory canal, which is swollen and almost completely occluded. An ear wick placed in the EAC facilitates delivery of topical antibiotic suspension and drainage of debris. (Courtesy of Frank Birinyi, MD.)

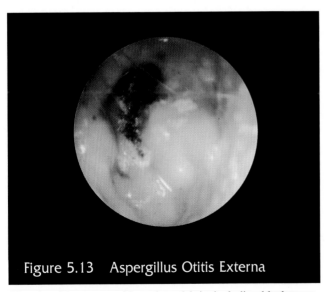

Figure 5.13   Aspergillus Otitis Externa

Chronic otitis externa with copious debris, including black spores from *Aspergillus niger,* cottony fungal elements, and wet debris. This patient had been treated with topical and systemic antibiotics. (Courtesy of C. Bruce MacDonald, MD.)

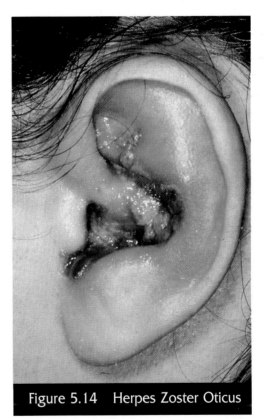

Figure 5.14   Herpes Zoster Oticus

The appearance of erythema and drainage coming from the EAC is seen in this patient with herpes zoster oticus. Otitis externa can have a similar appearance, but does not have vesicles, as seen in this patient. (Courtesy of Robin T. Cotton, MD.)

EXTERNAL AUDITORY CANAL FOREIGN BODY

Associated Clinical Features

A wide variety of objects find their way into an external auditory canal (EAC) of children and adults. Young children have objects placed in their ear by themselves or other children (Fig. 5.15). Very young children may not recall the event, but parents later note bleeding and drainage from the ear, irritability, hearing loss, and ear pulling. Adolescents and adults are more likely to present with insects or cotton swab tips in their ear (Fig. 5.16) and can recall the exact onset of symptoms. The physician should ask how the object entered the ear, what the object might be, and what attempts have been made to remove the object.

Differential Diagnosis

Cerumen impactions, cholesteatomas, and furuncles may resemble foreign bodies on otoscopy. Otitis externa can result from an occult EAC foreign body.

ED Treatment and Disposition

Topical anesthetic solutions make the patient more comfortable and cooperative with the examination and removal. Canal irrigation and debridement may be required to visualize a foreign object if it has caused a secondary otitis externa. Routine equipment for removal includes straight alligator forceps, right angle hooks, suction tips, and syringes with IV catheter tips. Mineral oil and topical anesthetics should be available for insect immobilization.

Insects should be immobilized before attempting extraction not only to minimize patient discomfort but also to prevent canal and tympanic membrane injury from a struggling insect. Viscous lidocaine, topical anesthetics and mineral oil suffocate insects and minimize patient discomfort.

Once the object has been removed, the EAC should be reexamined for other objects and secondary trauma. Ototopical steroid and antibiotic drops provide some pain relief and prevent secondary infection. Occasionally, narcotic analgesics are necessary for adequate pain control.

Clinical Pearls

1. For hard, round items such as popcorn seeds, beads, and metal objects, small suction tips can often remove the objects when forceps would push them deeper into the EAC.
2. Hydrophilic objects, such as vegetable matter, expand and become difficult to remove if they are exposed to water.
3. Several situations require early referral: if the object is in the inner third of the EAC or perforates the tympanic membrane; if there is significant inflammatory reaction; if the patient cannot cooperate with the removal; or if significant manipulation is required. Children may require conscious sedation or general anesthesia for removal of deep objects.
4. Button batteries require prompt removal or referal, as leakage may cause tissue destruction.

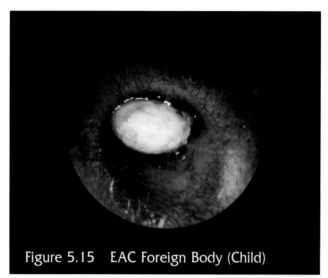

Figure 5.15   EAC Foreign Body (Child)

External auditory canal foreign body (bean) with a clear exudate surrounding the object. (Courtesy of Robin T. Cotton, MD.)

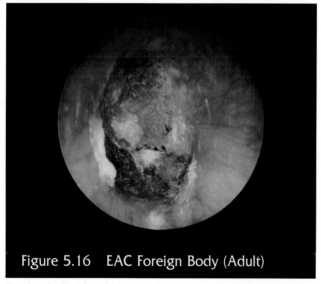

Figure 5.16   EAC Foreign Body (Adult)

Foreign body (tip of a cotton swab) impacted in an ear canal. (Courtesy of C. Bruce MacDonald, MD.)

Associated Clinical Features

Mastoiditis is a mastoid air cell infection or inflammation which usually results from extension of purulent otitis media with progressive destruction and coalescence of air cells. Medial erosion can cause cavernous sinus thrombosis, facial nerve palsy, meningitis, brain abscess, and sepsis. With the use of antibiotics for acute otitis media, the incidence of mastoiditis has fallen sharply.

Patients present with fever, chills, postauricular ear pain, and external auditory canal discharge. Patients may have tenderness, erythema, swelling, and fluctuance over the mastoid process; lateral displacement of the pinna (Fig. 5.17); erythema of the posterior-superior external auditory canal wall; and purulent otorrhea through a tympanic membrane perforation.

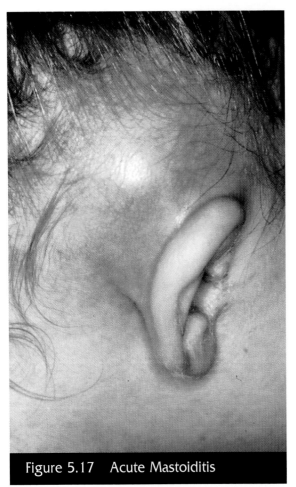

Figure 5.17   Acute Mastoiditis

Postauricular swelling and redness in a young girl with acute mastoiditis. (Courtesy of Robin T. Cotton, MD.)

Differential Diagnosis

Postauricular abscesses, furuncles, suppurative adenitis, lymphadenitis, and rarely, carcinomas of the mastoid can present with signs and symptoms of acute mastoiditis.

ED Treatment and Disposition

Initial evaluation includes a thorough head, neck, and cranial nerve examination. Radiographs of the mastoid process can demonstrate coalescence of the mastoid air cells, whereas head CT scans may reveal bony extension and intracranial involvement.

Penicillinase-resistant penicillins, amoxicillin-clavulanic acid, first-generation cephalosporins, and the newer macrolides are effective in mild cases of mastoiditis. Severe cases require parenteral semisynthetic penicillins, cephalosporins, or vancomycin. Mastoiditis requires close follow-up and prompt consultation.

Clinical Pearls

1. Most patients require admission for parenteral antibiotics to cover *Haemophilus influenzae, Moraxella catarrhalis,* streptococcal species, and *Staphylococcus aureus.*
2. Surgical irrigation and debridement, and possibly mastoidectomy, are reserved for refractory cases.
3. Delays in treatment and failure to ensure adequate follow-up can result in significant morbidity and mortality.

Associated Clinical Features

Perichondritis is an infection of the auricular cartilage. Perichondritis can result from trauma; traumatic hematoma; thermal injuries, typically frostbite; external auditory canal foreign bodies; chronic otitis media; otitis externa; skin infections; chronic mastoiditis; and surgical procedures on the ear. Destruction and necrosis of the auricular cartilage can lead to a flaccid, flat ear.

The microbiology of perichondritis reflects the source of infection. Infections of skin structures and trauma involve streptococci and staphylococci. Ear and mastoid sources frequently involve gram-negative organisms. Untreated perichondritis in the elderly diabetic, and immunocompromised, can lead to malignant external otitis.

Patients present with severe pain and diffuse swelling of the ear. Physical examination reveals an erythematous, swollen, warm, and tender pinna (Fig. 5.18). Advanced cases can present with necrosis of the ear cartilage and spreading cellulitis.

Differential Diagnosis

Periauricular cellulitis can mimic perichondritis but has facial involvement. Auricular hematomas follow direct trauma. Contact dermatitis can develop from topical ear medications and jewelry.

ED Treatment and Disposition

Immediate treatment of perichondritis is essential to preserve the external ear cartilage. Early perichondritis is treated by irrigation and debridement of any abscess, with administration of broad spectrum antibiotics such as penicillinase-resistant penicillins, amoxicillin-clavulanate, first-generation cephalosporins, or ciprofloxacin. Topical antibiotics are ineffective. A compressive mastoid and auricular dressing is beneficial. Strict follow-up is essential to prevent treatment failure and progression of infection. Advanced perichondritis requires high-dose parenteral antibiotics and early specialist referral for surgical irrigation and debridement.

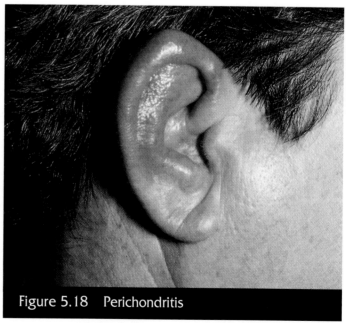

Figure 5.18   Perichondritis

The pinna is swollen and erythematous. No concomitant otitis externa, mastoiditis, or furuncle is noted. (Courtesy of Lawrence B. Stack, MD.)

Clinical Pearl

1. Early diagnosis and treatment is necessary to avoid permanent deformity of the pinna.

HERPES ZOSTER OTICUS
(RAMSAY HUNT SYNDROME)

Associated Clinical Features

Herpes zoster oticus (HZO), or Ramsay Hunt syndrome, is the second most common cause of facial paralysis, representing 3 to 12% of patients with facial paralysis. The syndrome consists of facial and neck pain, acoustic symptoms, and facial palsy associated with the reactivation of varicella zoster in the facial nerve and geniculate ganglion (Figs. 5.19 and 5.20, see also Fig. 5.14). Patients first note a pruritus, followed by pain out of proportion to the physical examination over the face and ear. Patients may note vertigo, hearing loss (sensorineural) from eighth cranial nerve involvement, tinnitus, rapid onset of facial paralysis, decrease in salivation, loss of taste sensation over the posterior-lateral tongue, and vesicles on the ear, external auditory canal, and face.

Differential Diagnosis

Cerebrovascular accidents develop acutely and do not produce facial or external auditory canal pain. Facial paralysis from temporal bone fractures is associated with antecedent trauma. Meniere's disease can be confused with early HZO but is painless and does not cause facial paralysis.

ED Treatment and Disposition

The diagnosis of HZO is based largely on history and physical examination. Tzanck preparations may be difficult because of vesicle location.

Oral acyclovir, 800 mg five times a day for 7 to 10 days, or famciclovir, 800 mg TID for 10 days, are the mainstays for HZO treatment. It is important to protect the involved eye from corneal abrasions and ulcerations by using lubricating drops. Other treatments, including steroids, have not been shown to improve postherpetic neuralgia.

Clinical Pearl

1. The prognosis for facial paralysis due to HZO is worse than that for Bell's palsy. Approximately 10 and 66% of patients with full and partial facial paralysis, respectively, recover fully. The prognosis improves if the symptoms of HZO are preceded by the vesicular eruption.

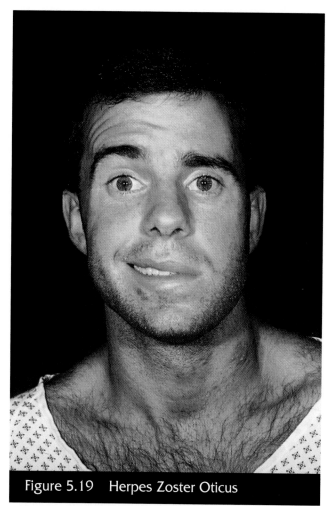

Figure 5.19   Herpes Zoster Oticus

Facial palsy in a young adult. Note the vesicular eruptions on the neck. (Courtesy of Frank Birinyi, MD.)

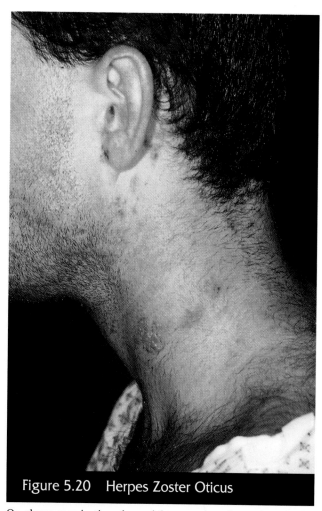

Figure 5.20   Herpes Zoster Oticus

On closer examination, the vesicles extend up the neck to the external auditory canal. (Courtesy of Frank Birinyi, MD.)

Associated Clinical Features

The seventh cranial nerve, or facial nerve, provides innervation of the facial muscles via the five branches of the motor root; innervates the submandibular, sublingual, and lacrimal glands, as well as the taste organs on the anterior two-thirds of the tongue; and provides sensation to the pinna of the ear. Seventh-nerve palsies may occur as an isolated finding or as part of a constellation of symptoms. Facial palsies are described as being either central or peripheral. Central seventh-nerve lesions occur before or proximal to the seventh-nerve nucleus in the pons. Lesions that occur distal to the nucleus are classified as peripheral lesions. The hallmark of central lesions is the sparing of the ipsilateral frontalis muscle (Fig. 5.21), since it receives innervation in the nucleus from both ipsilateral and contralateral motor cortices. Peripheral injuries involve the entire side of the face, including the forehead (Fig. 5.22).

The most common etiology of seventh-nerve dysfunction is Bell's palsy, an idiopathic facial nerve dysfunction. Bell's palsy is most likely a viral or postviral syndrome, with 60% of patients having a viral prodrome. Bell's palsy shows no age, sex, or racial predilection. The incidence is higher in pregnant women, diabetics, and in those with a family history of Bell's palsy. It is bilateral in less than 1% of patients.

Patients with Bell's palsy have an acute onset of facial weakness and may note numbness or pain on the ipsilateral face, ear, tongue, and neck, and a decrease or loss of ipsilateral tearing and saliva flow. Hearing in Bell's palsy is preserved.

The prognosis for facial nerve palsies is variable. Facial weakness compared with complete paralysis has a better prognosis for full recovery. Facial palsies due to herpes zoster have a protracted course, and many do not fully resolve. In comparison, 80% of patients with Bell's palsy due to other causes completely recover within 3 months. The recurrence rate of Bell's palsy is 7 to 10%.

Differential Diagnosis

Acoustic neuromas and central nervous system masses have gradual progression of symptoms and cause other neurologic findings. Neurologic disorders, such as Guillain-Barré syndrome, multiple sclerosis, neurosarcoid, and cerebral vascular accidents also cause additional neurologic sequelae. Temporal bone fractures are associated with trauma. The differential diagnosis also includes middle ear infections and parotid tumors.

ED Treatment and Disposition

Initial evaluation is directed by the history. The examination should include a thorough examination of the ear (including sensorineural or conductive hearing loss), the eye (including lacrimation), and the cranial nerves. Motor function of the seventh cranial nerve is evaluated by having the patient raise his or her eyebrows, smile, pucker, and frown. No single laboratory test is diagnostic. A screening head CT is of little value in the absence of additional findings on physical examination.

Most authors empirically recommend steroids for Bell's palsy. A typical regimen is prednisone, 60 mg a day for 10 days, then tapered. If treated within the first 3 weeks, steroids may decrease the sequelae of Bell's palsy. Facial nerve palsies due to Ramsay Hunt syndrome are treated with acyclovir (see Herpes Zoster Oticus). In all facial nerve palsies, eye lubricants and taping or patching of the eye at night help prevent keratitis and ulceration. Referral to a specialist should be made for follow-up care.

Clinical Pearls

1. Facial nerve paralysis is a symptom, not a diagnosis. The etiology of the paralysis is required before a diagnosis is made.
2. If a provisional diagnosis of Bell's palsy is made and no resolution of symptoms occurs, the diagnosis must be reconsidered. In patients misdiagnosed with Bell's palsy, tumors are the number one missed etiology.
3. Lacrimation is tested by the Schirmer's or litmus test. Asymmetry may indicate a lesion proximal to the geniculate ganglion.

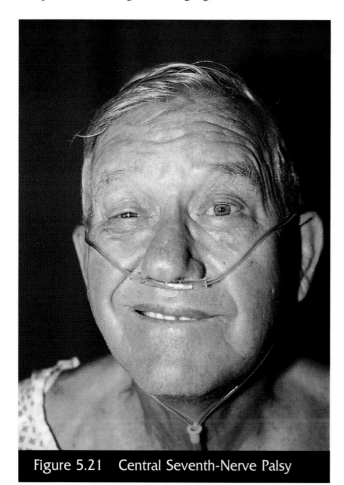

Figure 5.21   Central Seventh-Nerve Palsy

Central facial nerve paralysis with forehead sparing. (Courtesy of Frank Birinyi, MD.)

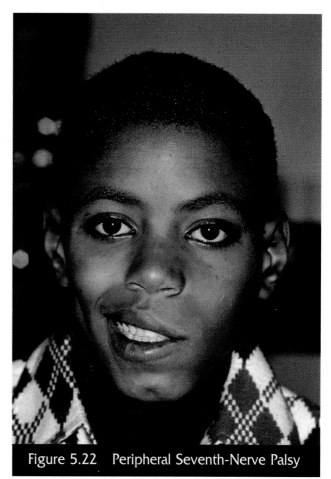

Figure 5.22   Peripheral Seventh-Nerve Palsy

A peripheral nerve paralysis involving the entire ipsilateral face, including the forehead is seen in this patient with Bell's palsy. (Courtesy of Robin T. Cotton, MD.)

Associated Clinical Features

Angioedema is clinically characterized by acute onset of well demarcated cutaneous swelling of the face, lips, and tongue; edema of the mucous membranes of the mouth, throat, or abdominal viscera; or nonpitting edema of the hands and feet. Angioedema is classified as either hereditary, allergic, or idiopathic. Whatever the cause, angioedema can be a life-threatening illness. Complications of angioedema range from dysphagia and dysphonia to respiratory distress, airway obstruction (Fig. 5.23), and death. Of special interest is angiotensin converting enzyme (ACE) inhibitor–induced angioedema. Angioedema due to ACE inhibitors has a predilection for lips (Fig. 5.24), face, tongue, and glottis involvement. Standard treatment practices for allergic urticaria often fail to improve ACE inhibitor–induced angioedema, and in those who do improve, rebound is frequently seen.

Differential Diagnosis

Anaphylaxis and asthma occur in patients with histories of similar events and involve the lower airways. Patients with epiglottitis, Ludwig's angina, and peritonsillar or retropharyngeal abscesses often have a preceding pharyngeal or odontogenic infection and present with systemic symptoms of infections, such as fever and chills.

ED Treatment and Disposition

Initial treatment of angioedema is airway management. Most patients do not require intervention, but frequent reassessment of the patient's airway is mandatory. Airway interventions include nasopharyngeal intubation, endotracheal intubation (often difficult due to lingual and oral obstruction), or nasotracheal intubation (either blindly or with fiberoptics), or a cricothyrotomy.

Acute angioedema is treated similarly to an allergic reaction. Depending on the severity of symptoms, it can be treated with steroids, antihistamines, both H_1 and H_2 blockers, and subcutaneous epinephrine. Chronic angioedema responds better to corticosteroids and H_2 blockers, but airway protection remains the primary focus of emergency treatment. Hereditary angioedema is more refractory to medical interventions, and epinephrine, corticosteroids, and antihistamines provide little relief.

Disposition depends on the severity and resolution of symptoms. Patients whose symptoms significantly improve and show no progression after 4 h of observation may be discharged home on a short course of oral steroids and antihistamines. Any medication which may have caused the angioedema should be discontinued. Angioedema with airway involvement requires admission to a monitored environment, with airway equipment always at the bedside.

Clinical Pearls

1. Do not underestimate the degree of airway involvement; act early to preserve airway patency.
2. Angioedema can also cause gastrointestinal and neurologic involvement.
3. Early response to medical intervention does not preclude rebound of symptoms to a greater extent than at presentation.
4. Patients who have been using ACE inhibitors for months or years can still develop angioedema.

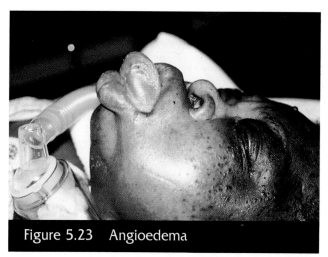

Figure 5.23   Angioedema

Severe angioedema of the face and tongue requiring emergent cricothyrotomy. (Courtesy of W. Brian Gibler, MD.)

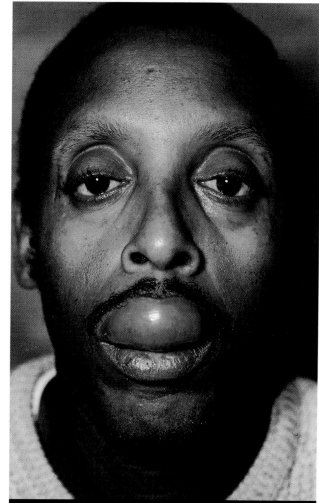

Figure 5.24   ACE Inhibitor–Induced Angioedema

Angioedema of the upper lip in a man taking an ACE inhibitor for 2 years. The patient had no previous episodes. (Courtesy of Kevin J. Knoop, MD, MS.)

Associated Clinical Features

Pharyngitis is an inflammation, and frequently an infection, of the pharynx and its lymphoid tissues, which make up Waldeyer's ring. Most causes of pharyngitis are infectious. Viral infections account for 90% of all cases. Common bacterial agents include group A beta hemolytic streptococci (GABHS, responsible for up to 50% of bacterial cases), other streptococci, *Mycoplasma pneumoniae, Neisseria gonorrhea,* and *Corynebacterium diphtheriae.* In immunocompromised patients and in patients on antibiotics, *Candida* species can cause thrush. Sore throats that last longer than 2 weeks should increase suspicion for either a deep-space neck infection or a neoplastic cause.

Patients with bacterial, and especially GABHS pharyngitis present with an acute onset of sore throat and fever, and frequently nausea, vomiting, headache, and abdominal cramping. On examination, patients may have a mild to moderate fever, an erythematous posterior pharynx and palatine tonsils, tender cervical lymphadenopathy, and palatal petechiae (Fig. 5.25). Classically, the tonsils have a white or yellow exudate with debris in the crypts; however, many patients may not have exudate on examination. Viral pharyngitis is typically more benign with a gradual onset, lower temperature, and less impressive erythema and swelling of the pharynx. Except for infectious mononucleosis (Fig. 5.26), which can take weeks to resolve, most cases of viral pharyngitis are self-limited with spontaneous resolution in a matter of days. Lingual and adenoid tonsillitis may also be present (Fig. 5.27).

Differential Diagnosis

Deep-space neck infections, diphtheria, epiglottitis, infectious mononucleosis, and Ludwig's angina are other infectious causes of sore throats that should be considered. Allergic rhinitis, angioedema, and pharyngeal neoplasms are noninfectious causes of similar pharyngeal symptoms. Foreign bodies and local pharyngeal trauma produce similar symptoms but usually have an antecedent event.

ED Treatment and Disposition

Treatment is largely symptomatic, except for antibiotics and rehydration. Current first-line antibiotic therapies are intramuscular benzathine penicillin or oral penicillin. Patients allergic to penicillin should receive erythromycin for primary prophylaxis against rheumatic fever. Other suitable antibiotics are macrolides and second-generation cephalosporins. Analgesics, antipyretics, and throat sprays or gargles can provide symptomatic relief.

Clinical Pearls

1. The physical examination should not end at the neck. Auscultation of the chest, palpation of the abdomen, and examination of the skin are also important.
2. Sore throats or chronic pharyngitis that lasts more than 2 weeks must be referred for further evaluation to rule out possible neoplastic or neurologic causes, especially in patients over 50 years old who have a smoking or chewing tobacco history.
3. Recurrent tonsillitis in children merits referral for possible adenoid tonsillectomy.

4. Amoxicillin should be avoided if infectious mononucleosis is a possibility, as a diffuse maculopapular rash will occur in up to 80%.

5. Pharyngitis itself may be a prodrome for other pathologic conditions, such as measles, scarlet fever, and influenza.

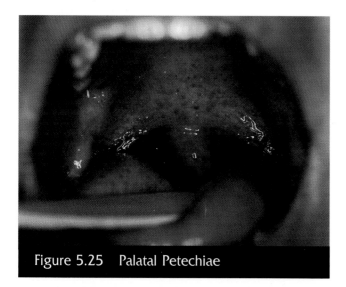

Figure 5.25   Palatal Petechiae

Palatal petechiae and erythema of the tonsillar pillars in a patient with streptococcal pharyngitis. (Courtesy of Kevin J. Knoop, MD, MS.)

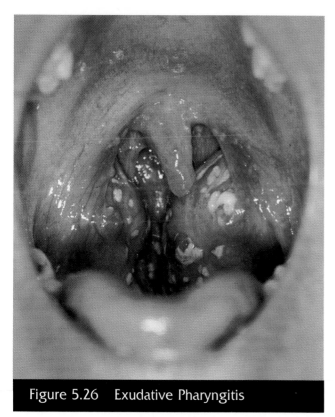

Figure 5.26   Exudative Pharyngitis

Exudative pharyngitis showing erythema and tonsillar exudate in a patient with viral mononucleosis. (Courtesy of George L. Murrell, MD.)

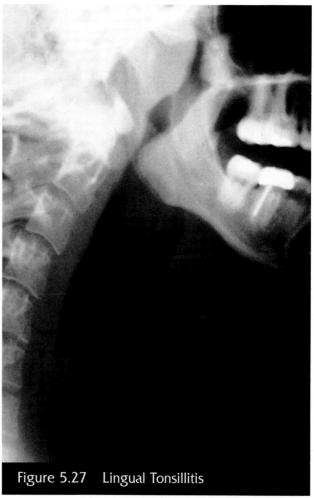

Figure 5.27   Lingual Tonsillitis

A radiograph showing lingual and adenoid tonsillitis. (Courtesy of Edward C. Jauch, MD, MS.)

Associated Clinical Features

Peritonsillar abscess, or quinsy, is the most common deep neck infection. Although most occur in young adults, immunocompromised and diabetic patients are at increased risk. Most abscesses develop as a complication of tonsillitis or pharyngitis, but they can also result from odontogenic spread, recent dental procedures, and local mucosal trauma. They recur in 10 to 15% of patients.

The pathogens involved are similar to tonsillitis, especially streptococcal species, but many infections are polymicrobial and involve anaerobic bacteria. Patients present with a fever, severe sore throat that is often out of proportion to physical findings, localization of symptoms to one side of the throat, trismus, drooling, dysphagia, dysphonia, and ipsilateral ear pain.

During the early stages, the tonsil and anterior pillar are erythematous, appear full, and may be shifted medially (Fig. 5.28). Later, the uvula and soft palate are shifted to the contralateral side (Fig. 5.29). The tonsil may feel fluctuant and tender on palpation.

Differential Diagnosis

Ludwig's angina, odontogenic neck infections, peritonsillar cellulitis, and retropharyngeal abscesses can be confused with peritonsillar abscesses. Angioedema has a rapid onset of symptoms, whereas oral neoplasms develop slowly.

ED Treatment and Disposition

Most patients with signs of an abscess can have a needle aspiration performed as the sole surgical drainage procedure and can expect a satisfactory outcome. Alternative surgical drainage procedures, including incision and drainage, and abscess tonsillectomy, can be performed by an otolarynogologist or oral surgeon. Most can be managed as outpatients on oral antibiotics following drainage. Patients who are immunocompromised, have airway involvement, appear toxic, or cannot tolerate oral intake require admission for rehydration, parenteral antibiotics, and specialty consultation.

Studies to date are divided on the incidence of penicillin-resistant organisms in peritonsillar abscess. Although penicillin alone is arguably a good first choice, penicillin and metronidazole, amoxicillin with clavulanate, clindamycin, or third-generation cephalosporins are also suitable antibiotic choices.

Clinical Pearl

1. The value of culturing aspirates is questionable, with a review of several studies showing no clinical benefit from the cultures unless the patient is immunocompromised.

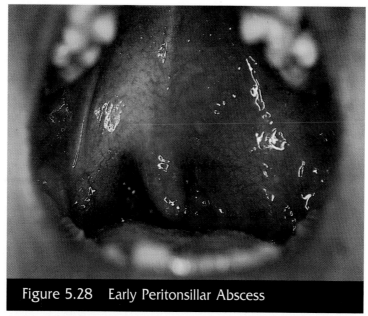

Figure 5.28   Early Peritonsillar Abscess

Acute peritonsillar cellulitis with erythema and fullness of the anterior pillar and soft palate. Trismus is not present in this patient. (Courtesy of Kevin J. Knoop, MD, MS.)

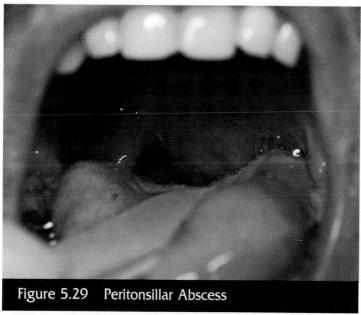

Figure 5.29   Peritonsillar Abscess

Acute peritonsillar abscess showing medial displacement of the uvula, palatine tonsil, and anterior pillar. Some trismus is present as demonstrated by patient's inability to maximally open the mouth. (Courtesy of Kevin J. Knoop, MD, MS.)

Associated Clinical Features

The uvula is the fleshy midline extension of the soft palate that hangs from the roof of the mouth. The two most common causes of uvular enlargement are infections and angioedema, although most causes of uvular edema are idiopathic. Regardless of the cause, most patients with uvular edema or uvulitis complain of a sore throat, gagging sensation, or a foreign body sensation in the back of their mouths.

The infectious etiologies of uvulitis are bacterial, including *Haemophilus influenzae* and streptococci; fungal, such as *Candida albicans;* and viral. Infections of the uvula are typically extensions from adjacent infections, such as epiglottitis, tonsillitis, peritonsillar abscesses, and pharyngitis.

With infectious uvulitis, patients note fever, odynophagia, trismus, facial pain, hoarseness, neck pain, and headache. On examination the uvula is red, firm, swollen, and very tender to palpation. When associated with peritonsillar abscesses, the uvula is displaced to the contralateral side of the mouth.

Angioedema of the uvula, known as Quincke's disease, can be hereditary, acquired, or idiopathic. Medications, allergens, thermal stimuli, pressure, and iatrogenic or accidental trauma can initiate angioedema. In addition to the swollen uvula (Fig. 5.30), patients may note pruritus, urticaria, and wheezing. With uvular edema, the angioedema may involve the face, tongue, and oropharynx. Airway compromise is more common in angioedema of the uvula. The uvula with angioedema appears pale, boggy, and edematous, resembling a large white grape (uvular hydrops).

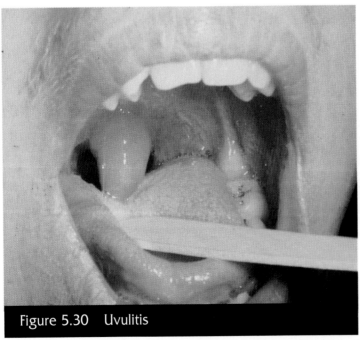

Figure 5.30   Uvulitis

Angioedema of the uvula, known as Quincke's disease. (Courtesy of Lawrence B. Stack, MD.)

Differential Diagnosis

Benign polyps and neoplasms cause asymmetry of the palate or uvula. Cellulitis and peritonsillar abscesses may also cause uvular distortion.

ED Treatment and Disposition

Most cases of uvulitis are benign and self-limited. Angioedematous uvulitis is treated similarly to any angioedema. Administration of steroids, antihistamines, both H_1 and H_2 blockers, and epinephrine, either subcutaneously or nebulized, may provide symptomatic relief. For infectious uvulitis, antibiotic coverage is dictated by the primary source of infection. For odontogenic infections, pharyngitis, or tonsillitis with uvulitis, penicillin, clindamycin, or amoxicillin with clavulanate are effective. Epiglottitis associated with uvulitis requires potent *H. influenzae* coverage, such as third-generation cephalosporins. Admission is based on severity of airway compromise and accompanying infections.

Clinical Pearls

1. Although the incidence of concomitant epiglottis has decreased dramatically, any airway symptom dictates an evaluation of the hypopharynx, either with a soft-tissue lateral neck radiograph or fiber-optic nasopharyngoscope, or by direct laryngoscopy.
2. If the uvula itself is causing enough airway compromise, uvular decompression by longitudinal incisions or a partial uvulectomy can be performed.
3. If the possibility of hereditary angioedema is considered, referral for evaluation is warranted.

Associated Clinical Features

Epiglottitis is an inflammation of the supraglottic structures including the epiglottis, aryepiglottic folds, arytenoids, and periepiglottic soft tissues. Bacterial epiglottitis, a rare but potentially fatal infection, is caused primarily by *Haemophilus influenzae,* but *Streptococcus pneumoniae, Staphylococcus aureus,* and β hemolytic streptococcus have been isolated. The advent of the *H. influenzae* B vaccination for infants has changed what used to be a disease primarily of children, with a peak age range from 2 to 6 years of age, to one found increasingly in adults. Bacterial epiglottitis occurs most commonly in the winter and spring but may occur at any time.

Patients with acute epiglottitis appear quite ill. They present with sore throat, fever, drooling, severe dysphagia, dyspnea, muffled or hoarse voice, and occasionally stridor. Patients with severe respiratory distress assume the "tripod" position: sitting upright with the neck extended, arms supporting the trunk, and the jaw thrust forward. This position maximizes airway patency and caliber. Patients may have a prodromal viral illness, but many have a sudden onset and rapid progression to respiratory distress. The course and symptoms are more variable in adults.

Differential Diagnosis

Croup, bacterial tracheitis, lingual tonsillitis, and retropharyngeal abscesses are other infectious causes of respiratory distress. Angioedema and foreign bodies cause a sudden onset of acute respiratory distress without antecedent illnesses.

ED Treatment and Disposition

Airway management is paramount. Children should be calmed, comforted by a parent, and allowed to assume whatever position they feel is most comfortable. Anesthesiology and ENT should be consulted immediately. Indications for intubation are clinical, but severe stridor and respiratory distress are clear reasons to intervene. Nasotracheal intubation in children is preferred but not when performed blindly. Needle cricothyrotomy can provide temporary oxygenation until a surgical airway is performed.

Radiographs of the neck may reveal the classic "thumb" sign, a thickened epiglottis on the lateral soft-tissue neck radiograph (Fig. 5.31). Visualization of the epiglottis is possible in the stable adult patient via direct and indirect laryngoscopy and fiber-optic nasopharyngoscopy (Fig. 5.32). The airway orifice may be difficult to see because of the extreme distortion of tissues. In children, the top of the swollen epiglottis may be visualized on careful oral examination, whereas pharyngoscopy is typically reserved for an experienced anesthesiologist or otolaryngologist in a controlled setting.

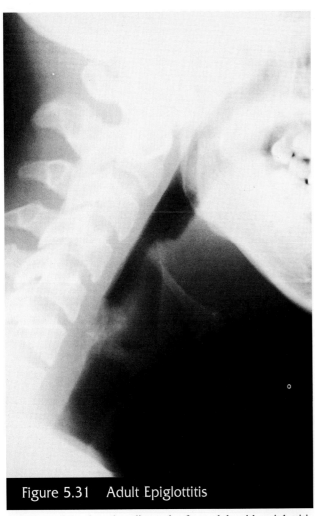

Figure 5.31 Adult Epiglottitis

Soft-tissue lateral neck radiograph of an adult with epiglottitis demonstrating the classic "thumb" sign of a swollen epiglottis. (Courtesy of Kevin J. Knoop, MD, MS.)

The mainstay of epiglottitis treatment is antibiotics. Second- and third-generation parenteral cephalosporins, ampicillin with sulbactam and trimethoprim with sulfamethoxazole, have proven efficacy in treating epiglottitis.

Steroids or epinephrine, either nebulized or subcutaneous, may provide some improvement in edema. Recently, helium and oxygen gas mixtures, which, owing to their lower density compared to air, improve the work of breathing and flow rates, have shown promise in delaying or even preventing intubation in some patients.

Clinical Pearls

1. Transport of patients with suspected epiglottitis must be done by an experienced transport team. The airway must be secured before transport of all but the most stable patient.
2. During intubation, pushing on the patient's chest may cause a bubble to form at the airway orifice guiding placement of the tube.

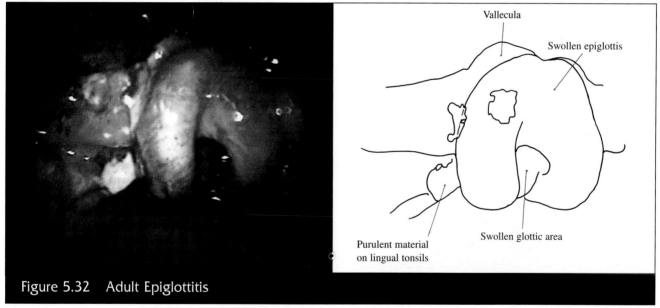

Figure 5.32   Adult Epiglottitis

Fiber-optic laryngoscopy showing red, edematous epiglottis and glottic area with marked airway compromise in an adult with epiglottitis. (Courtesy of Timothy L. Smith, MD.)

Associated Clinical Features

Ranulas are mucoceles (mucous retention cysts) that develop in the floor of the mouth, arising from obstructed sublingual or submandibular ducts, or smaller minor salivary glands. At first the cysts are small and barely noticeable, but over time they can expand outward or deeper into the neck (plunging ranula). Large cysts can displace the tongue forward and upward, making the patient uncomfortable. Contrary to sialolithiasis, patients may not always notice an increase in swelling associated with eating. Physical examination reveals a soft, minimally tender translucent cyst with dilated veins running over its surface (Fig. 5.33). Unlike carcinomas, no ulceration is noted, and ranulas are generally softer.

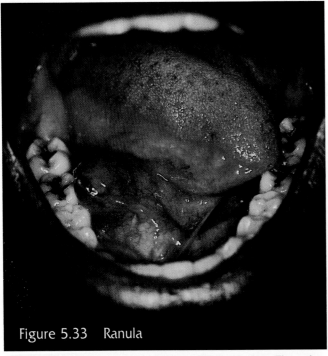

Figure 5.33   Ranula

Sublingual ranula, or mucocele, lateral to Wharton's duct. The patient was asymptomatic except for being aware of the lesion. (Courtesy of Kevin J. Knoop, MD, MS.)

Differential Diagnosis

Torus mandibularis is a hard bony growth off the lingual surface of the mandible. Obstructed major salivary glands are often painful and intermittent. Carcinomas of the mouth are slower growing and firm. Abscesses and local cellulitis also produce sublingual swelling.

ED Treatment and Disposition

Recognition by the physician is essential for proper referral. Definitive treatment is excision or marsupialization, although needle aspiration of the cyst can provide temporary relief. Unless secondarily infected, no antibiotic coverage is required.

Clinical Pearls

1. Most ranulas are painless and are incidental findings on routine examinations.
2. Ranulas often recur, requiring total excision of the offending salivary gland.

Associated Clinical Features

Sialoadenitis is a general term describing inflammation of any salivary gland. The three major salivary glands are the parotid, submandibular, and sublingual. There are also numerous smaller salivary glands that empty into the oral cavity, and all are capable of becoming inflamed. Salivary gland disorders have a broad spectrum of causes, including acute and chronic infections; metabolic, systemic, and endocrine disorders; infiltrative processes; obstructions; allergic inflammation; and neoplastic diseases. Key features in the history are the duration and course of the symptoms, complaints of pain, and unilateral or bilateral location.

Both viral and bacterial infections of the salivary gland can lead to enlarged, swollen, painful masses. Suppurative sialoadenitis is most commonly caused by *Staphylococcus aureus* and is found in patients who are elderly, diabetic, or have poor oral hygiene. It may follow episodes of dehydration, such as surgery or debilitation. Viral sialoadenitis, such as mumps parotitis, occurs with a concomitant viral illness and is usually bilateral, whereas bacterial infections are primarily unilateral.

Obstructive sialoadenitis occurs from a stone or calculus in the salivary gland or duct, most commonly in the submandibular gland. The flow of saliva is obstructed, causing swelling, pain, and firmness. Patients with sialolithiasis note general xerostomia and recurrent worsening of swelling and pain during mealtime.

A thorough head and neck examination is essential, especially a bimanual examination of the major salivary glands. In suppurative sialoadenitis, purulent drainage may be expressed from the submandibular duct (Wharton's) or parotid duct (Stensen's), and the glands are very tender and painful to examination (Figs. 5.34 to 5.37). Sialolithiasis can manifest as enlargement of the ducts with minimal saliva expressed on stripping and, rarely, a palpable or visible stone (Fig. 5.38) or duct thickening. Facial radiographs are of limited utility.

Differential Diagnosis

Tumors of the face and oropharynx, particularly primary salivary neoplasms and secondary lymphatic metastases, develop slowly and produce firm, minimally tender nodules and clear saliva. Cutaneous and odontogenic infections, angioedema variants, and lymphadenitis can mimic sialoadenitis.

ED Treatment and Disposition

Treatment of suppurative sialoadenitis requires antibiotics with staphylococcal coverage, rehydration, proper oral hygiene, and oc-

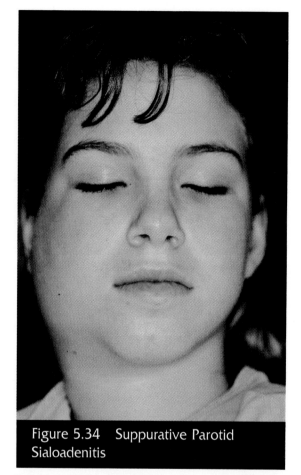

Figure 5.34   Suppurative Parotid Sialoadenitis

Painful swelling over the right parotid initially had clear saliva from Stensen's duct. (Courtesy of Kevin J. Knoop, MD, MS.)

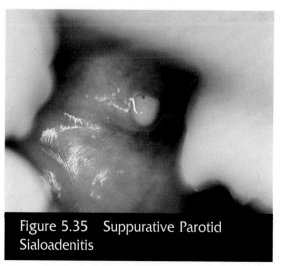

Figure 5.35   Suppurative Parotid Sialoadenitis

After applying firm pressure on the cheek, purulent discharge is seen coming from Stensen's duct. (Courtesy of Kevin J. Knoop, MD, MS.)

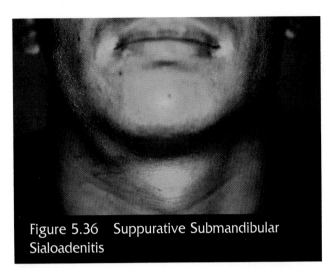

Figure 5.36   Suppurative Submandibular Sialoadenitis

Unilateral submandibular swelling. (Courtesy of Jeffery D. Bondesson, MD.)

casionally surgical irrigation and drainage. Obstructive sialoadenitis is rarely an emergency. Most salivary stones pass spontaneously without complication, and patients can be discharged home on lozenges to stimulate salivary secretions and expel the stone. Prompt follow-up of sialoadenitis is essential to prevent possible morbidity and mortality associated with infections or neoplasms.

Clinical Pearls

1. Examine secretions of both mouth and eyes, and elicit any history of dry eyes, keratoconjunctivitis, cutaneous lesions, or rheumatoid arthritis to establish the diagnosis of a systemic disorder.
2. Medications such as antihistamines, psychotropic drugs, and those possessing atropine-like side effects can cause xerostomia.
3. Lack of improvement on antibiotics suggests an abscess or multiple loculated abscesses that require drainage.

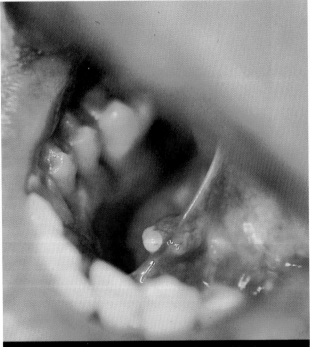

Figure 5.37   Suppurative Submandibular Sialoadenitis

After applying firm pressure, purulent discharge is seen coming from Wharton's duct. (Courtesy of Jeffery D. Bondesson, MD.)

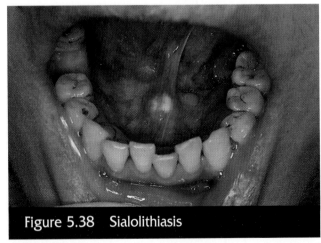

Figure 5.38   Sialolithiasis

A stone is seen at the orifice of Wharton's duct. (Courtesy of David P. Kretzschmar, DDS., MS.)

Associated Clinical Features

Sinusitis is an inflammation of the paranasal sinuses. Sinusitis can be classified as acute, subacute, or chronic; purulent or sterile; and allergic or nonallergic.

Maxillary sinusitis is the most common form of sinusitis and is associated with paranasal face pain, maxillary dental pain, purulent rhinorrhea (Fig. 5.39), retroocular pain, and conjunctivitis. Ethmoid sinusitis is more common in children and produces a low-grade fever and periorbital pain. Frontal sinusitis can cause a severe headache above the eyes, which is exacerbated by leaning forward, a low-grade fever, upper lid edema, and rhinorrhea. Sphenoid sinusitis is fortunately rare. Patients classically complain of a vertex headache and retroocular pain. Due to its intracranial location, sphenoid sinusitis can involve several cranial nerves, the pituitary gland, and cavernous sinus. Involvement of all sinus cavities is referred to as pansinusitis. Important complications of sinusitis include periorbital and orbital cellulitis and Pott's puffy tumor (Figs. 5.40 and 5.41). Patients with Pott's puffy tumor (an osteomyelitis of the cranium from direct extension of a frontal sinusitis) present with a boggy, tender swelling above the eye.

A careful history is important in patients presumed to have sinusitis. Recent steroid use, prodromal viral illness, dental work, and facial trauma are important temporal events. A history of septal deviation or defects, cystic fibrosis, smoking, and cocaine use increase the risk of sinusitis.

Imaging modalities include transillumination of the maxillary sinuses, plain radiographs, CT, and MRI. CT is the most sensitive and specific technique and allows for better delineation of the sphenoid and ethmoid sinuses.

Common bacterial isolates are *Haemophilus influenzae*, *Streptococcus pneumoniae* (together representing 60 to 70% of all bacterial causes), *Streptococcus pyogenes*, *Staphylococcus aureus*, and *Moraxella catarrhalis*. Immunocompromised patients are susceptible to fungal infections.

Differential Diagnosis

Other infections, including facial cellulitis, early herpes zoster, odontogenic infections, and otitis media may produce similar signs and symptoms. Neoplasms and trigeminal neuralgia should also be considered.

ED Treatment and Disposition

For acute bacterial sinusitis, amoxicillin, macrolides, and trimethoprim-sulfamethoxazole are appropriate agents. Refractory cases or immunocompromised patients require broader spectrum antibiotics such as amoxicillin with clavulanate, clarithromycin, and second- or third-generation cephalosporins. Treatment for up to 3 weeks may be necessary.

Decongestants reduce local edema, increase air movement within the sinuses, and decrease local secretions. A short course of topical oxymetazoline or phenylephrine as well as oral pseudoephedrine for 10 days helps minimize secretions and assists in maintaining ostia patency. Humidifed air, steam, or saline nasal sprays also facilitate drainage. Patients should be strongly encouraged to stop smoking.

Steroids are not used in the acute case of sinusitis but do have a role in the subacute and chronic forms. Inhaled steroids, such as triamcinolone, used daily, decrease local inflammation and, when used with decongestants, allow greater drug delivery.

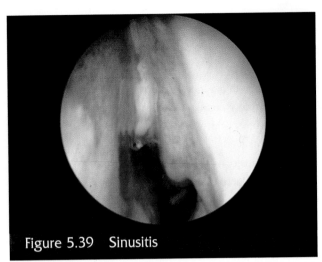

Figure 5.39   Sinusitis

Purulent drainage from maxillary sinus ostium in a patient with maxillary sinusitis. Drainage may not always be apparent, since the ostium may be occluded from swelling and inflammation. (Courtesy of Robin T. Cotton, MD.)

Referral or follow-up by an otolaryngologist or primary care provider should be made for all patients within 3 weeks for routine cases. Patients with co-morbid illnesses or more complicated sinusitis should be admitted for parenteral antibiotic therapy and supportive care.

Clinical Pearls

1. Chronic sinusitis may be due to mucoid retention cysts or polyps, which are often visible on plain radiographs. Refer these patients for possible surgery.
2. Physicians must consider fungal etiologies in patients with co-morbid illnesses.

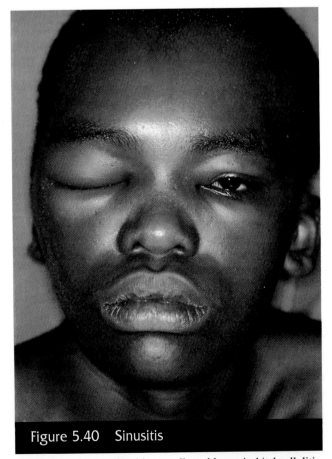

Figure 5.40   Sinusitis

Adolescent with pansinusitis complicated by periorbital cellulitis. The patient was also found to have osteomyelitis of frontal cortex (Pott's puffy tumor). (Courtesy of Robin T. Cotton, MD.)

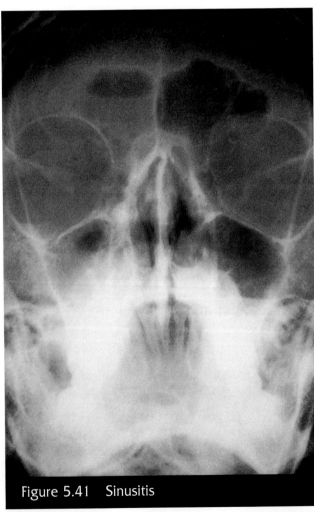

Figure 5.41   Sinusitis

Waters view of the patient in Fig. 5.40 showing air-fluid level in right frontal and bilateral maxillary sinuses. (Courtesy of Robin T. Cotton, MD.)

ORAL TRAUMA

CHAPTER 6

MOUTH

Edwin D. Turner
Edward C. Jauch
Sarah J. Gahm

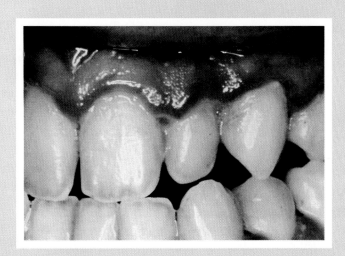

Associated Clinical Features

Tooth subluxation refers to the loosening of a tooth in its alveolar socket. Traumatic oral injury is a common mechanism by which dental subluxation occurs; however, infection and chronic periodontal disease may also produce loosening of teeth. Gingival lacerations and alveolar fractures are commonly associated with dental subluxations. Subluxated, or loosened, teeth are diagnosed by applying gentle pressure to the teeth with a tongue blade or fingertip. Mild displacement may also be noted (Fig. 6.1). Blood along the crevice of the gingiva, where the tooth meets the gingiva, is also a sign of subluxation. Various degrees of tooth mobility may be noted on examination.

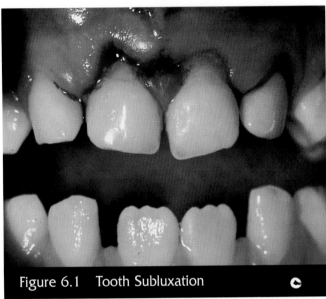

Figure 6.1   Tooth Subluxation

Note the presence of blood along the crevice of the gingival margin of both central incisors—an indication of subluxation following trauma. Mild displacement of the subluxated teeth is noted. (Courtesy of James F. Steiner, DDS.)

Differential Diagnosis

Dental impaction and alveolar ridge fracture should be considered and ruled out clinically and with radiographs.

ED Treatment and Disposition

1. *Primary teeth:* If the subluxated tooth is forced into close proximity to the underlying permanent tooth, extraction by a dentist or oral surgeon is indicated. Otherwise, the patient should be instructed to follow a soft diet for 1 to 2 weeks, allowing the tooth to reimplant.

2. *Permanent teeth:* If the tooth is unstable, it should be temporarily immobilized. This may be accomplished with gauze packing, a figure-eight suture around the tooth and an adjacent tooth, aluminum foil, or a special periodontal dressing (COE-pak). The patient should be referred for dental follow-up.

Clinical Pearls

1. Any evidence of tooth mobility following trauma is a subluxation by definition.
2. Always consider the possibility of an associated underlying alveolar fracture.

Associated Clinical Features

Impacted or intruded teeth result when a tooth is forced deeper into the alveolar socket or surrounding tissues as a result of trauma (Fig. 6.2). The force causing the impaction may be directly on the incisal or occlusal surface of the tooth. The tooth appears shorter than its contralateral partner. The primary dentition is more prone to impaction than permanent teeth. An impacted tooth may be partially visible or completely hidden by the gingiva and buried in the alveolar process. Completely impacted teeth may erroneously be considered avulsed until a radiograph demonstrates the intruded position. The apex of a completely impacted permanent central incisor may be driven through the alveolar bone into the floor of the nostril causing a nosebleed. The apex of the incisor may be noted on examination of the nostril floor. Primary dentition apices tend to be driven into the thin vestibular bone. Other associated injuries include possible alveolar fractures, dental crown or root fractures, as well as oral mucosal and gingival lacerations. Dental pulp necrosis occurs in 15 to 50% of cases.

Differential Diagnosis

Tooth avulsion and fractures should be considered in the differential diagnosis because of a similar mechanism of injury. Completely impacted teeth may simulate an avulsed tooth in appearance. Laterally luxated teeth may appear shortened and angulated and may also simulate partially impacted teeth. Traumatic injury to gingiva around a normal erupting tooth may be mistaken for an impaction. Impacted teeth tend to emit a high metallic sound on percussion test with a metallic instrument, similar to ankylosed teeth. Normal teeth do not produce a metallic sound, whereas subluxated teeth produce a dull sound on percussion. Radiographs also aid in differentiating these dental injuries.

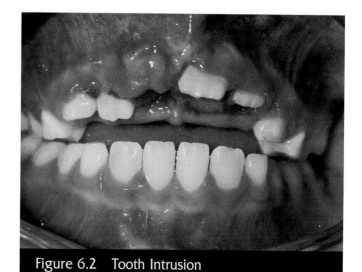

Figure 6.2   Tooth Intrusion

This impaction injury with multiple anterior maxillary tooth involvement shows various degrees of tooth impaction. Also note the complete absence of a central incisor. This may indicate a complete intrusion into the alveolar socket or an avulsion of the tooth. Radiographic studies are required when a tooth's location is in question. (Courtesy of James F. Steiner, DDS.)

Treatment and Disposition

Primary teeth which are impacted usually reerupt and reposition spontaneously within 1 to 6 months. Surgical intervention is indicated if spontaneous reduction does not occur within this time frame. Any intruded primary tooth whose apex is displaced toward or impacts on the follicle of its permanent successor should be extracted. These patients should have dental follow-up and be monitored clinically and radiographically for 1 year. Permanent teeth do not reerupt. Surgical reduction is indicated to prevent complications such as external root resorption and loss of supporting bone. Orthodontic repositioning and splinting is generally carried out over 3 to 4 weeks. Follow-up for a minimum of 1 year is recommended.

Clinical Pearls

1. An undiagnosed impacted tooth is predisposed to infection and tends to have a poor cosmetic result.
2. The maxillary incisors are the most commonly affected teeth.
3. Only the immature primary teeth will reerupt; the permanent teeth do not.

Associated Clinical Features

Avulsion is the total displacement of a tooth from its socket (Fig. 6.3). There is usually a history of trauma; however, infectious etiologies can also cause an avulsion. Complete disruption of the periodontal ligament fibers from the affected tooth occurs as a result. Various degrees of bleeding from the socket and surrounding gingiva may be noted. Depending on the mechanism of injury, there may be an associated underlying alveolar fracture. Prompt inquiry into the location of any unaccountable tooth should be made. Radiographic evaluation to rule out aspiration or soft-tissue entrapment is indicated when the tooth's location is in question.

Differential Diagnosis

Complete tooth impactions may appear to be an avulsion. Dental fractures with retained tooth fragments in the alveolar socket may also simulate an avulsion. Radiographs should be taken to rule out an intrusion or dentoaveolar fracture.

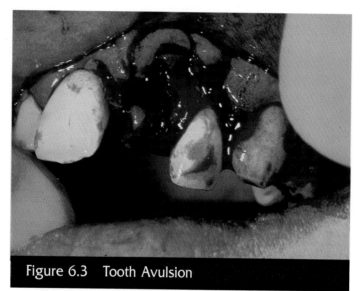

Figure 6.3   Tooth Avulsion

Avulsion injury with angulation and displacement of teeth from the alveolar socket. (Courtesy of James F. Steiner, DDS.)

ED Treatment and Disposition

Permanent teeth should be replaced in their sockets as soon as possible. The tooth should first be rinsed with saline, but not scrubbed, and the root should not be handled. Successful reimplantation depends on the survival of periodontal ligament fibers, which are attached to the root of the avulsed tooth. The tooth should be placed in the socket and emergent dental consultation obtained. Antibiotics against mouth flora (penicillin, clindamycin) should be administered, as well as tetanus prophylaxis. If not replaced, the avulsed tooth should be stored in the mouth of the patient or parent, or in a container of milk. Normal saline can be used, but water should not be used. A commercial kit called the "Tooth Preserving System" contains Hank's solution, which is the ideal storage medium for the avulsed tooth until reimplantation. Primary teeth are not reimplanted, but the patient should be referred to a dentist for follow-up, since procedures are sometimes needed to maintain space in the mouth until the permanent tooth erupts.

Clinical Pearls

1. Reimplantation of primary avulsed teeth in patients younger than 6 years may interfere with eruptions of permanent teeth because of ankylosing and fusion to the bone.
2. Successful reimplantation of an avulsed tooth is best achieved within the first 30 min after an avulsion.
3. For every minute a tooth is out of the socket, a 1% chance of successful reimplantation is lost.

Associated Clinical Features

Anatomically, each tooth has a crown and root portions. Externally the crown is covered with white enamel and the root portion with cementum. The cementoenamel junction (cervical line) is where the crown and root meet. The yellow-to-tan dentin is the second innermost layer and composes the bulk of the tooth. The red-to-pink pulp tissue is located in the center of the tooth and furnishes the neurovascular supply to the tooth. The Ellis classification system is used to describe tooth fractures (Fig. 6.4):

Ellis class I: Involves the enamel only (Fig. 6.5).

Ellis class II: Involves the enamel plus exposure of the dentin (Fig. 6.6). The patient may complain of temperature sensitivity.

Ellis class III: Fracture extends into the pulp. A pink or bloody discoloration on the fracture surface is diagnostic of this type of fracture (Fig. 6.7). The patient may have severe pain, but may also have no pain, due to loss of nerve function.

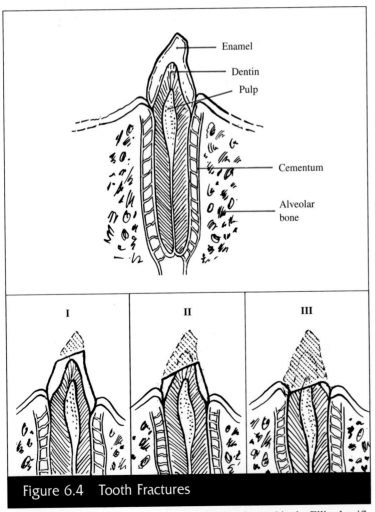

Figure 6.4 Tooth Fractures

Enamel, dentin, and pulp are the anatomic landmarks used in the Ellis classification of tooth fractures.

Differential Diagnosis

Subluxation, alveolar fracture, avulsion, or a traumatic impaction are in the differential. Dental fractures may also be occult and occur below the gum line or at the level of root. Radiographic evaluation will aid in differentiating these conditions.

ED Treatment and Disposition

Ellis class I: Pain control should be initiated. Rough tooth edges may be smoothed with an emery board. Immediate dental referral within 24 h is indicated when soft-tissue injury is caused by sharp pieces of the tooth.

Ellis class II: Patients under 12 years of age have less dentin than older patients and are at risk for infection of the pulp. They should have a calcium hydroxide dressing placed, coverage with gauze or aluminum foil, and see a dentist within 24 h. Older patients should be advised to see a dentist within 24 to 48 h.

Ellis class III: This is considered a dental emergency, and immediate dental consultation is indicated. Delay in treatment may result in severe pain and abscess formation.

Clinical Pearls

1. The anterior teeth are most commonly involved because of more direct exposure to trauma.
2. Consider child abuse when dental injuries occur in young children.

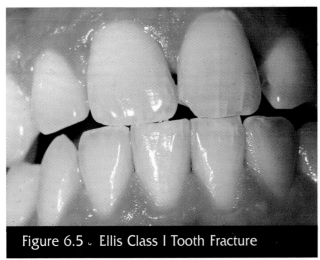

Figure 6.5 Ellis Class I Tooth Fracture

Note the fracture of the left upper central incisor. The sole involvement of the enamel is consistent with an Ellis type I injury. (Courtesy of James F. Steiner, DDS.)

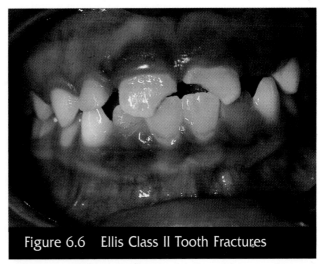

Figure 6.6 Ellis Class II Tooth Fractures

Bilateral maxillary central incisor injuries with exposed enamel and dentin consistent with an Ellis class II fracture. (Courtesy of James F. Steiner, DDS.)

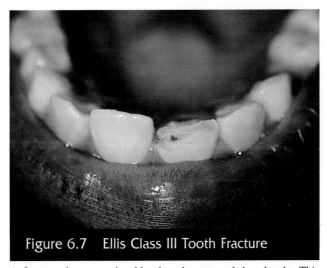

Figure 6.7 Ellis Class III Tooth Fracture

A fracture demonstrating blood at the exposed dental pulp. This sign is pathognomonic for an Ellis class III fracture. (Courtesy of Kevin J. Knoop, MD, MS.)

Associated Clinical Features

The alveolus is the tooth-bearing segment of the mandible and maxilla. Fracture of the alveolar process tends to occur more often in the thinner maxilla than in the mandible. However, the most common type of mandible fracture is an alveolar fracture. The anterior alveolar processes are at greatest risk for fracture due to more direct exposure to trauma (Fig. 6.8). Exposed pieces of bone may be noted in alveolar fractures. Various degrees of tooth mobility and gingival bleeding may be noted. Both subluxation and avulsion of teeth may be associated with underlying alveolar fractures of the mandible or maxilla.

Differential Diagnosis

Fractures of the mandible and maxilla may both present with pain, deformity, malocclusion, and bleeding, which may resemble an alveolar fracture. Gingival lacerations with significant tissue damage may be associated with an underlying fracture and should be considered.

ED Treatment and Disposition

Preservation of as much viable tissue as possible is important. Do not remove any segment of alveolus firmly attached to the mucoperiosteum. Significant cosmetic deformity may result from alveolar bone loss. The involved alveolar segment should have a saline-soaked gauze applied with gentle direct pressure. Any avulsed teeth should also be preserved. The patient's tetanus status should be addressed. Antibiotic therapy with penicillin or a cephalosporin should also be considered, particularly if bony fragments are exposed. Oral surgery consultation should be obtained for possible wire stabilization, arch bar fixation, and follow-up.

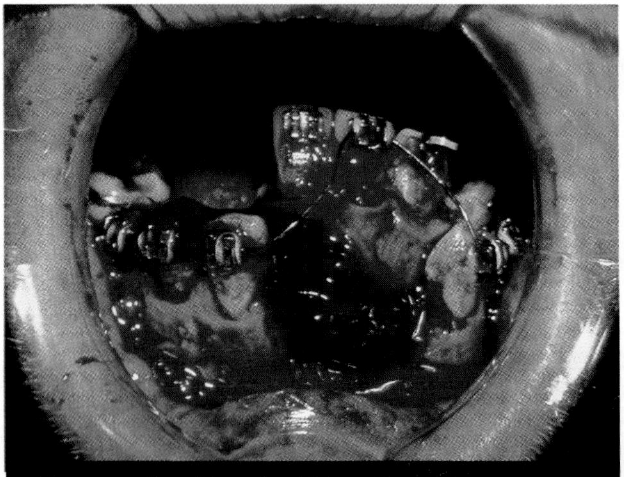

Figure 6.8   Alveolar Ridge Fracture

Note the exposed alveolar bone segment and associated multiple tooth involvement. Attempts should be made to maximally preserve all viable tissue. (Courtesy of James F. Steiner, DDS.)

Clinical Pearls

1. Always consider the possibility of an associated cervical spine injury when evaluating patients with facial trauma.
2. If an avulsed tooth is associated with an alveolar fracture, the clinician should inquire about its location. If unaccounted for, then consider the possibility of aspiration or soft-tissue entrapment.

Associated Clinical Features

Dislocation generally results from direct trauma to the chin while the mouth is open, or more commonly in predisposed individuals after a vigorous yawn. Opening the mouth excessively wide while eating or laughing may also result in dislocation. Acute dislocation occurs when the mandibular condyles displace forward and become locked anterior to the articular eminence. Muscle spasm contributes to prevention of spontaneous relocation. Weakness of the temporal mandibular ligament, an overstretched joint capsule, and a shallow articular eminence are predisposing factors. Patients usually present with an inability to close an open mouth (Fig. 6.9). Other associated symptoms include pain, discomfort, and facial swelling near the temporal mandibular joint (TMJ). Difficulty speaking and swallowing is common. Anterior dislocations are most common; however, posterior dislocation may occur with significant force in association with a basilar skull fracture. Unilateral dislocation results in deviation of the mandible to the unaffected side (Fig. 6.10).

Differential Diagnosis

Temporal mandibular joint hemarthrosis, dystonic reactions, and hysterical dislocation can mimic the true process of TMJ dislocation. Unilateral or bilateral mandible fractures should also be strongly considered, particularly if there is a history of facial trauma.

ED Treatment and Disposition

Acute reduction of pain, muscle spasm, and anxiety is achieved using reassurance, analgesics, and muscle relaxants. Panorex or TMJ x-ray films (pre- and post-reduction) are obtained to exclude a fracture (Fig. 6.11). The patient is typically treated in the sitting position. While facing the patient, the physician grasps the angles of the mandible with both hands. The thumbs are wrapped in gauze for protection and rest on the occlusive surfaces of the molars while downward and backward pressure is applied until the condyle slides back into the articular eminence. Instruct the patient to avoid excessively wide mouth opening while eating and yawning for 3 to 4 weeks. Apply warm compresses to the TMJ areas. A soft diet for 1 week is advised, as is the use of nonsteroidal anti-inflammatory drugs as needed. Dental follow-up should be arranged.

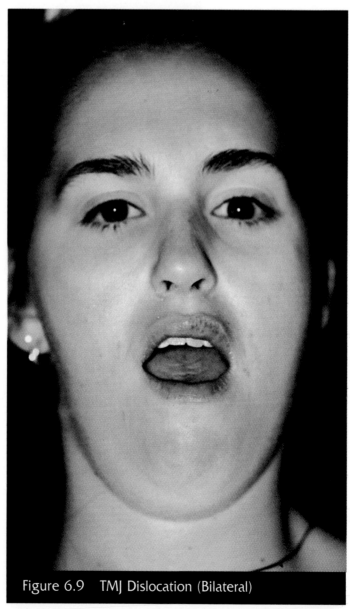

Figure 6.9   TMJ Dislocation (Bilateral)

This patient awoke from sleep with the inability to close her mouth. Note the dry lips and tongue secondary to prolonged exposure. (Courtesy of Warren K. Russell, MD.)

Clinical Pearls

1. Approximately 70% of the general population can subluxate the mandible partially and then spontaneously reduce it.
2. TMJ dysfunction secondary to a neuroleptic or antipsychotic medication–related dystonic reaction is treated with diphenhydramine or benztropine.
3. When trauma is the cause of TMJ dislocation, maintain a high index of suspicion for cervical spine injury.

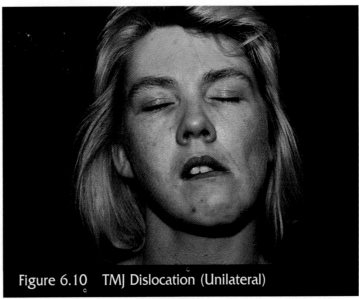

Figure 6.10   TMJ Dislocation (Unilateral)

Note the asymmetric jaw deviation toward the unaffected side. Always consider the possibility of an associated underlying fracture or cervical spine injury. (Courtesy of Kevin J. Knoop, MD, MS.)

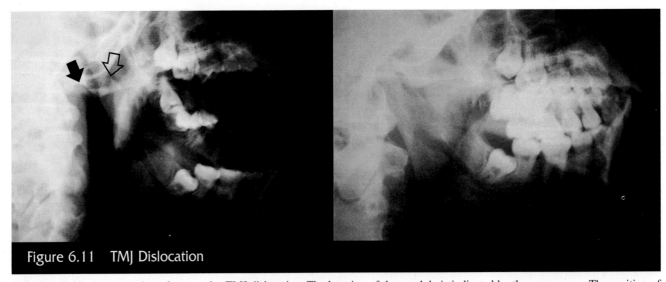

Figure 6.11   TMJ Dislocation

A. Radiographic demonstration of an anterior TMJ dislocation. The location of the condyle is indicated by the open arrow. The position of the mandibular notch is indicated by the closed arrow. *B.* Postreduction radiograph showing normal positioning of the condyle in the mandibular notch. (Courtesy of Edwin D. Turner, MD.)

Associated Clinical Features

Tongue lacerations are usually the result of oral trauma and tongue biting (Fig. 6.12). Injuries to the tongue or mouth floor can cause serious hemorrhage and potential airway compromise. Careful examination of the intraoral-oral cavity for associated injuries is necessary. Specifically, the injury or absence of teeth should be ascertained. Dorsal tongue lacerations may be associated with a concurrent ventral laceration sustained from the mandibular teeth. Closely inspect the wound for possibly entrapped dental elements.

Differential Diagnosis

Superficial tongue abrasions, oral mucosal, and gingival lacerations may all bleed profusely and cause difficulty localizing the exact source. Any of the aforementioned lacerations may also accompany a tongue laceration. A detailed examination of the entire oral cavity is indicated.

ED Treatment and Disposition

Most lacerations to the tongue do not mandate surgical repair. A generous blood supply results in spontaneous repair of most tongue defects. An exception to this rule is lacerations involving the tip where rapid healing may produce a "forked tongue." Lacerations greater than 1 cm in length or those involving a lateral margin are usually best stabilized by a few well-placed sutures; 4-0 black silk or chromic suture should be used. Deep tongue lacerations should have layered closure with absorbable suture. Laceration repair, if opted for in children, is best carried out in a controlled environment under appropriate anesthesia. Anesthesia of the anterior two-thirds of the tongue may be obtained using a regional inferior alveolar nerve block, which also blocks the lingual nerve on the ipsilateral side. Patients with tongue lacerations involving the floor of the mouth or having persistent bleeding may have tongue swelling and airway compromise as a result. Oral surgical consultation for hospital admission with airway surveillance may be indicated.

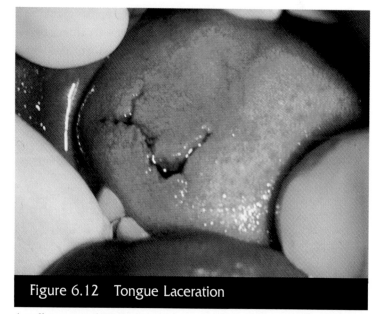

Figure 6.12   Tongue Laceration

A stellate tongue laceration that does not require suturing is shown. The ventral aspect of the tongue should be examined for additional lacerations sustained from the mandibular teeth. (Courtesy of James F. Steiner, DDS.)

Clinical Pearls

1. If repair is elected, use an absorbable or braided suture material. Multiple well secured knots should be placed, as tongue motion tends to untie suture material.

2. Extensive complex tongue lacerations are at risk for infection and should be prophylactically treated with oropharyngeal antibiotics.

Associated Clinical Features

Anatomically, the vermilion border of the lips represents a transition area from mucosal tissue to skin. Lip lacerations involving the vermilion border (Fig. 6.13) present a unique clinical situation, since inadequate repair may cause an unacceptable cosmetic result. Marked tissue edema is frequently noted with most lip trauma, which may distort the anatomy. Vermilion border lacerations may be partial or full thickness through the lip to the mucosal surface. An associated underlying gingival or dental injury is a common finding.

Differential Diagnosis

Vermilion border lip hematomas, abrasions, and soft-tissue swelling may mimic a true laceration involving the vermilion border. Careful examination of the facial and mucosal surfaces of the lip help differentiate these entities.

ED Treatment and Disposition

Accurate vermilion margin reapproximation is the goal of lip repairs. An unapproximated vermilion margin of 2 mm or greater results in a cosmetic deformity and occasionally a puckering defect. A regional block of the mental or infraorbital nerve is recommended for anesthesia to avoid additional tissue edema and anatomic distortion produced by local infiltration. After closure of the deeper tissue, the first skin suture is always placed at the vermilion border to reestablish the anatomic margin. Using 5-0 or 6-0 nylon, suturing should continue along the vermilion surface until the moist mucous membrane is noted. Deep or through-and-through lacerations involving the vermilion border should be closed in layers. The deep muscular and dermal layer may be closed with 3-0 or 4-0 chromic or Vicryl sutures, and the skin with 6-0 nylon sutures. Mucosal layers are loosely reapproximated with 4-0 absorbable suture or silk. The patient should be given wound care instructions. Follow-up for wound evaluation and possible suture removal in 5 to 7 days should be arranged.

Clinical Pearls

1. A vermilion border with as little as 2 mm of malalignment may produce a cosmetically noticed defect.
2. Always place the first skin suture in the vermilion border in any lip laceration involving this area.

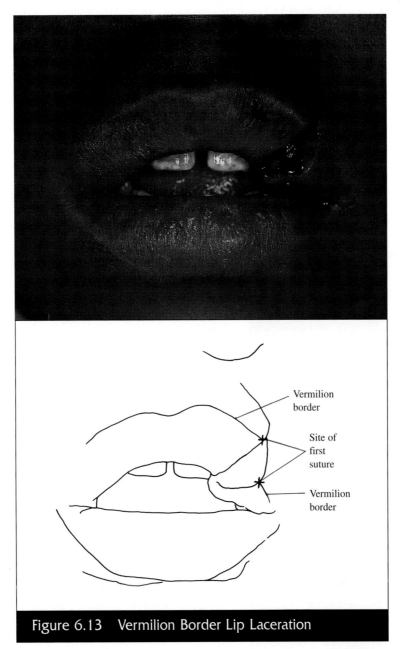

Figure 6.13   Vermilion Border Lip Laceration

A lip laceration with disruption of the vermilion border. Wound repair begins at the vermilion-skin junction for a good cosmetic result. (Courtesy of Kevin J. Knoop, MD, MS.)

Odontogenic Infections

Associated Clinical Features

Gingival abscesses tend to involve the marginal gingiva, and result from entrapment of food and plaque debris in a gingival pocket with subsequent staphylococcal, streptococcal, anaerobic, or mixed bacteria overgrowth leading to abscess formation. Localized swelling, erythema, tenderness, and possible fluctuance in the space between the tooth and the gingiva (the so-called pocket) is the usual location. There may be spontaneous purulent drainage from the gingival margin, or an area of pointing may be seen. In cases of acute gingival abscess formation, pus may be expressed from the gingival margin by gentle digital pressure. When the gingival abscess involves the deeper supporting periodontal structures, it is referred to as a periodontal abscess (Fig. 6.14).

These may present as a fluctuant vestibular abscess or with a draining sinus that opens onto the gingival surface.

Differential Diagnosis

Periapical abscesses are deep and not obvious on inspection. They usually present as tenderness to percussion or pain with chewing over the involved tooth, unlike gingival abscesses. A parulis may also simulate a gingival abscess; however, a parulis represents the cutaneous manifestation of a deeper periapical abscess. Unlike a parulis or periapical abscesses, gingival abscesses are not usually associated with dental caries or fillings. Pericoronal abscesses tend to involve the gingiva overlying a partially erupted third molar and should be considered in the differential diagnosis.

ED Treatment and Disposition

The initial management is a small incision with drainage and warm saline irrigation. Removal of entrapped food and debris is performed. Oral antibiotic therapy with penicillin or clindamycin is recommended. Analgesics should be provided along with dental follow-up. The patient's tetanus status should be addressed.

Clinical Pearls

1. Patients with gingival abscesses are usually afebrile.
2. Consider more extensive abscess formation and oral disease processes in the febrile toxic-appearing patient.
3. Patients with chronic deep periodontal abscesses complain of dull gnawing pain as well as a desire to bite down on and grind the tooth.

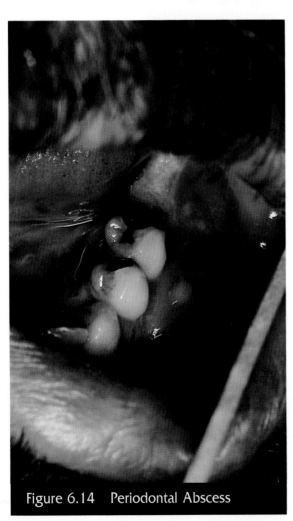

Figure 6.14 Periodontal Abscess

Localized gingival swelling, erythema, and fluctuance are seen in this periodontal abscess with spontaneous purulent drainage. (Courtesy of Kevin J. Knoop, MD, MS.)

Associated Clinical Features

Acute pain, swelling, and mild tooth elevation is characteristic of a periapical abscess. Exquisite sensitivity to percussion or chewing on the involved tooth is a common sign. The involved tooth may have had a root canal treatment, a filling, or a dental carie. Periapical abscesses may enlarge over time and "point" internally on the lingual or buccal mucosal surfaces, or extraorally with swelling and redness of the overlying skin. Occasionally these lesions may tract up to the alveolar periosteum and gingival surface to form a parulis ("gumboil"). Radiographically, these abscesses appear as well circumscribed areas of radiolucency at the dental apex or along the lateral aspect of the root (Fig. 6.15). Early acute periapical abscesses may not demonstrate any radiographic changes. Both deep periodontal and periapical abscesses may have sinuses draining purulent material onto the gingival surface. If the infection is allowed to progress, it can erode through the nearest cortical bone, manifesting itself in a variety of locations (Fig. 6.16).

Differential Diagnosis

Gingival or deep periodontal abscess, buccal space abscess, and unilateral sublingual, parapharyngeal, and submandibular space abscesses should all be considered in the differential diagnosis. All the aforementioned may present with oral pain, tenderness, facial swelling, and possible fever. Panorex films, dental radiographs, or a CT scan may aid in making the diagnosis.

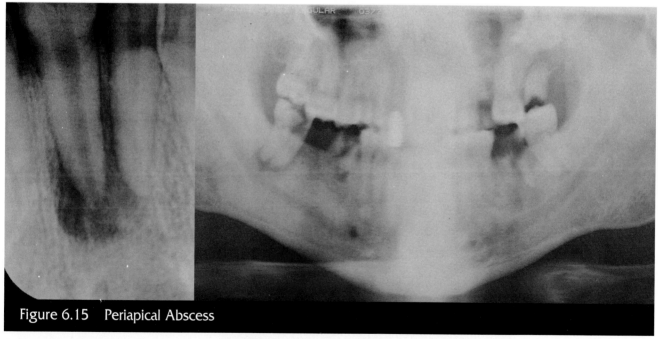

Figure 6.15　Periapical Abscess

A. Note the well defined radiolucent area at the apex and lateral root of the tooth in this radiograph. (Courtesy of James L. Kretzschmar, DDS, MS.) *B.* This Panorex film shows several areas consistent with periapical abscesses. (Courtesy of David P. Kretzschmar, DDS, MS.)

ED Treatment and Disposition

NSAIDs or oral narcotics for pain should be administered as well as oropharyngeal antibiotic therapy. A regional nerve block may be performed with a local anesthetic agent for more immediate temporary relief. Administer tetanus toxoid if indicated. Dental consultation or follow-up in 1 to 2 days is recommended for endodontic evaluation or possible extraction of the involved tooth. Incision and drainage with saline irrigation and prompt referral constitutes the initial treatment of a parulis.

Clinical Pearls

1. More than one tooth may be involved simultaneously.
2. Exquisite tenderness and pain on tooth percussion is a key feature on physical examination and identifies the involved tooth.
3. Periapical abscesses are almost always associated with carious or nonviable teeth.

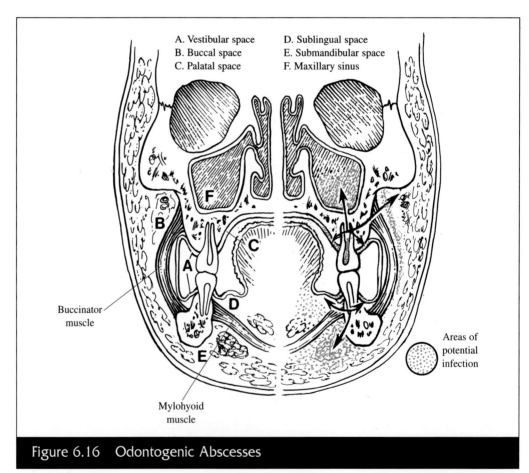

A. Vestibular space   D. Sublingual space
B. Buccal space   E. Submandibular space
C. Palatal space   F. Maxillary sinus

Buccinator muscle

Mylohyoid muscle

Areas of potential infection

Figure 6.16   Odontogenic Abscesses

As infection progresses from the pulp at the tooth apex, it erodes through the bone and can express itself in a variety of places. This illustration notes several possible locations or spaces. (Adapted with permission from Cummings C, Schuller D (eds): *Otolaryngology Head and Neck Surgery,* 1st ed. Chicago, Mosby-Year Book, 1986.)

Associated Clinical Features

A partially erupted or impacted third molar (wisdom tooth) is the most common site of pericoronitis and pericoronal abscesses. The accumulation of food and debris between the overlying gingival flap and crown of the tooth sets up the foci for pericoronitis and subsequent abscess formation. The gingival flap becomes irritated and inflamed. The area is also repeatedly traumatized by the opposing molar tooth and may interfere with complete jaw closure as swelling and tenderness increases. The inflamed gingival process may eventually become infected and form a fluctuant abscess (Fig. 6.17). Foul taste, inability to close the jaw, and fever may occur. Swelling of the cheek and angle of the jaw as well as localized lymphadenopathy are also characteristic. More advanced disease may spread posteriorly to the base of the tongue and oropharyngeal area. Potential spread into the deep cervical spaces is also an important concern with extensive processes.

Differential Diagnosis

Ludwig's angina, peritonsillar abscess, gingival abscess, buccal space abscess, and a severe periapical abscess may all present similar to a pericoronal abscess. Ludwig's angina and peritonsillar abscesses are in fact potential sequelae of acute pericoronitis and pericoronal abscesses.

ED Treatment and Disposition

Superficial incision and drainage with warm saline irrigation may be performed initially in the emergency department. Adequate analgesia and antibiotic coverage should be provided. Consultation or referral to an oral and maxillofacial surgeon for follow-up is indicated for possible extraction of the involved teeth.

Clinical Pearls

1. Pericoronitis and abscess formation rarely occur in the pediatric population and tend to be late adolescent and adult processes.
2. The mandibular third molar is the most commonly involved tooth.
3. Airway compromise is a potential complication with posterior extension of a pericoronal abscess.

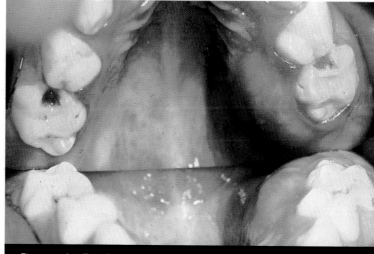

Figure 6.17   Pericoronal Abscess

Note the inflammed fluctuant gingival tissue approximating the incompletely erupted third molar. (Courtesy of James F. Steiner, DDS.)

Associated Clinical Features

The buccal space lies anatomically between the buccinator muscle and the overlying superficial fascia and skin. The maxillary second and third molar teeth are the usual source of infection contributing to buccal space abscesses. Infection from the involved teeth erodes through the maxillary alveolar bone superiorly into the buccal space (Fig. 6.18). Rarely, the third mandibular molar may be the source. In this instance, the infection erodes through the mandibular alveolar bone inferiorly into the buccal space. These patients present with unilateral facial swelling, redness, and tenderness to the cheek (Fig. 6.19). Trismus is generally not present.

Differential Diagnosis

Canine space abscess, parapharyngeal abscess, facial cellulitis, Ludwig's angina, and masticator space abscess formation are all conditions that may resemble buccal space abscesses. Inspection of all the maxillary and third mandibular molar teeth is essential to help make the diagnosis. CT scan can aid in localizing the space involved.

ED Treatment and Disposition

Parenteral antibiotic therapy with penicillin or a third-generation cephalosporin is recommended. Antibiotic coverage for anaerobic organisms may also be added to the treatment regimen. NSAIDs or mild oral narcotic analgesics should be provided as indicated. Dental or oral surgical consultation is necessary for intramural abscess drainage and endodontic therapy versus extraction of the involved molar teeth.

Clinical Pearls

1. Ovoid cheek swelling with sparing of the nasolabial fold helps to identify buccal space abscesses and differentiates it from canine space abscesses.
2. Odontogenic infections of the second or third maxillary molars is the most common source for buccal space abscesses.

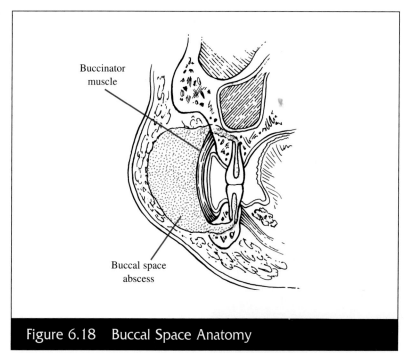

Figure 6.18 Buccal Space Anatomy

The buccal space lies between the buccinator muscle and the overlying skin and superficial fascia. This potential space may become involved by maxillary or mandibular molars. (Adapted with permission from Cummings C, Schuller D (eds): *Otolaryngology Head and Neck Surgery,* 2d ed. Chicago, Mosby-Year Book, 1993.)

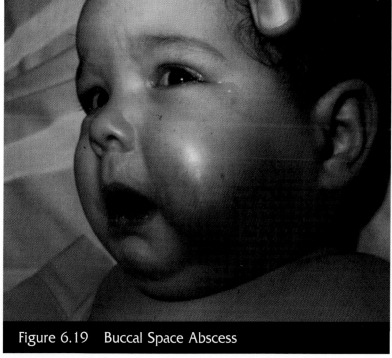

Figure 6.19 Buccal Space Abscess

Note the ovoid cheek swelling with sparing of the nasolabial fold. This finding along with accompanying redness and tenderness helps to identify buccal space abscess formation. (Courtesy of Michael J. Nowicki, MD.)

Associated Clinical Features

The canine space lies between the anterior surface of the maxilla and levator labii superioris muscle of the face. The origin of these abscesses can be from upper anterior teeth and bicuspids, although it is almost exclusively from the maxillary canine tooth. Erosion of maxillary tooth infection through the alveolar bone into the canine space leads to abscess formation, although cutaneous infections from the upper lip and nose are a rare source. Unilateral facial redness, pain, and swelling lateral to the nose with obliteration of the nasolabial fold is characteristic (Fig. 6.20). Severe upper lip and lower eyelid swelling may cause eye closure and drooling at the corner of the mouth.

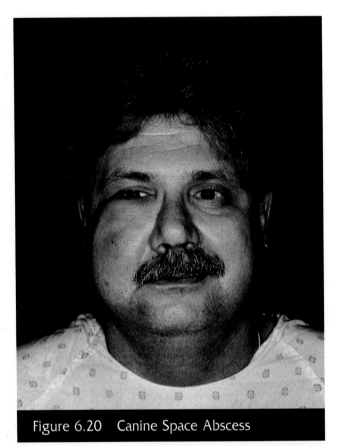

Figure 6.20   Canine Space Abscess

Unilateral facial swelling lateral to the nose with associated redness and the typical loss of the nasolabial fold is shown. The maxillary canine tooth is usually the source of this process. (Courtesy of Frank Birinyi, MD.)

Differential Diagnosis

Buccal space infection, facial cellulitis, and maxillary sinusitis may present with various clinical features similar to canine space abscesses. Examination of the anterior maxillary teeth may provide very helpful clues to the origin and diagnosis of canine space abscesses. CT scan and sinus x-rays may aid in defining these lesions.

ED Treatment and Disposition

Parenteral antibiotic therapy is to include anaerobic coverage indicated for treatment. Dental or oral surgical consultation for intramural incision and drainage represents the most definitive treatment for canine space abscesses. Extraction or endodontic treatment of the involved anterior maxillary teeth is usually necessary.

Clinical Pearls

1. The maxillary canine (cuspid) teeth are the most common source for canine space abscesses.
2. Although these patients may drool when significant upper lip swelling is present, they typically do not have trismus, dysphagia, or odynophagia.

Associated Clinical Features

Ludwig's angina is defined as bilateral cellulitis of the submandibular and sublingual spaces (see Fig. 6.16) with associated tongue elevation (Figs. 6.21 and 6.22). A characteristic painful brawny induration is present rather than fluctuance in the involved tissue. The posterior mandibular molars represent the usual odontogenic origin for the infection. *Streptococcus, Staphylococcus,* and *Bacteroides* species are the most common offending pathogens. Affected individuals are usually 20 to 60 years old with a male predominance. These patients are usually febrile and may demonstrate trismus, dysphonia, and odynophagia. Dysphagia and drooling are secondary to tongue displacement and oropharyngeal swelling. Potential airway compromise or spread of the infection to the deep cervical layers and the mediastinum is possible.

Differential Diagnosis

Peritonsillar abscesses, epiglottititis, and parapharyngeal and retropharyngeal abscesses all have clinical features similar in presentation to Ludwig's angina. Oropharyngeal examination is often uncomfortable and difficult in all the aforementioned conditions. Such examinations, however, are contraindicated if epiglottitis is suspected.

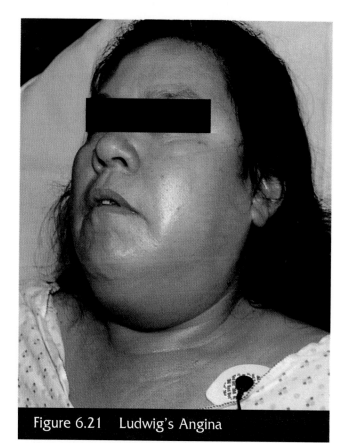

Figure 6.21   Ludwig's Angina

Note the diffuse submandibular swelling and fullness. Direct palpation of this area would reveal a characteristic brawny induration. Potential airway compromise is a key concern in all patients with Ludwig's angina. (Courtesy of Jeffrey Finkelstein, MD.)

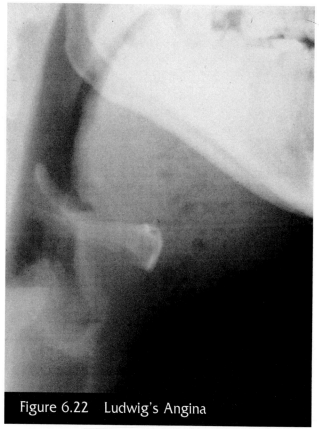

Figure 6.22   Ludwig's Angina

Note the presence of subcutaneous gas in the abscessed submandibular area on this radiograph of a patient with Ludwig's angina. (Courtesy of Edward C. Jauch, MD, MS.)

ED Treatment and Disposition

Acute laryngospasm with airway compromise is a potential life-threatening complication and concern with Ludwig's angina; therefore, plans for definitive airway management should be prepared. Up to one third require intubation or surgical airway placement. Parenteral antibiotic therapy can be initiated with penicillin or a third-generation cephalosporin. Coverage for anaerobic organisms should also be provided with clindamycin or metronidazole. The role of steroids is controversial and ill-defined for potential airway edema in this setting. Parenteral analgesic should be given as needed. The definitive treatment is intraoperative surgical drainage of the abscess. CT or MRI can be used to identify abscess location. Admission to the intensive care unit is indicated for airway surveillance and management. Oral and maxillofacial surgical or otolaryngologic consultation is prudent.

Clinical Pearls

1. The second mandibular molar is the most common site of origin for Ludwig's angina.
2. Admission of these patients to the intensive care unit is almost always indicated because of the potential for airway compromise.
3. Intraoperative surgical incision and drainage is the definitive treatment.
4. Brawny submandibular induration and tongue elevation are common and characteristic clinical findings.

Associated Clinical Features

The parapharyngeal space is also known as the lateral pharyngeal or pharyngomaxillary space. Anatomically it is a pyramid-shaped space with its apex at the hyoid bone and base at the base of the skull. Laterally it is bound by the internal pterygoid muscle and parotid gland with the superior pharyngeal constrictor muscle medially. The posterior aspect of this space is in close proximity with the carotid sheath and cranial nerves IX through XII. Presenting symptoms include fever, dysphagia, odynophagia, drooling, and ipsilateral otalgia. Unilateral neck and jaw angle facial swelling, in association with rigidity and limited neck motion, is common (Fig. 6.23). Potentially disastrous complications that have been associated with infections of this space include: cranial neuropathies, jugular vein septic thrombophlebitis, and erosion into the carotid artery. The origin of parapharyngeal abscesses may be from infected tonsils, sinuses and teeth, or lymphatic spread.

Differential Diagnosis

Buccal space abscess, Ludwig's angina, peritonsillar and retropharyngeal abscesses, and parotitis represent clinical conditions to consider. A CT scan provides more specific information and aids in making the diagnosis.

ED Treatment and Disposition

Preparations for definitive airway management via endotracheal intubation or a surgically obtained airway is vital. Early recognition and anticipation of other potentially disastrous complications should be considered and managed appropriately. Broad spectrum antibiotic coverage for mixed aerobic and anaerobic infections should be initiated. Otolaryngologic or oral surgical consultation is warranted for definitive intraoperative incision and drainage of the abscess.

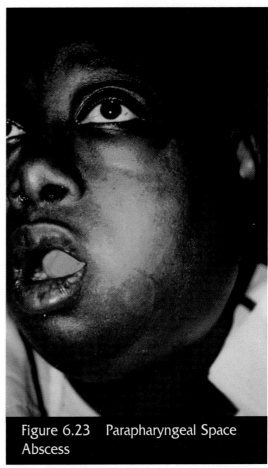

Figure 6.23   Parapharyngeal Space Abscess

Unilateral facial, jaw angle, and neck swelling is seen in this patient. Nuchal rigidity may also be present. (Courtesy of Sarah J. Gahm, MD.)

Clinical Pearls

1. Suspected oropharyngeal abscesses in association with neuropathy in cranial nerves IX through XII is pathognomonic of parapharyngeal abscesses.
2. Bacterial pharyngitis represents the most common source of parapharyngeal abscesses.

Oral Conditions

TRENCH MOUTH (ACUTE NECROTIZING ULCERATIVE GINGIVITIS)

Associated Clinical Features

Painful, severely edematous interdental papillae is characteristic of acute necrotizing ulcerative gingivitis (ANUG). Other associated features include the presence of ulcers with an overlying grayish pseudomembrane and "punched out" appearance (Fig. 6.24). The inflamed gingival tissue is very friable, necrotic, and represents an acute destructive disease process of the periodontium. Fever, malaise, and regional lymphadenopathy are commonly associated signs. Patients may also complain of foul breath and a strong metallic taste. Poor hygiene, emotional stress, smoking, and immunocompromised states all may contribute to predisposition for ANUG. Anaerobic *Fusobacterium* and spirochetes are the predominate bacterial organisms involved. The anterior incisor and posterior molar gingival regions are the most commonly affected oral tissue.

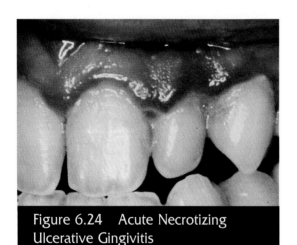

Figure 6.24 Acute Necrotizing Ulcerative Gingivitis

Note the inflamed, friable, and necrotic gingival tissue. An overlying grayish pseudomembrane or punched out ulcerations of the interdental papillae are pathognomonic. (Courtesy of David P. Kretzschmar, DDS, MS.)

Differential Diagnosis

Acute herpetic gingivostomatitis, aphthous stomatitis, desquamative gingivitis, gonococcal and streptococcal gingivostomatitis, and chronic periodontal disease all represent oral diseases which may mimic ANUG. Differentiating these oral conditions from one another is based primarily on history and a thorough oropharyngeal examination.

ED Treatment and Disposition

Initial management includes warm saline irrigation. Systemic analgesics and topical anesthetics such as viscous lidocaine may facilitate oral hygiene measures. Antibiotic treatment is initiated immediately with oropharyngial coverage. Dilute 1.5 to 2% hydrogen peroxide oral rinses is also helpful. Follow-up with a dentist or periodontist in 1 to 2 days is recommended. Patients with more advanced disease may require admission and oral surgical consultation.

Clinical Pearls

1. Dramatic relief of symptoms within 24 h of initiating antibiotics supportive treatment is characteristic.
2. Periodontal abscesses and underlying alveolar bone destruction are common complications of ANUG and dental follow-up.
3. There is no evidence that ANUG is a communicable disease.
4. Gingivitis is a nontender inflammatory disorder.

Associated Clinical Features

Bulimia nervosa is an eating disorder thought to be psychological in origin with significant associated physical complications. This disorder is characterized by binge eating with self-induced vomiting, laxative use, dieting, and exercise to prevent weight gain. Patients with bulimia are at significant risk for dental enamel and dentin damage as a result of repeated episodes of vomiting. Chronic exposure to regurgitated acidic gastric contents represents the main mechanism of injury, which is aggravated by tongue movement. The lingual dental surfaces are most commonly affected (Fig. 6.25). In severe cases, all surfaces of the teeth may be affected. Buccal dental surface erosions may be noted as a result of excessive consumption of fruit (i.e., lemons) and juices by some bulimic patients. Trauma to the oral and esophageal mucosa may also result from induced vomiting. The quantity, buffering capacity, and pH of both the resting and stimulated saliva are found to be reduced. Salivary gland enlargement, most commonly the parotid, may occur in bulimic persons as well. Unexplained elevation of serum amylase, hypokalemia, esophagitis, menstrual irregularities, and fluctuating weight are other complications noted with bulimia.

Differential Diagnosis

Included in the differential diagnosis of acid tooth erosion are conditions that involve vomiting, such as pregnancy, stricture or spasm of the esophagus, and gastrointestinal tract peristalsis disturbances. Xerostomia is a condition of excessive mouth dryness (associated with Sjögren's syndrome) and can also accelerate the process of enamel loss. Conditions resulting in short-term episodes of vomiting do not have severe destructive effects on the dentition. Dental abrasions and erosions, singly or in combination, may result in a considerable loss of tooth structure. Tooth erosions may be brought about by the use of tobacco (Fig. 6.26), eating betel nuts, dentifrice, bruxism, abnormal swallowing, and clenching.

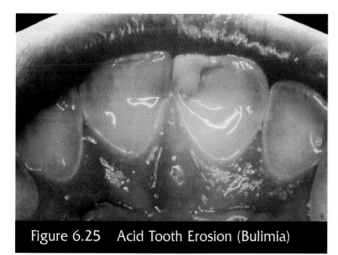

Figure 6.25   Acid Tooth Erosion (Bulimia)

Erosive dentin exposure of the maxillary teeth secondary to chronic vomiting. The involvement of the lingual dental surfaces is characteristic of bulimia. (Courtesy of David P. Kretzschmar, DDS, MS.)

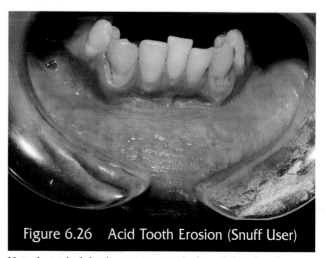

Figure 6.26   Acid Tooth Erosion (Snuff User)

Note the typical dentin exposure on the buccal dental surfaces resulting from prolonged snuff use and its accompanying acid erosion. (Courtesy of David P. Kretzschmar, DDS, MS.)

ED Treatment and Disposition

Dental treatment should begin with vigorous oral hygiene to prevent further destruction of tooth structures. Regular professional fluoride treatments to cover exposed dentin should be instituted as well as pain treatment. With the exception of temporary cosmetic procedures, definitive dental treatment should be deferred until the patient is adequately stabilized psychologically. The initial emergency management of patients with bulimia should address any medical complication of the disorder like hypokalemia, metabolic acidosis, and its associated cardiac, renal, and CNS effects. Hospitalization to stabilize medical complications and provide nutritional support may be indicated. A multidisciplinary team approach is necessary, and should involve psychiatry, internal medicine, and dental consultation as needed.

Clinical Pearls

1. The lingual surfaces of the teeth are the most commonly involved tooth surfaces.
2. Attrition or bruxism tends to cause enamel loss from occlusal and incisal dental surfaces.
3. The labial and buccal surfaces of the teeth tend to show enamel loss from repeat or prolonged chemical contact (e.g., lemon sucking or tobacco products).

Associated Clinical Features

White, flaky, curdlike plaques covering the tongue and buccal mucosa with an erythematous base is typical of thrush (Fig. 6.27). These lesions tend to be painless; however, painful inflammatory erosions or ulcers may be noted, particularly in adults. Decreased oral intake secondary to pain is common. Colonization of surface epithelium by *Candida* may be opportunistic as a result of an altered oral milieu. Predisposing factors include antibiotic use, corticosteroids, radiation to the head and neck, extremes of ages, patients with immunologic deficiencies, and chronic irritation (e.g., denture use and xerostomia).

Differential Diagnosis

Hairy leukoplakia, lingual lichen planus, flecks of milk or food debris, and liquid antacid adhering to the tongue may be confused with candidiasis. Hairy leukoplakia cannot be brushed off with a tongue depressor. This helps differentiate this process from thrush or residue from ingested materials. Microscopic examination of the removed specimen for the presence of hyphae in potassium hydroxide mount will aid in the identification of *Candida*.

ED Treatment and Disposition

Nystatin oral tablets, nystatin suspension, or clotrimazole oral troches are usually adequate therapy. Topical analgesic cocktails may also provide comfort for patients (e.g., Maalox™, diphenhydramine, viscous lidocaine oral rinse).

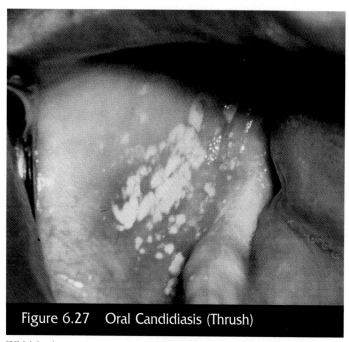

Figure 6.27   Oral Candidiasis (Thrush)

Whitish plaques are seen here on the buccal mucosa. These plaques are easily removed with a tongue blade, differentiating them from lichen planus or leukoplakia. (Courtesy of James F. Steiner, DDS.)

Clinical Pearls

1. Thrush is most common in premature infants and immunosuppressed patients.
2. In young adults thrush may be the first sign of AIDS; a history of HIV risk factors should be elicited.

Associated Clinical Features

Hairy leukoplakia is usually found on the tongues of HIV-positive individuals. It tends to appear on the lateral aspect as corrugated white patches of hairlike projections (Fig. 6.28). It may occasionally occur on the dorsal surface of the tongue and oral mucosa. Although the exact etiology of hairy leukoplakia is unknown, there is a strong association with Epstein-Barr virus (EBV) infection of the oral mucosa. The lesion is asymptomatic.

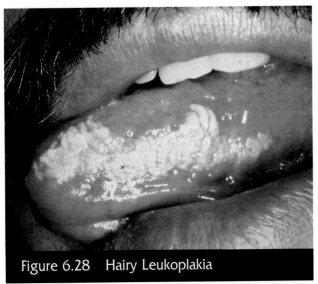

Figure 6.28   Hairy Leukoplakia

The corrugated white patch on the lateral tongue border is a characteristic finding with hairy leukoplakia. This material is firmly attached and cannot be readily removed. (Courtesy of James F. Steiner, DDS.)

Differential Diagnosis

Thrush, lichen planus, food debris, and repeated inadvertent biting of the lateral tongue borders tend to produce lesions that may be misdiagnosed as leukoplakia.

ED Treatment and Disposition

Referral for HIV testing and counseling should be arranged. Treatment is solely for cosmetic reasons. Acyclovir and topical retinoids have both produced satisfactory clinical improvement.

Clinical Pearls

1. More than 60% of hairy leukoplakia patients develop AIDS within 2 years, and 80% in 3 years.
2. Hairy leukoplakia cannot be scraped off the tongue or oral mucosa.

Associated Clinical Features

Kaposi's sarcoma is the most common AIDS-related malignancy. For unknown reasons, it is more common in homosexual men with HIV than in other HIV-positive groups. The most common intraoral site for Kaposi's sarcoma is the palate (Fig. 6.29). It may, however, be found anywhere in the mouth or in different locations of the body (See also Fig. 13.45). It appears as vascularlike, flat, bluish-red patches with irregular borders. Kaposi's sarcoma alone is generally not associated with a significant morbidity or mortality.

Differential Diagnosis

Ecchymosis, hemangioma, purpura, lymphoma, and oral nevus formation all represent oral conditions which may mimic Kaposi's sarcoma.

ED Treatment and Disposition

Referral for HIV testing, counseling, and biopsy of the lesion is the recommended management. Radiation and chemotherapy are generally reserved for cosmetically disfiguring, extensive, and very painful lesions.

Clinical Pearls

1. Kaposi's sarcoma is the most common cutaneous manifestation of AIDS.
2. Kaposi's sarcoma is the second most common overall manifestation of AIDS, *Pneumocystis carinii* being the first.

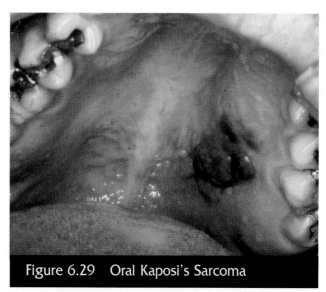

Figure 6.29   Oral Kaposi's Sarcoma

Note the typical bluish-red coloration and the irregular borders commonly found with these lesions. The palate is the most common intraoral location for Kaposi's sarcoma. (Courtesy of James F. Steiner, DDS.)

Associated Clinical Features

Oral herpes simplex may present acutely as a primary gingivostomatitis, or as a recurrence. Painful vesicular eruptions on the oral mucosa, tongue, palate, vermilion borders, and gingiva are highly characteristic (Fig. 6.30). A 2- to 3-day prodromal period of malaise, fever, and cervical adenopathy is common. The vesicular lesions rupture to form a tender ulcer with yellow crusting and an erythematous margin. Pain may be severe enough to cause drooling and odynophagia, which can discourage eating and drinking, particularly in children. The disease tends to run its course in a 7- to 10-day period with resolution of the lesions without scarring. Recurrent herpes labialis may present with an aura of burning, itching, or tingling prior to vesicle formation. Oral trauma, sunburn, stress, and any variety of febrile illnesses can precipitate this condition.

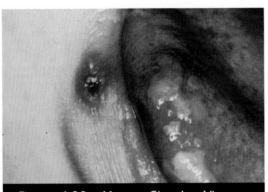

Figure 6.30   Herpes Simplex Virus (HSV) Stomatitis

Note the vermilion border and lingual lesions that are common in this condition. A prodromal period of fever, malaise, and cervical adenopathy may herald the onset of these painful ulcerations. (Courtesy of James F. Steiner, DDS.)

Differential Diagnosis

Oral erythema multiforme or Stevens-Johnson syndrome, aphthous lesions, oral pemphigus, and hand-foot-mouth (HFM) syndrome are in the differential diagnosis. It should be noted that aphthous ulcers tend to occur on movable oral mucosa and rarely on immovable mucosa (i.e., hard palate and gingiva). The vermilion border is a characteristic location for herpes labialis as opposed to aphthous lesions. Posterior oropharyngeal ulcerations with associated hand and foot lesions help to define HFM syndrome. Painful hemorrhagic oral ulcers in association with anorectal and conjunctival lesions aid in identifying erythema multiforme or Stevens-Johnson syndrome. Oral pemphigus is commonly found in elderly patients. Cutaneous skin bullae and several weeks of vague constitutional symptoms are also characteristic of pemphigus. A thorough history is invaluable in differentiating the aforementioned disorders.

ED Treatment and Disposition

Supportive care with rehydration and pain control are the mainstays of therapy. Temporary pain relief may be achieved with topical analgesics. Viscous lidocaine, 2%, may be used as an oral rinse, 5 mL every 3 to 4 h. Oral acyclovir, 200 mg capsules five times per day, may be useful in adults with primary infections. Topical acyclovir ointment may also be of use by preventing viral spreading and acting as a lubricant to prevent lip cracking and bleeding. Secondary infection of herpetic lesions should be treated with oral penicillin or erythromycin.

Clinical Pearls

1. Oral herpetic lesions tend to occur commonly on the vermilion border, gingiva, and hard palate.
2. Fatal viremia and systemic involvement may occur in infants and children with herpetic gingivostomatitis.
3. Primary acute oral herpetic infection occurs most commonly in children and young adults.
4. Corticosteroid use is contraindicated in herpetic gingivostomatitis because of potential worsening of the condition.

Associated Clinical Features

Aphthous ulcers are painful mucosal lesions varying in size from 1 to 15 mm. A prodromal burning sensation in the affected area may be noted 2 to 48 h before an ulcer is noted. The initial lesion is a small, white papule, which ulcerates and enlarges over the subsequent 48 to 72 h (Fig. 6.31). The lesions are typically round or ovoid with a raised yellow border and surrounding erythema. Multiple aphthous ulcers may occur on the lips, tongue, buccal mucosa, floor of the mouth, or soft palate (Fig. 6.32). Spontaneous healing of lesions occurs in 7 to 10 days without scarring. The exact etiology of aphthous lesions is unknown. Deficiencies of vitamin B_{12}, folic acid, and iron and viruses have all been implicated. Stress, local trauma, and immunocompromised states have all been cited as possible precipitating factors.

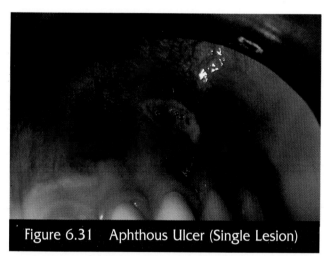

Figure 6.31   Aphthous Ulcer (Single Lesion)

Raised yellow borders with surrounding erythema are typical of aphthous ulcers. (Courtesy of James F. Steiner, DDS.)

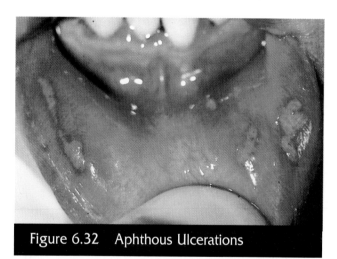

Figure 6.32   Aphthous Ulcerations

Note the multiple ulcers of various sizes located on the lip and gingival mucosa. These lesions rarely occur on the immobile oral mucosa of the gingiva or hard palate. (Courtesy of James F. Steiner, DDS.)

Differential Diagnosis

Primary or recurrent herpetic oral lesions may present with a near identical prodrome and similar appearance to aphthous ulcerations. Herpetic lesions, unlike aphthous ones, tend to occur on the gingiva, hard palate, and vermilion border. Oral erythema multiforme may also present similar to aphthous stomatitis; however, like oral herpes, it may tend to present with multiple vesicles in the early stages. Stevens-Johnson syndrome represents a severe form of erythema multiforme characterized by hemorrhagic anogenital and conjunctival lesions as well as oral lesions. Herpangina results from coxsackie and echo viruses with oral ulcerations typically involving the posterior pharynx. Oral pemphigus should also be considered in the differential. Behçet's syndrome can present with recurrent oral lesions, but also demonstrates genital ulcers and uveitis.

ED Treatment and Disposition

Supportive care, rehydration, and pain control constitutes the focus of therapy. A topical anesthetic agent such as 2% viscous lidocaine as an oral rinse every 3 to 4 h is palliative. Protective dental paste (Orabase) may be applied every 6 h to prevent irritation of lesions. Triamcinolone acetonide in an emollient dental paste applied three to four times daily may also reduce pain and promote healing of the lesions.

Clinical Pearls

1. Aphthous ulcers may be associated with Crohn's disease.
2. Women are more commonly affected by aphthous lesions than men.
3. The first aphthous episode occurs most commonly in the second decade of life.
4. Aphthous lesions almost never occur on the gums or hard palate.

Associated Clinical Features

Reddened, hypertrophied lingual papillae, called strawberry tongue, is associated primarily with scarlet fever, which is caused by group A streptococcus. The tongue initially appears white with the erythematous papillae sticking through. After several days, the white coating is lost and the tongue appears bright red (Fig. 6.33). Other signs of group A streptococcal infection include fever, an exudative pharyngitis, a scarlatiniform rash, and the presence of Pastia's lines (petechial linear rash in the skin folds).

Differential Diagnosis

Kawasaki syndrome may also present with an injected pharynx and a erythematous strawberrylike tongue. It is essential to make the distinction between streptococcal infection and Kawasaki syndrome, since the latter is associated with a high incidence of coronary artery aneurysm if left untreated. Also consider toxic shock syndrome (TSS), in which one-half to three-fourths of patients tend to have pharyngitis with a strawberry-red tongue. Patients with TSS also have skin rashes as with scarlet fever; however, the rash in TSS is macular and "sunburnlike." Erythema multiforme can also be associated with fever, pharyngeal erythema, and lingual lesions; however, it has a more distinct pathognomonic cutaneous rash called target, or iris, lesions.

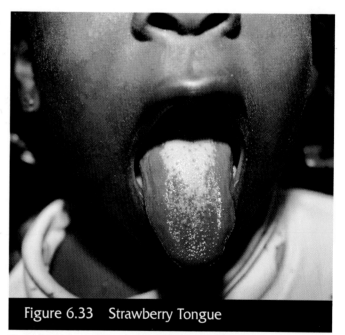

Figure 6.33   Strawberry Tongue

Note the white exudate with bulging red papillae. The white coating is eventually lost after several days, and the tongue then appears bright red. (Courtesy of Michael Nowicki, MD.)

ED Treatment and Disposition

Penicillin or erythromycin is the drug of choice for group A streptococci. Pharyngeal cultures are useful for confirming the diagnosis. Antistreptolysin O (ASO) titers can be used for confirmation in the convalescent stage if the diagnosis is in question.

Clinical Pearls

1. A course, palpable, sandpaperlike rash of the skin is highly characteristic of scarlet fever.
2. Strawberry tongue initially appears white in color, with prominent red papillae bulging through the white exudate. After several days, the tongue becomes completely beefy red.

Associated Clinical Features

Koplik's spots are oral lesions pathognomonic for measles. They appear 1 to 2 days before the generalized measles rash. The spots are bright red with a tiny bluish-white center. They are most often seen on the buccal mucosa opposite the posterior teeth (Figs. 6.34 and 14.19). By the second or third day, the spots coalesce. The patient generally complains of prodromal symptoms such as fever, conjunctivitis, cough, and malaise for 1 to 2 days before the Koplik's spots appear.

Differential Diagnosis

Before the onset of rash, the syndrome may be mistaken for any number of viral syndromes. Aphthous lesions, herpes simplex virus, and lesions from herpangina should be considered. Forschheimer's spots are nonspecific pinpoint petechiae found on the soft palate of some patients with rubella (German measles). Koplik's spots, however, are nonpetechial, nonulcerated lesions and are nontender.

ED Treatment and Disposition

Measles is a highly contagious infection transmitted by respiratory droplets. Almost all unprotected household contacts are either infected or at considerable risk for infection. Supportive care including rest, antipyretics, and fluids is usually adequate. For more definitive treatment recommendations see Chapter 14.

Clinical Pearls

1. Measles is now an unusual infection because of routine vaccination.
2. Koplik's spots may occur on any mucosal surface in the oral cavity except the tongue.
3. The oral mucosa opposite the first and second molars is the most common location for these lesions.
4. Koplik's spots are nontender and do not cause odynophagia.

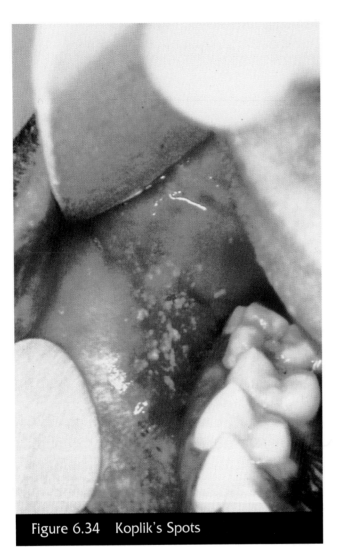

Figure 6.34   Koplik's Spots

The presence of bright red buccal mucosal spots with a whitish center near the molars is most consistent with Koplik's spots. (Courtesy of Michael J. Nowicki, MD.)

Associated Clinical Features

Tori are benign nodular overgrowths of the cortical bone. Although their physical appearance can be somewhat alarming to those unfamiliar with this entity, there is generally no need for concern. These bony protuberances occur in the midline of the palate where the maxilla fuses (Fig. 6.35). Tori may also be located on the mandible, typically on the lingual aspect of the molar teeth. Tori are covered by a thin epithelium, which is easily traumatized and ulcerated. These ulcerations tend to heal very slowly because of the poor vascularization of the tori. Torus palatinus, in particular, is slow growing and may occur at any age; however, it is most commonly noted prior to age 30 in adults. Torus palatinus affects females twice as frequently as males.

Differential Diagnosis

There are a variety of oral conditions that may be confused with mandibular or palatal tori. Gingival fibromatosis, fibroma formation secondary to irritation, granulomas, abscesses, and oral neurofibromatosis located on the palate may all be similar in appearance to torus palatinus. Nodular bony enlargement in the oral cavity may also result from fibrous dysplasia, osteomas, and Paget's disease. Biopsies, oral radiographs, and CT scans may aid in differentiating these conditions.

ED Treatment and Disposition

Tori are a normal structural variant and do not represent any inflammatory or neoplastic process. Therefore, they are of no clinical significance and require no treatment unless associated with a complication. Tori may enlarge enough to interfere with eating or speaking and impair proper fitting of dental prosthesis. For some patients the mere presence of torus palatinus may be bothersome and undesirable. Oral and maxillofacial consultation is indicated when complications call for surgical excision of the lesion. Reassurance is otherwise all that is indicated. However, elective removal can be undertaken for the overly anxious patient who is preoccupied with or annoyed by their presence.

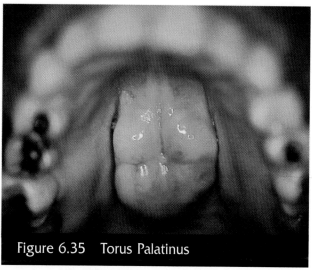

Figure 6.35 Torus Palatinus

Note the nodular appearance and characteristic central palatal location. Abrasions and ulcerations can occur on the thin overlying epithelium secondary to trauma by food and oral objects. (Courtesy of Kevin J. Knoop, MD, MS.)

Clinical Pearls

1. Torus palatinus almost always occurs in the midline of the hard palate.
2. Both torus palatinus and torus mandibularis are nontender and otherwise asymptomatic.

CHAPTER 7

CHEST AND ABDOMEN

Stephen Corbett
Lawrence B. Stack
Kevin J. Knoop

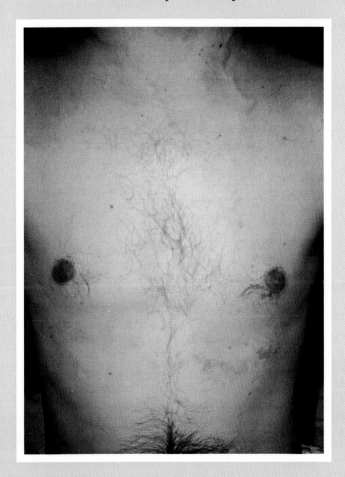

Associated Clinical Features

Traumatic asphyxia is due to a sudden increase in intrathoracic pressure against a closed glottis. The elevated pressure is transmitted to the veins, venules, and capillaries of the head, neck, extremities, and upper torso, resulting in capillary rupture. Survivors demonstrate plethora, ecchymoses, petechiae (Figs. 7.1 and 7.2), and subconjunctival hemorrhages. Severe cases may produce CNS injury with seizures, posturing, and paraplegia.

Differential Diagnosis

Sudden traumatic compression of the superior vena cava produces obstruction similar to that seen in the superior vena cava syndrome. Both demonstrate a violaceous discoloration of the face and neck. History will confirm the diagnosis.

ED Treatment and Disposition

Treatment is supportive with attention to other concurrent injuries. Long-term morbidity is related to the associated injuries.

Clinical Pearls

1. Facial petechiae are known as Tardieu's spots.
2. Be alert for associated rib and vertebral fractures.

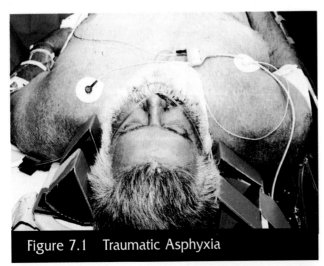

Figure 7.1   Traumatic Asphyxia

This 45-year-old male was pinned when the truck he was working under fell on his chest. He was unable to breathe for 3 to 4 min until his coworkers rescued him. The violaceous coloration of the shoulders, face, and upper chest is apparent. (Courtesy of Stephen Corbett, MD.)

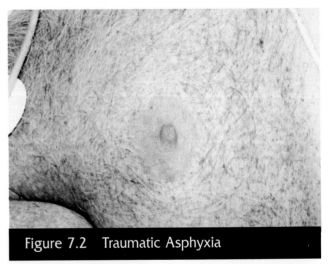

Figure 7.2   Traumatic Asphyxia

A closer view showing the petechial nature of this rash. The patient was observed in the hospital overnight and recovered completely. (Courtesy of Stephen Corbett, MD.)

Associated Clinical Features

A tension pneumothorax results when air is able to enter, but not exit, the pleural space. Air in the pleural space accumulates and compresses the ipsilateral lung and vena cava with rapid decrease in cardiac output. The contralateral lung may suffer VQ mismatch. Subcutaneous air, tracheal deviation, jugulovenous distention (JVD), and diminished or hyperresonant ipsilateral breath sounds can be clues. Subcutaneous emphysema may be visible on the neck and chest and is easily diagnosed by palpation. The released air from a tension pneumothorax can be heard escaping from a needle thoracostomy.

Differential Diagnosis

Cardiac tamponade, congestive heart failure with pulmonary edema, esophageal intubation, and anaphylaxis should be considered.

ED Treatment and Disposition

Treatment requires rapid recognition of the tension pneumothorax, frequently without benefit of chest radiographs. A large-bore needle (at least 14 gauge) should be placed over the superior rib surface of the second interspace in the midclavicular line (Fig. 7.3). A rush of air with improvement of vital signs confirms the diagnosis. A syringe loaded with sterile saline allows visualization of air return, but is not mandatory. If there is no immediate improvement, do not hesitate to place a second needle in the next interspace. A chest tube should be placed as soon as possible. Ventilation with appropriate inspiratory/expiratory ratio would prevent further occurrences.

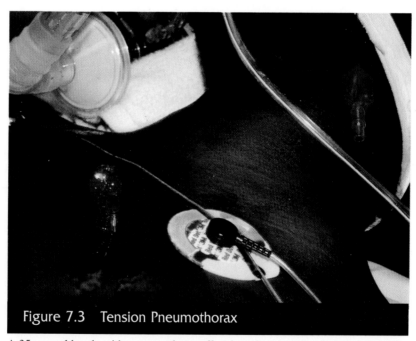

Figure 7.3   Tension Pneumothorax

A 35-year-old male with severe asthma suffered respiratory arrest during transport by ambulance. He was intubated on arrival, but soon became hard to ventilate and developed subcutaneous emphysema followed by hypotension. Needle thoracostomy produced a rush of air and bubbling from the needle with stabilization of vital signs. (Courtesy of Stephen Corbett, MD.)

Clinical Pearls

1. Do not overventilate patients with obstructive pulmonary disease. "Stacking" breaths trap air in the lungs and predisposes to bleb rupture and pneumothorax. The pathophysiology of this disease requires a prolonged expiratory phase.
2. The diagnosis of a tension pneumothorax is made clinically and should be treated immediately with a needle thoracostomy, and ultimately a tube thoracostomy.

CARDIAC TAMPONADE WITH PERICARDIOCENTESIS

Associated Clinical Features

Beck's triad of acute cardiac tamponade includes jugulovenous distention (JVD) from an elevated central venous pressure (CVP), hypotension, and muffled heart sounds. In trauma, only one-third of patients with cardiac tamponade demonstrate this classic triad, although 90% have at least one of the signs. The simultaneous appearance of all three physical signs is a late manifestation of tamponade and usually seen just prior to cardiac arrest. Other symptoms include shortness of breath, orthopnea, dyspnea on exertion, syncope, and symptoms of inadequate perfusion.

Differential Diagnosis

Patients with a chronic pericardial effusion have an elevated CVP and a small quiet heart, but are relatively asymptomatic and without hypotension.

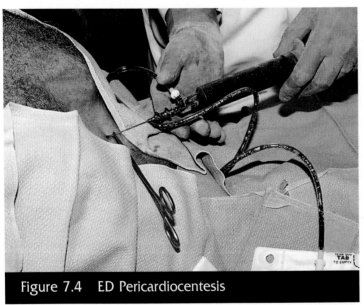

Figure 7.4   ED Pericardiocentesis

A positive pericardiocentesis in a patient with a sudden onset of shortness of breath and electrical alternans. (Courtesy of Lawrence B. Stack, MD.)

ED Treatment and Disposition

The clinical diagnosis of tamponade requires suspicion and a careful evaluation of the signs and imaging techniques when available. Two-dimensional echocardiography represents the ultimate standard for diagnosis. ED pericardiocentesis (Fig. 7.4) is a diagnostic and resuscitative procedure in patients with suspected cardiac tamponade. Goals of ED pericardiocentesis include identification of pericardial effusion and removing blood from the pericardial space to relieve the tamponade.

Clinical Pearls

1. An electrical alternans seen on a 12-lead ECG suggests pericardial effusion.
2. Beck's triad for acute cardiac tamponade is a late manifestation and is seen in only 30% of traumatic patients.

Associated Clinical Features

ED thoracotomy is a resuscitative procedure performed in penetrating chest trauma patients who have lost signs of life in the presence of prehospital or ED personnel. Resuscitative thoracotomy (Fig. 7.5) in the ED has specific goals once the chest is opened: relief of cardiac tamponade, supporting cardiac function (internal cardiac compressions, cross-clamping the aorta to improve coronary perfusion, and internal defibrillation), and controlling hemorrhage from the heart, pulmonary vessels, thoracic wall, and great vessels.

Differential Diagnosis

Few conditions present which require immediate ED thoracotomy. A trauma patient who has lost vital signs prior to arrival of prehospital personnel is deceased and not a candidate for this procedure.

ED Treatment and Disposition

Patients with penetrating thoracic trauma who lose their vital signs en route to the ED should receive an immediate thoracotomy on arrival by the most experienced provider. Patients with penetrating thoracic trauma whose blood pressure cannot be maintained above 70 mmHg with aggressive fluid and blood management should be considered for ED thoracotomy. Blunt trauma patients who lose their vital signs en route to the ED should not receive an ED thoracotomy, since they rarely survive. Notification of surgical support should be done as soon as possible.

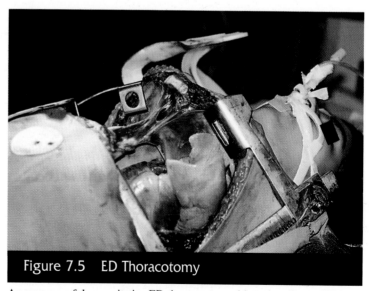

Clinical Pearls

1. Injuries potentially responsive to resuscitative ED thoracotomy include cardiac tamponade, pulmonary parenchymal and tracheobronchial injuries, large-vessel injuries, air embolism, and penetrating heart injuries.

2. Resuscitative ED thoracotomy should be performed immediately once the indications have been met, since the likelihood of survival is greater when performed earlier in the resuscitation.

Figure 7.5 ED Thoracotomy

An unsuccessful resuscitative ED thoracotomy with pericardiotomy in a patient with penetrating chest trauma who lost signs of life in the field after the paramedics arrived at the scene. (Courtesy of Alan B. Storrow, MD.)

Associated Clinical Features

Diagnostic peritoneal lavage (DPL) was introduced in 1965 as a simple, fast, and reliable technique to identify hemoperitoneum in blunt and penetrating abdominal trauma patients. It is performed by placing a catheter into the peritoneum, aspirating for gross blood, and introducing 1 L of crystalloid if the initial aspiration is negative (Fig. 7.6). The lavage fluid is then withdrawn and white and red blood counts are performed. Interpretation of the results is based on the type of trauma. A "grossly positive" DPL is evident when 10 cc of blood is obtained on the initial aspiration. The procedure is considered positive in blunt abdominal trauma when $>100,000$ RBC/mm^3 or >500 WBC/mm^3 are present in the lavage fluid. In penetrating abdominal trauma the procedure is considered positive when $>10,000$ RBC/mm^3 are present (up to 100,000 RBC/mm^3 is used by some). Lavage fluid containing intestinal contents is evidence of perforating bowel injury.

Indications for DPL in blunt trauma include equivocal examination with significant abdominal trauma, unreliable examination (intoxication, spinal trauma, head injury), unexplained hypotension with suspected abdominal injury, and when serial examinations are not possible (patients going to the operating room for other injuries).

Indications for DPL in penetrating trauma include patients in whom the need for celiotomy is unclear, tangential wounds in which peritoneal penetration is uncertain, stab wounds in which there are no peritoneal signs or signs of peritoneal penetration, and low chest wounds to identify diaphragmatic injury.

Contraindications to DPL include any condition in which a celiotomy is clearly indicated, since this would delay definitive treatment.

Differential Diagnosis

Injuries which may not be diagnosed with DPL include subcapsular liver or spleen hematomas, hollow viscous injuries, ruptured diaphragm, and ruptured bladder. Retroperitoneal injuries are not diagnosed with DPL.

ED Treatment and Disposition

A positive DPL is an indication for celiotomy. Patients with negative DPL's are observed or discharged based on a variety of factors including injury mechanism, co-morbid disease states, and concurrent traumatic injuries sustained.

Clinical Pearls

1. Intraperitoneal blood (30 cc) will typically give a DPL result of $\geq 100,000$ RBC/mm^3.
2. Controversy exists over the positive cell count in penetrating abdominal trauma, since the range for a positive result can vary between centers from 1000 to 100,000 RBC/mm^3.
3. If a patient is being transferred to another facility, a sample of the DPL fluid should accompany the patient.

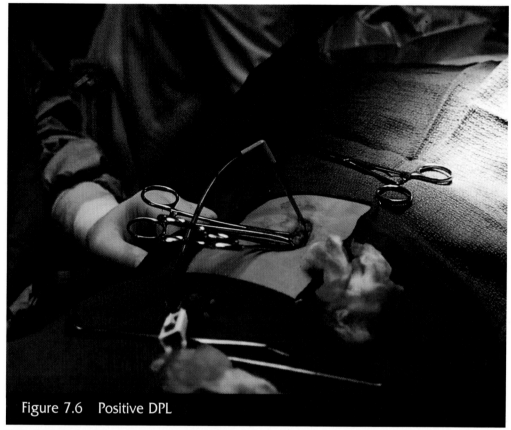

Figure 7.6   Positive DPL

DPL fluid obtained from this patient with blunt trauma was microscopically positive. Initial aspiration was negative. (Courtesy of Kevin J. Knoop, MD, MS.)

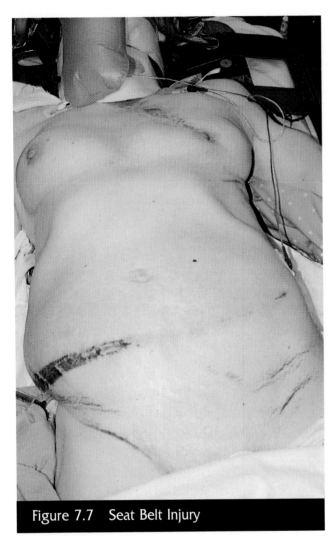

Figure 7.7   Seat Belt Injury

Ecchymosis from the three-point seat belt is clearly seen. The injuries identified are multiple rib fractures and multiple small bowel wall hematomas. (Courtesy of Stephen Corbett, MD.)

Associated Clinical Features

Seat belts have reduced the mortality and the severity of injuries following motor vehicle accidents; however, they occasionally produce injury. Injuries caused by the standard three-point restraint harness (Fig. 7.7) are most commonly rib fractures. Injuries caused by the older lap belts include abdominal injuries such as bowel contusion or perforation.

Differential Diagnosis

A careful primary and secondary survey identifies most injuries caused by seat belt use. Difficult diagnosis occurs in the case of bowel perforation or diaphragmatic rupture in which signs and symptoms may not occur until hours or days after the initial injury.

ED Treatment and Disposition

Patients with a mechanism for significant trauma, or with other injuries requiring admission, should be admitted for observation or definitive treatment. Patients discharged home from the ED should be given appropriate precautions to monitor for a delayed injury presentation.

Clinical Pearls

1. Maintain a high suspicion for intraabdominal injury when ecchymosis from seat belts is seen in the trauma patient.
2. When lap belt bruises are present, there is a higher incidence of bowel injury.

Associated Clinical Features

Evisceration of abdominal contents (Fig. 7.8) usually occurs after a stab or slash wound to the abdomen. It is an indication for celiotomy (laparotomy). Other indications for celiotomy in penetrating abdominal trauma include peritoneal injury, unexplained shock, evidence of blood in the stomach, bladder, or rectum, and loss of bowel sounds.

Differential Diagnosis

Superficial laceration without peritoneal penetration, laceration with peritoneal penetration but no visceral injury, and laceration with peritoneal penetration and visceral injury may present with a similar mechanism and need to be differentiated. Consideration of the anatomic boundaries of the abdomen (Fig. 7.9) is important in differentiating abdominal injuries from penetrating chest or retroperitoneal injuries.

ED Treatment and Disposition

Initial stabilization (intravenous fluid resuscitation, oxygen, and monitoring), obtaining appropriate laboratory studies including a blood type and crossmatching, and resource mobilization (notifying surgical team, operating room, and anesthesiology) are important steps in the initial management of penetrating abdominal trauma. In most cases, definitive treatment is celiotomy.

Clinical Pearls

1. Indications for celiotomy after stab wounds to the abdomen include evisceration; peritoneal signs; unexplained hypotension; blood in the stomach, bladder, or rectum; and loss of bowel sounds.
2. Selected patients with stab wounds to the abdomen and peritoneal penetration may be conservatively observed for delayed complications.
3. As many as 20% of patients with stab wounds to the abdomen can be discharged from the ED based on a negative wound exploration.

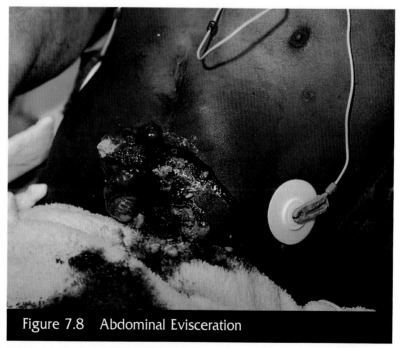

Figure 7.8   Abdominal Evisceration

Self-induced evisceration with bowel perforation and spillage of food particles is clearly seen in this photograph. This patient went directly to the operating room. (Courtesy of Lawrence B. Stack, MD.)

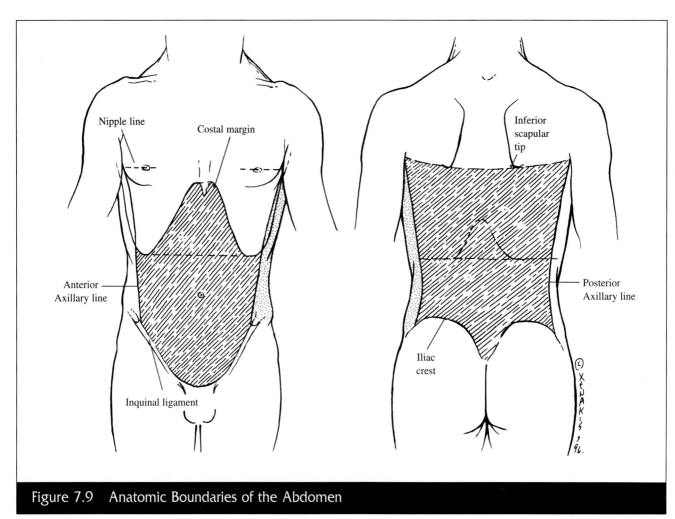

Figure 7.9   Anatomic Boundaries of the Abdomen

Anterior abdomen: Anterior costal margins superiorly, laterally by the anterior axillary lines and inferiorly by the inguinal ligaments.

Low chest: Nipple line (fourth intercostal space) anteriorly, and inferior scapular tip (seventh intercostal space) to inferior costal margins.

Flank: (Shaded blue) Anterior axillary line anteriorly, posteriorly by the posterior axillary line, inferiorly by the iliac crest, and superiorly by the inferior scapular tip. The back is bounded laterally by the posterior axillary lines.

Back: Inferior scapular tip to iliac crest and posterior axillary lines.

Ultrasonographic examination of the trauma patient offers several advantages over current imaging techniques. The examination is inexpensive, noninvasive, easy to interpret, and can be completed within minutes of the patient's ED arrival. It compares favorably with both diagnostic peritoneal lavage and computed tomography in its ability to detect hemoperitoneum. Sonographic examinations, however, do not reliably identify specific organ injury. CT is better in this regard. Although algorithms to determine the most appropriate role for ultrasound in trauma resuscitation are currently being tested, it does appear that the rapid initial sonographic examination is a useful screen for chest and abdominal injury.

A standard trauma examination consists of four views (Fig. 7.10): subxiphoid, right upper quadrant, left upper quadrant, and pelvis. Typically, each view can be completed within 1 min and be performed concurrently with resuscitative procedures.

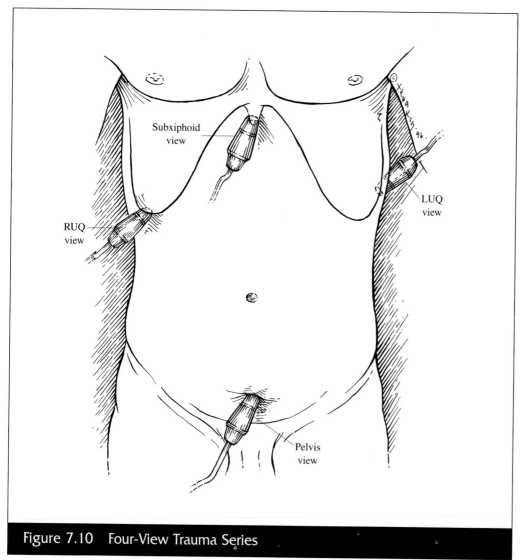

Figure 7.10 Four-View Trauma Series

Ultrasound transducer positions for rapidly detecting pericardial fluid or hemoperitoneum.

Subxiphoid View

The subxiphoid view allows examination of the heart for the presence of cardiac activity and pericardial fluid. Differentiating among the various causes of hypotension in the patient with trauma to the chest is often difficult. Pericardial fluid, when present, is immediately apparent (Fig. 7.11) as the hypoechoic stripe follows the contour of the heart. One of the most significant contributions of the bedside ultrasound is the identification of pericardial fluid.

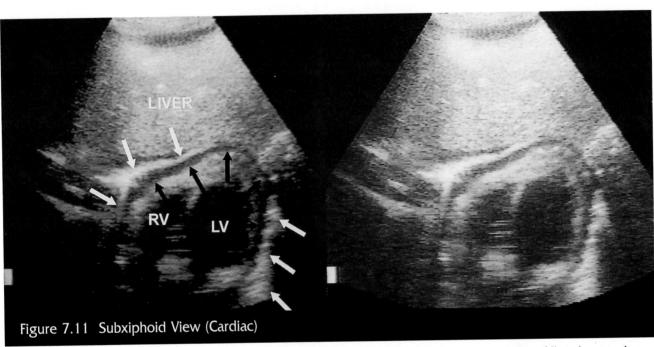

Figure 7.11 Subxiphoid View (Cardiac)

When imaging the heart in the subxiphoid view, the ultrasound beam frequently passes through a small portion of liver that extends over the midline. When correlating the image with anatomic structures, the patient's right is on the left of the image, the patient's left is on the right of the image, the patient's anterior is to the top of the image, and the patient's posterior is to the bottom of the image. The pericardium has a bright, hyperechoic signal (*white arrows*). A pericardial effusion is seen as a hypoechoic (dark) stripe (*black arrows*) between the myocardium and the pericardium. Liver, right ventricle (RV), left ventricle (LV), and a small portion of the interventricular septum are also seen. (Courtesy of Stephen Corbett, MD.)

Right Upper Quadrant View

Examination of the right upper quadrant is performed by placing the transducer in the intercostal space between the anterior axillary and midaxillary lines and consists of an oblique view of the diaphragm, liver, and Morison's pouch and a coronal view of the kidney and pericolic gutter. Morison's pouch is the potential space between the liver and the right kidney. Fluid is easily identified as a dark (hypoechoic) stripe between these two structures (Fig. 7.12). Fluid may also be seen above the diaphragm in the case of hemothorax, below the diaphragm, around the liver, or in the pericolic gutter in the case of hemoperitoneum.

Left Upper Quadrant View

Examination of the left upper quadrant is performed by placing the transducer in the intercostal space between the midaxillary and posterior axillary lines and consists of an oblique view of the diaphragm, spleen, and kidney with a coronal view of the kidney and pericolic gutter. The splenorenal recess, analogous to Morison's pouch on the right, is a potential space created by the peritoneal reflection between the kidney and spleen (Fig. 7.13). The splenorenal recess, however, is not as large as Morison's pouch owing to a relatively small spleen and more superior location of the left kidney. Fluid seen in the splenorenal recess and Morison's pouch can be augmented by placing the patient in the Trendelenburg position.

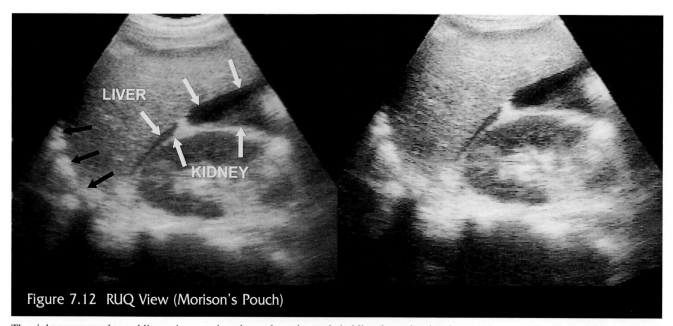

Figure 7.12 RUQ View (Morison's Pouch)

The right upper quadrant oblique view requires the probe to be angled obliquely so the signal passes between ribs. The axilla is to the left, the feet to the right, lateral to the top, and medial to the bottom of the image. Hypoechoic blood between the liver and kidney is seen in Morison's pouch (*white arrows*). The hyperechoic signal of the diaphragm is also seen (*black arrows*). (Courtesy of Stephen Corbett, MD.)

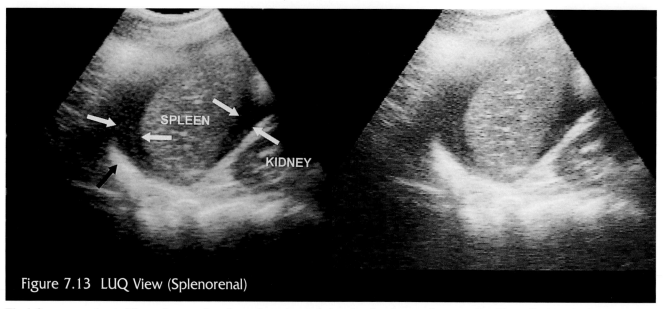

Figure 7.13 LUQ View (Splenorenal)

The left upper quadrant oblique view requires the probe to be angled so the signal passes between ribs. The axilla is to the left, the feet to the right, lateral to the top, and medial to the bottom of the image. Fluid seems to completely surround the spleen (*white arrows*). There is blood present between the diaphragm (*black arrow*) and spleen. There is also blood in the splenorenal recess, the potential space between the spleen and the left kidney. (Courtesy of Stephen Corbett, MD.)

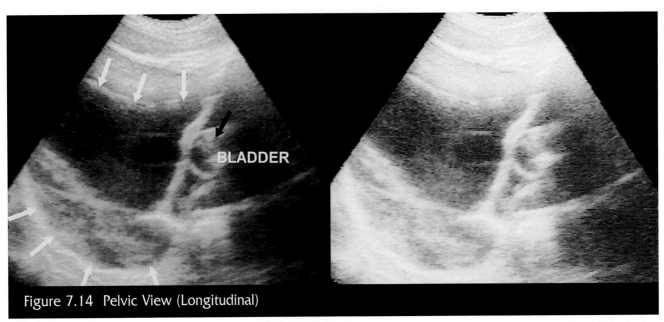

Figure 7.14 Pelvic View (Longitudinal)

The longitudinal view of the pelvis is obtained by placing the probe in the midline just cephalad to the symphysis pubis with the marker dot directed to the patient's left. The patient's head is to the left, feet to the right, anterior to the top, and posterior to the bottom on the photograph. The partially collapsed bladder with the catheter balloon inside (*black arrow*) is seen to the right. Blood, visualized as hypoechoic fluid, is seen over the dome of the bladder anteriorly and in Douglas' pouch posteriorly (*white arrows*). (Courtesy of Stephen Corbett, MD.)

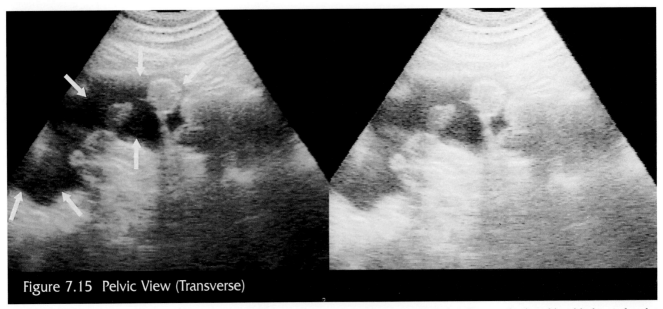

Figure 7.15 Pelvic View (Transverse)

The transverse view of the pelvis is obtained by placing the probe in the midline just cephalad to the symphysis pubis with the marker dot directed cephalad. Fluid outlines loops of bowel with their mesenteric attachments (*arrows*) just superior to the dome of the bladder (not seen). (Courtesy of Stephen Corbett, MD.)

Pelvic View

Pelvic views are obtained by placing the probe in the midline just cephalad to the symphysis pubis with the probe oriented in the longitudinal and transverse planes. The pelvis is the most dependent area of the body in the supine position and is the most sensitive location for detection of early intraperitoneal hemorrhage. The potential space in the rectouterine area (Douglas' pouch) is a common site for such fluid (Fig. 7.14). Under normal circumstances, bowel is not well visualized on ultrasound because the combination of intraluminal fluid and gas creates a mixed signal without distinctive features. When there is fluid in the peritoneum, the bowel is outlined and more easily seen (Fig. 7.15).

Clinical Pearls

1. The smallest detectable hypoechoic stripe in Morison's pouch represents approximately 500 cc of free peritoneal fluid.
2. Subcutaneous air that often accompanies pneumo- and hemothorax may prevent adequate visualization of deeper structures.
3. The ultrasound cannot reliably distinguish blood from other fluids such as urine, ascites, or lavage fluid.
4. Bedside ED ultrasonography of the heart is advocated by some authors in all patients with hypotension of unknown cause to identify potentially reversible etiologies such as cardiac tamponade.

Chest and Abdominal Conditions

RESPIRATORY RETRACTIONS

Associated Clinical Features

Increased respiratory effort may be manifest by increased respiratory rate, increased chest wall excursion, and retractions of the less rigid structures of the thorax. Retractions of the sternum (Fig. 7.16), suprasternal notch (Fig. 7.17), and intercostal retractions reflect increased respiratory effort. This may be due to obstructive disease such as asthma, or tracheal obstruction, pneumonia, or restrictive disease. The presence of stridor, wheezing, or rhonchi will help distinguish the cause.

Differential Diagnosis

Asthma, chronic obstructive pulmonary disease, emphysema, epiglottitis, croup, foreign body aspiration, esophageal foreign body, bacterial tracheitis, posterior pharyngeal abscess, and anaphylaxis are all conditions that must be considered in a patient with retractions.

ED Treatment and Disposition

An aggressive search for the cause of the retractions is required to direct therapy. Rapid evaluation of the airway for patency, and breathing for oxygenation should be done immediately on presentation. High-flow oxygen by face mask is appropriate for patients in respiratory distress. Preparations for securing an airway should be underway for those patients in severe distress or respiratory failure. Routine measures for the mildly symptomatic patient depend on the cause of the retractions. For asthma or chronic obstructive pulmonary disease (COPD) exacerbations, nebulized β_2 agonists and steroid therapy may be appropriate. Patients with croup may require nebulized normal saline and possibly epinephrine or dexamethasone as initial therapy. Foreign body aspiration requires consultation for confirmation of the suspected diagnosis and removal.

Clinical Pearls

1. Retractions are best observed with the patient at rest and their chest exposed.
2. Retractions from obstructive airway disease can be intercostal and supraclavicular, and are usually accompanied by nasal flaring, increased expiratory phase, and increased respiratory rate.

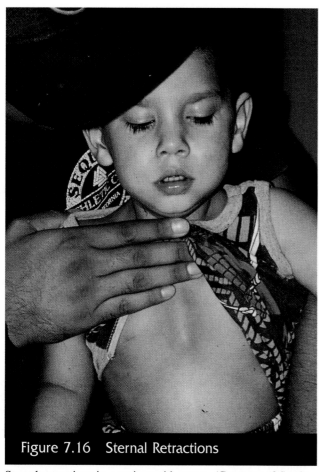

Figure 7.16 Sternal Retractions

Sternal retractions in a patient with croup. (Courtesy of Stephen Corbett, MD.)

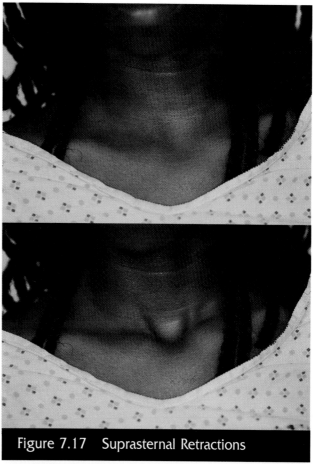

Figure 7.17 Suprasternal Retractions

Suprasternal retractions in an adolescent with severe asthma. (Courtesy of Kevin J. Knoop, MD, MS.)

Associated Clinical Features

This symptom complex develops from venous drainage obstruction of the upper body resulting in increased venous pressure, which leads to collateral circulation dilation. Superior vena cava syndrome (SVCS) is most commonly caused by malignant mediastinal tumors. Dyspnea; swelling of the face, upper extremities, and trunk; chest pain, cough, or headache may be present. Physical findings include dilation of collateral veins of the trunk and upper extremities, facial edema and erythema (plethora), cyanosis, and tachypnea (Fig. 7.18).

Differential Diagnosis

Malignancy, pericarditis, pericardial tamponade, tuberculosis, and congestive heart failure should be considered.

ED Treatment and Disposition

Radiation therapy is the treatment of choice for most malignant mediastinal tumors causing SVCS. Administration of corticosteroids and diuretics initiated in the ED may provide temporary relief pending definitive therapy.

Clinical Pearls

1. SVCS is most commonly caused by malignant mediastinal tumors.
2. Treatment of most mediastinal tumors causing SVCS is radiation therapy.
3. CT scan of the chest is the diagnostic modality of choice for patients with SVCS.

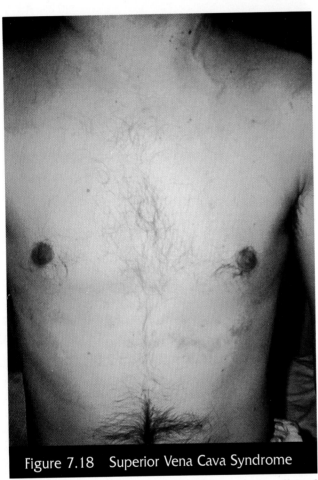

Figure 7.18 Superior Vena Cava Syndrome

A 27-year-old man with SVCS. Note the prominent collateral veins of the chest and neck. (Courtesy of William K. Mallon, MD)

Associated Clinical Features

Pancoast's tumor involves the apical lung and may affect contiguous structures such as the brachial plexus, sympathetic ganglion, vertebrae, ribs, superior vena cava, and recurrent laryngeal nerve (more common for left-sided tumors). Horner's syndrome, extremity edema, nerve deficits, hoarseness, and superior vena cava syndrome may result. Erosion of tumor through the chest wall can cause compression of venous outflow with resultant jugulovenous distention (JVD) (Fig. 7.19).

Differential Diagnosis

Virchow's node of abdominal carcinoma, lymphoma, vascular abnormalities, and tuberculosis should be considered.

ED Treatment and Disposition

Treatment depends on the staging and type of tumor. The superior vena cava syndrome can be treated acutely with radiation and diuretics. Thrombolytic therapy has been used successfully in some cases of acute vena caval thrombosis.

Clinical Pearls

1. Thrombosis may cause acute decompensation with edema, plethora, and airway collapse.
2. Prompt radiation therapy can be lifesaving in cases of vena caval obstruction.

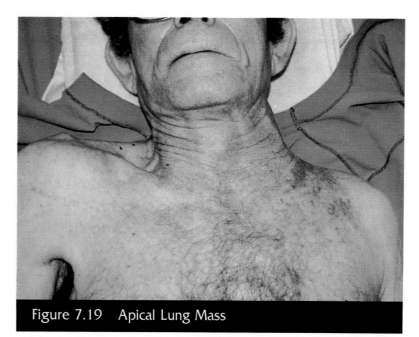

Figure 7.19   Apical Lung Mass

A 68-year-old male cigarette smoker complained of cough and weight loss. A chest radiograph shows a left apical tumor. There is erosion of the tumor into the chest wall with an indurated supraclavicular and infraclavicluar mass. Moderate JVD is apparent, suggesting venous outflow obstruction. (Courtesy of Stephen Corbett, MD.)

Associated Clinical Features

Central venous (right atrial) pressure is reflected by the distention of the internal or external jugular veins. Normal pressure is less than 3 cm of distention above the sternal angle of Louis. Distention greater than 4 cm should be considered abnormal. Evaluation begins by raising the head of the supine patient 30 to 60 deg. The highest point of venous pulsation at the end of normal expiration is measured from the sternal angle of Louis. The presence of jugulovenous distention (JVD) (Fig. 7.20) should prompt an immediate search for possible pulmonary or cardiac pathology. The presence of crackles, murmurs, rubs, percussed hyperresonance, or crepitus may help disclose the etiology.

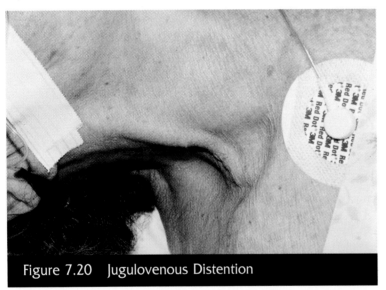

Figure 7.20 Jugulovenous Distention

An engorged external jugular vein is noted as it crosses the sternocleidomastoid muscle into the posterior triangle of the neck and disappears beneath the clavicle to join the brachiocephalic vein and the superior vena cava. This patient has severe congestive heart failure requiring intubation. (Courtesy of Stephen Corbett, MD.)

Differential Diagnosis

Causes of JVD include right ventricular failure, left ventricular failure, biventricular failure, parenchymal lung disease, pulmonary hypertension, pulmonic stenosis, restrictive pericarditis, superior vena cava syndrome, pulmonary embolus, tricuspid valve outflow obstruction, tension pneumothorax, increased circulating blood volume, and atrial myxoma. Temporary venous engorgement may result from Valsalva maneuver, positive pressure ventilation, and Trendelenburg position.

ED Treatment and Disposition

Treatment varies depending on the cause. Preload reduction may help in cases of congestive heart disease. Reversal of a traumatic etiology with needle thoracostomy or pericardiocentesis may be required.

Clinical Pearls

1. Right-sided myocardial infarction may produce JVD with clear lung fields.
2. JVD may be absent in the presence of the above-listed causes if hypovolemia is present.

Associated Clinical Features

Veins of the abdomen normally are scarcely visible within the abdominal wall. Engorged veins, however, are often visible through the normal abdominal wall. Engorged veins forming a knot in the area of the umbilicus are described as caput medusae (Fig. 7.21). The extent of associated findings depends on the underlying etiology. It is usually secondary to liver cirrhosis, with subsequent portal hypertension and development of circulation circumventing the liver.

Differential Diagnosis

Emaciation, inferior vena caval obstruction, superior vena caval obstruction, portal vein obstruction, and superficial abdominal vein thrombosis can cause engorged abdominal veins.

ED Treatment and Disposition

Treatment is directed at the underlying cause. This finding, by itself, doesn't require acute treatment.

Clinical Pearl

1. Caput medusae has the same clinical significance as the more common pattern of venous engorgement.

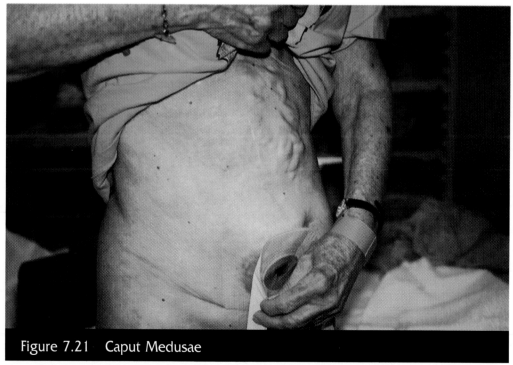

Figure 7.21   Caput Medusae

This elderly female with alcoholic cirrhosis has engorged abdominal veins in the knotted appearance consistent with caput medusae. (Courtesy of Gary Schwartz, MD.)

Associated Clinical Features

A hernia is a tissue protrusion through an abnormal body cavity opening. Most abdominal wall hernias occur at the groin and umbilicus. Incarceration is defined as the inability to reduce the protruding tissue to its normal position. Strangulation occurs when the blood supply of the hernia's contents is obstructed and tissue necrosis ensues. An *incisional* hernia (Fig. 7.22) may be manifest clinically by a mass or palpable defect adjacent to a surgical incision and can be reproduced by having the patient perform Valsalva's maneuver. Obesity and wound infection, which interfere with wound healing, predispose to the formation of incisional hernias. The defect of an *indirect* inguinal hernia (Fig. 7.23) is the internal (abdominal) inguinal ring, and may be manifest in either sex by a bulge over the midpoint of the inguinal ligament that increases in size with Valsalva's maneuver. A fingertip placed into the external ring through the inguinal canal may palpate the defect. A *direct* hernia (Fig. 7.24) may be manifest by a bulge midway adjacent to the pubic tubercle and may be felt by the pad of the finger placed in the inguinal canal. The defect is in the posterior wall of the inguinal canal. Direct inguinal hernias are usually painless and occur in males.

Nausea and vomiting may be present if incarceration with bowel obstruction occurs. Strangulation can lead to fever, peritonitis, and sepsis.

Differential Diagnosis

Tumor, aneurysm, lymphadenopathy, bowel obstruction, ascites, lipoma, femoral hernia, hydrocele, testicular torsion, and epididymitis may have similar presentations.

ED Treatment and Disposition

When patients present without clinical evidence of strangulation (fever, leukocytosis, systemic signs of toxicity), reduction should be attempted. In the presence of these signs, prompt surgical consultation is warranted for surgical reduction. Reduction in the ED is facilitated with systemic analgesia (as most patients present with significant pain), placing the patient in the supine position, and applying a cold pack to the hernia. Routine consultation for operative repair is indicated in asymptomatic patients with reducible hernias.

Clinical Pearls

1. Acutely strangulated or incarcerated hernias require immediate surgical evaluation.
2. Direct inguinal hernias are usually painless.
3. Evaluation and treatment of concomitant exacerbating conditions (cough, constipation, vomiting) prevents recurrences.

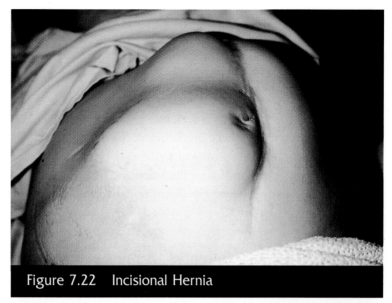

Figure 7.22   Incisional Hernia

An incisional hernia in an obese female. (Courtesy of Stephen Corbett, MD.)

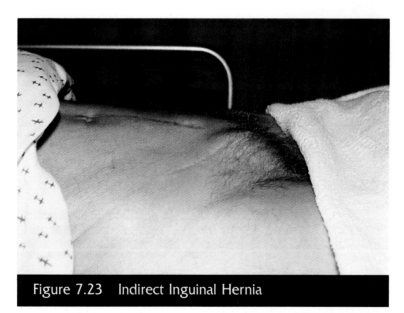

Figure 7.23   Indirect Inguinal Hernia

A recurrent indirect inguinal hernia in a female patient. (Courtesy of Frank Birinyi, MD.)

Associated Clinical Features

The umbilicus is a common site of abdominal hernias. Predisposing conditions in adults most commonly include ascites and prior abdominal surgery. The size of the defect determines the symptomatology and incidence of incarceration, with smaller defects resulting in more pronounced symptoms and an increased incidence of incarceration. Pain is located in the area of the fascial defect. Contents of the hernia may be palpable and tender. Symptoms of obstruction (nausea, vomiting, and abdominal distention) may be present. If the hernia becomes strangulated (Fig. 7.25), erythema of the overlying skin with fever and hypotension may occur.

Differential Diagnosis

An omphalocele, gastroschisis, or urachal duct may present as an umbilical mass.

ED Treatment and Disposition

Reduction is attempted in the stable patient without clinical evidence of strangulation. Treatment of any predisposing conditions (i.e., abdominal paracentesis in the patient with tense ascites) may cause spontaneous reduction and avoid progression of the hernia to strangulation. Routine consultation for elective repair is indicated in asymptomatic patients with reducible hernias.

Clinical Pearls

1. Umbilical hernias in children usually resolve without treatment.
2. Umbilical hernias in adults usually become worse and require elective repair.

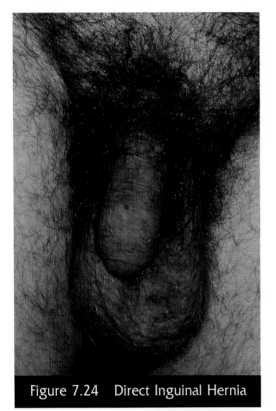

Figure 7.24   Direct Inguinal Hernia

A direct inguinal hernia. Note the bulge adjacent to the left pubic tubercle. (Courtesy of Daniel L. Savitt, MD.)

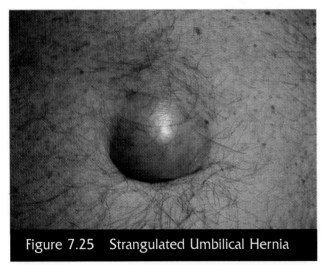

Figure 7.25   Strangulated Umbilical Hernia

The overlying skin of a strangulated umbilical hernia is erythematous and tender. (Courtesy of Lawrence B. Stack, MD.)

Associated Clinical Features

When the vestigial urachal duct is not obliterated during development, drainage can occur from the bladder to the umbilicus (Fig. 7.26). Cysts can often be palpated between the umbilicus and pubis. Besides drainage and pain, infection of the duct or cyst may occur. Rarely, adenocarcinoma may form in these remnants.

Differential Diagnosis

Omphalocele, prune belly syndrome, exstrophy of the bladder, gastroschisis, and umbilical hernias are other abdominal wall abnormalities in children.

ED Treatment and Disposition

Acute treatment is usually not required unless an infection is evident. Routine urologic consultation for surgical revision is indicated. A retrograde study with radiopaque dye will outline the patent duct.

Clinical Pearl

1. This finding should prompt a careful search for other urogenital anomalies.

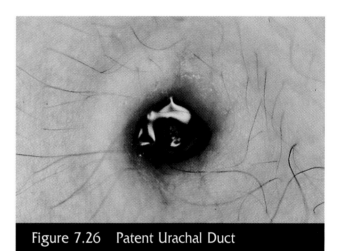

Figure 7.26   Patent Urachal Duct

This 19-year-old male presents to the ED with fluid draining from the umbilicus. Clear fluid (urine) is seen draining from the umbilicus, suggestive of a patent urachal duct. (Courtesy of Kevin J. Knoop, MD, MS.)

SISTER MARY JOSEPH NODE (NODULAR UMBILICUS)

Associated Clinical Features

A Sister Mary Joseph node is a metastasis manifesting as periumbilical lymphadenopathy secondary to abdominal carcinoma (Fig. 7.27). Cancers of the colon may cause pain, change in bowel habits, anemia, and obstruction. In general, left-sided cancers cause obstruction, whereas right-sided tumors may have significant metastases before they create signs and symptoms. These metastases typically involve peritoneal and omental spread with distant metastases to the liver. Spread to the umbilicus is colloquially known as the Sister Mary Joseph node.

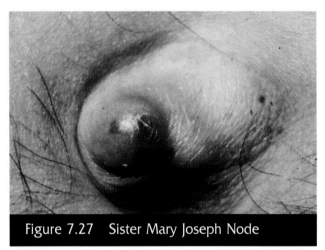

Figure 7.27   Sister Mary Joseph Node

Sister Mary Joseph nodule of patient with gastric carcinoma. (Courtesy of Department of Dermatology, Naval Medical Center, Portsmouth, VA.)

Differential Diagnosis

Other umbilical masses to consider are hernias, ascites, and urachal cysts.

ED Treatment and Disposition

Prompt referral for staging and treatment of the tumor is indicated. Other signs and symptoms (from obstruction, blood loss, malnutrition, and pain) should be addressed and treated.

Clinical Pearl

1. Virchow's node, presenting as a supraclavicular mass, also heralds bowel carcinoma.
2. A Sister Mary Joseph node is commonly due to gastric carcinoma.

Associated Clinical Features

Abdominal distention may be a symptom, often described by the patient as the feeling of being bloated, or a sign, an obvious protuberance of the patient's abdomen that may or may not be out of proportion to the rest of the body. Other findings vary widely, depending on the cause. In obesity, the abdomen is uniformly rounded while an increase in girth and fat concurrently accumulates in other parts of the body. In patients with ascites, there may be shifting dullness, a fluid wave, bulging flanks, or hepatomegaly. In patients with neoplasms, there may be a palpable mass. In gravid patients, fetal heart tones may be present and fetal motion may be felt. In patients with excess gas from bowel obstruction, there may be absent or high-pitched bowel sounds and absence of bowel movements or flatus.

Differential Diagnosis

Numerous conditions present with abdominal distention. Obesity, ascites, pregnancy, neoplasms, aneurysm, tympanites (excess gas), organomegaly, and feces are important etiologies to consider in the differential.

The profile of the fluid-filled abdomen of ascites (Fig. 7.28) is a single curve from xiphoid process to pubic symphysis. The umbilicus may be everted, and there may be prominent superficial abdominal veins. Other physical findings suggestive of ascites include shifting dullness and a fluid wave.

The pregnant abdomen profile (Fig. 7.29) shows the outward curve is more prominent in the lower half of the abdomen. The umbilicus may be everted in the last trimester of pregnancy. Prominent abdominal wall veins may also be seen. The presence of fetal heart tones confirms the diagnosis.

The abdominal profile of a patient with a leaking abdominal aortic aneurysm (Fig. 7.30) shows a mottled abdominal wall reflective of hypoperfusion of this structure. There may be a curve of the midabdomen to either side of the aorta, more often on the left. Palpation of a pulsatile mass supports the diagnosis. Ultrasound or CT scan of the abdomen will confirm the diagnosis.

Excess abdominal air (Fig. 7.31) can be located in the lumen of the stomach or intestines, or free in the peritoneum. This abdomen profile is a single curve from the xiphoid process to the pubic symphysis. Nausea, vomiting, decreased bowel sounds, and colicky pain are present in a small bowel obstruction. Large bowel obstruction may be accompanied by feculent vomiting and absent flatus production.

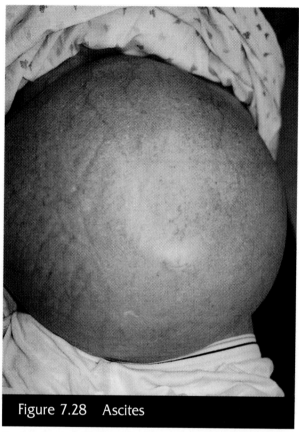

Figure 7.28   Ascites

Ascites in an alcoholic male. Note the everted umbilicus and prominent superficial abdominal veins. (Courtesy of Alan B. Storrow, MD.)

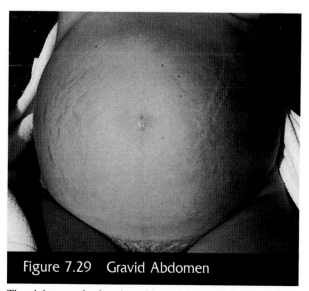

Figure 7.29   Gravid Abdomen

The abdomen of a female at 39 weeks gestation. Note the abdominal wall striae, everted umbilicus, and prominent superficial abdominal wall veins. (Courtesy of Stephen Corbett, MD.)

ED Treatment and Disposition

Treatment varies widely depending on the cause; thus emergent management is directed at determining the etiology. Life-threatening causes (aneurysm, obstruction, neoplasms) require stabilization and referral for definitive treatment.

Clinical Pearl

1. The six "f's" can categorize conditions causing abdominal distention: fat, flatus, fetus, fluid, feces, fatal growth.

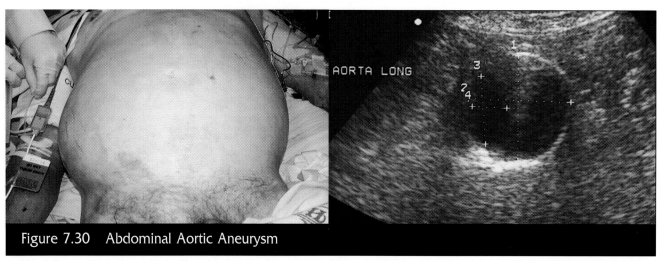

Figure 7.30   Abdominal Aortic Aneurysm

A. The abdomen of a patient with leaking abdominal aortic aneurysm. Note the mottled abdominal wall and the prominent curvature of the right side of the abdomen. (Courtesy of Stephen Corbett, MD.) *B.* Abdominal aortic aneurysm seen on ultrasound in another patient. (Courtesy of Sally Santen, MD.)

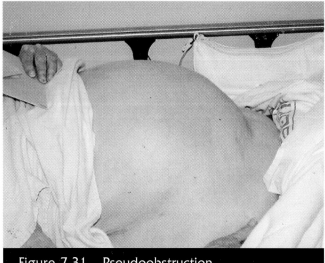

Figure 7.31   Pseudoobstruction

An 85-year-old female was brought from a nursing home with a complaint of abdominal distention and pain for 1 to 2 days. An eventual diagnosis of Ogilvie's syndrome, or pseudoobstruction of the large bowel, was made. This is usually seen in debilitated patients and can be treated with decompression. (Courtesy of Stephen Corbett, MD.)

Associated Clinical Features

Intertrigo is a dermatitis occurring on apposed surfaces of skin such as the creases of the neck, folds of the groin and armpit, or a panniculus (Fig. 7.32). It is characterized by a tender, red plaque with a moist macerated surface. A candidal infection may result and often becomes secondarily infected with skin flora. Erythema, fissures, burning, itching, exudates, and fever may also accompany intertrigo.

Differential Diagnosis

Necrotizing fasciitis of the abdominal wall, cellulitis, and *Candida albicans* infection should be considered.

ED Treatment and Disposition

Local care and good personal hygiene are recommended. Intravenous antibiotics initiated in the ED directed against skin flora are recommended if secondarily infected.

Clinical Pearl

1. Consider necrotizing fasciitis of the abdominal wall if the patient appears septic.

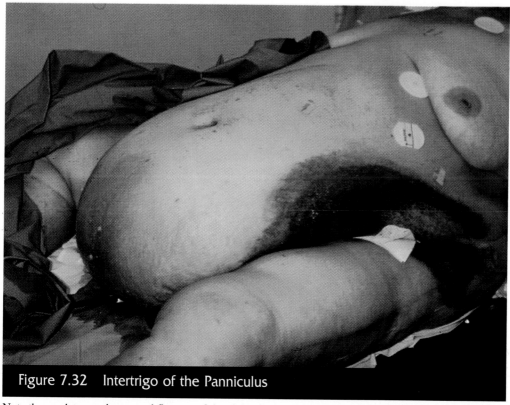

Figure 7.32   Intertrigo of the Panniculus

Note the exudate, erythema, and fissures of the abdominal wall. This patient also had fever, which suggests secondary infection. (Courtesy of Lawrence B. Stack, MD.)

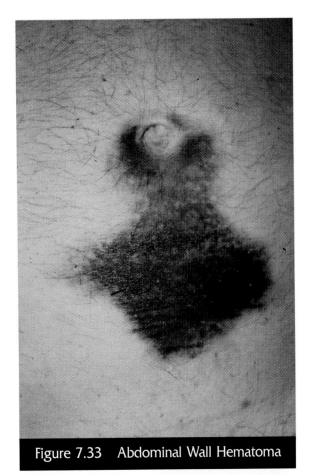

Figure 7.33 Abdominal Wall Hematoma

This 50-year-old male with chronic obstructive pulmonary disease developed right lower quadrant pain after an episode of coughing. A repeat examination on the second visit showed clearly visible ecchymosis. There was no coagulopathy and amylase was normal. A CT scan revealed a 10- by 8-cm hematoma in the right rectus abdominous sheath. (Courtesy of Stephen Corbett, MD.)

Associated Clinical Features

Mild trauma may produce hematomas of the rectus sheath (Fig. 7.33). This injury results in intense abdominal pain which can mimic an acute abdomen. The diagnosis is made by physical examination since the ecchymosis is not always visible. Palpation of the abdominal wall reveals a tender mass that is accentuated by contraction of the rectus. Ultrasound and CT scan may confirm the diagnosis.

Differential Diagnosis

Multiple causes of abdominal pain must be considered in the differential diagnosis. Careful examination with supplemental imaging studies, if needed, helps with the diagnosis. Two classic signs of retroparitoneal bleeding are Grey Turner's sign (flank ecchymosis) and Cullen's sign (periumbilical ecchymosis). Hemorrhagic pancreatitis and ruptured ectopic pregnancy should be considered respectively.

ED Treatment and Disposition

Assuming there is no underlying blood dyscrasia or coagulopathy, rectus sheath hematomas usually resolve in 1 to 2 weeks.

Clinical Pearl

1. Fothergill's sign is enhancement of a rectus sheath hematoma when the abdominal wall is tensed. The mass should not cross the midline and should be easier to palpate with abdominal muscle contractions. Intraabdominal masses are more difficult to palpate with such contractions.

Associated Clinical Features

Abdominal striae are linear, depressed pink or bluish scarlike lesions (Fig. 7.34) that may later become silver or white. They are caused by weakening of the elastic cutaneous tissues from chronic stretching. They most commonly occur on the abdomen, but are also seen on the buttocks, breasts, and thighs. Striae are commonly seen in obesity, pregnancy, Cushing's syndrome, and chronic topical corticosteroid treatment. In Cushing's syndrome, a state of adrenal hypercorticism, the skin becomes fragile and easily breaks from normal stretching.

Differential Diagnosis

Obesity, pregnancy, Cushing's syndrome, and chronic topical corticosteroid treatment should be considered.

ED Treatment and Disposition

This finding seldom presents as a condition requiring acute treatment; thus, attention is directed to determining and treating the underlying cause.

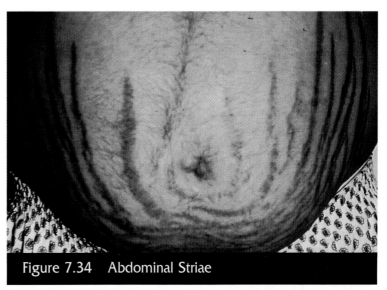

Figure 7.34   Abdominal Striae

These striae are from a patient with recent weight gain, moon facies, and altered mental status. The patient was diagnosed with Cushing's syndrome. (Courtesy of Geisinger Medical Center, Dept. of Emergency Medicine, Danvill Pennsylvania.)

Clinical Pearls

1. Recent striae (pink or blue) with moon facies, hypertension, renal calculi, osteoporosis, and psychiatric disorders are suggestive of Cushing's syndrome.
2. The striae caused by pregnancy typically fade with time, unlike those associate with Cushings syndrome.

CHAPTER 8

UROLOGIC CONDITIONS

Jeffrey D. Bondesson

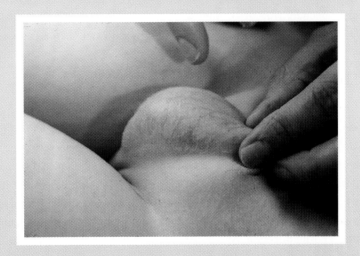

Associated Clinical Features

These patients are most often young men (average age 16 to 17.5 years) who present complaining of the sudden onset of pain in one testicle. The pain is then followed by swelling of the affected testicle, reddening of the overlying scrotal skin, lower abdominal pain, nausea, and vomiting. An examination reveals a swollen, tender, retracted testicle (Fig. 8.1) that often lies in the horizontal plane (bell clapper deformity) (Fig. 8.2). The spermatic cord is frequently swollen on the affected side. Delayed presentations may present with the entire hemiscrotum swollen, tender, and firm (Fig. 8.3). The urine is usually clear with a normal urinalysis. In one-third of cases there is a peripheral leukocytosis.

Differential Diagnosis

Alternative diagnoses that should be considered include acute epididymitis, torsion of the testicular appendix (Fig. 8.4), trauma, acute orchitis (mumps), hydrocele, spermatocele, varicocele, hernia, and tumor. A good history and physical examination helps narrow the diagnosis.

ED Treatment and Disposition

Urologic consultation should be obtained immediately and preparation made to go to the operating room without delay. Doppler ultrasound or technetium scanning may be helpful if they will not delay surgery. In the interim, detorsion may be attempted if the patient is seen within a few hours of onset: the affected testicle should initially be opened like a book, that is, the right testicle turned counterclockwise when viewed from below, and the left testicle turned clockwise when viewed from below. Pain relief should be immediate. Decreased pain should prompt additional turns (as many as three) to complete detorsion; increased pain should prompt detorsion in the opposite direction. Ancillary studies should not delay operative intervention, since testicular infarction will occur within 6 to 12 h after torsion.

Clinical Pearls

1. The cremasteric reflex is almost always absent in testicular torsion.
2. Patients may report similar, less severe episodes that spontaneously resolved in the recent past.
3. Half of all torsions occur during sleep.
4. Abdominal or inguinal pain is sometimes present without pain to the scrotum.
5. The age of presentation has a bimodal pattern, since torsion is also more prevalent during infancy.

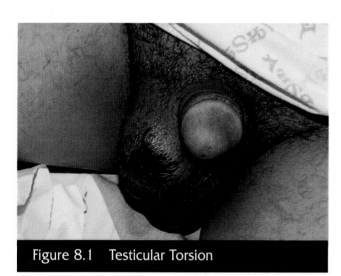

Figure 8.1   Testicular Torsion

Swollen, tender hemiscrotum, with erythema of scrotal skin and retracted testicle. (Courtesy of Stephen Corbett, MD.)

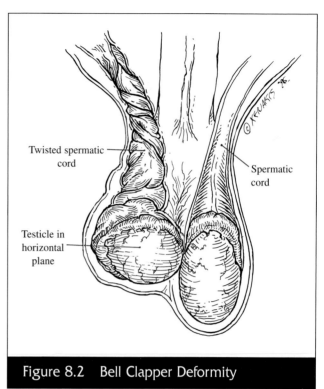

Figure 8.2   Bell Clapper Deformity

A bell clapper deformity in testicular tortion results from the twisting of the spermatic cord and causes the testis to be elevated with a horizontal lie. The lack of fixation of the tunica vaginalis to the posterior scrotum predisposes the freely movable testis to rotation and subsequent torsion. An elevated testis with a horizontal lie may be seen in asymptomatic patients at risk for torsion.

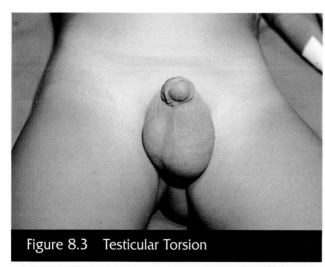

Figure 8.3   Testicular Torsion

Swollen, tender scrotal mass. (Courtesy of Patrick McKenna, MD.)

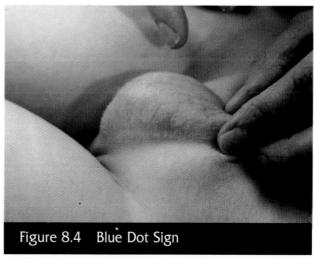

Figure 8.4   Blue Dot Sign

A blue dot sign is caused by torsion of the testicular appendix. It is best seen with the skin held taut over the testicular appendix. (Courtesy of Javier A. Gonzalez del Rey, MD.)

Associated Clinical Features

Acute epididymitis causes pain in the scrotum on the affected side, with referred pain to the groin, inguinal canal, or lower abdominal quadrant. The onset of pain is gradual, occurring over hours. When the patient presents early in the course, a tender, indurated, edematous epididymis can be palpated separately from the nontender testis. Late presentations will have generalized scrotal swelling and pain, making examination and differentiation more difficult (Fig. 8.5). The urinalysis will reveal pyuria or bacteriuria half of the time, and the peripheral white blood cell count is frequently elevated. Patients can present with fever and signs of sepsis.

Differential Diagnosis

Torsion of the testis, torsion of the testicular appendix, orchitis, trauma, tumor, or hernia may present in a similar fashion. Nuclear isotope scanning or ultrasound may be helpful by demonstrating increased testicular and epididymal blood flow.

ED Treatment and Disposition

Treatment is usually outpatient (NSAID's, scrotal support), and based on the most likely causative organism. Younger men (under 35 years) tend to have the sexually transmitted organisms of *Chlamydia trachomatis* and *Neisseria gonorrhoeae* as the most frequent offenders, whereas older men tend to have infections caused by bacteria commonly associated with urinary tract infections, that is, *Escherichia coli, Enterococcus* species and *Pseudomonas aeruginosa.* Adolescents and children should be referred for urologic evaluation to rule out congenital anomalies, which are common in nongonococcal infections in this age group. A history of recent urinary tract instrumentation or urinary tract infection should be sought. Febrile patients should be considered for admission and IV antibiotics.

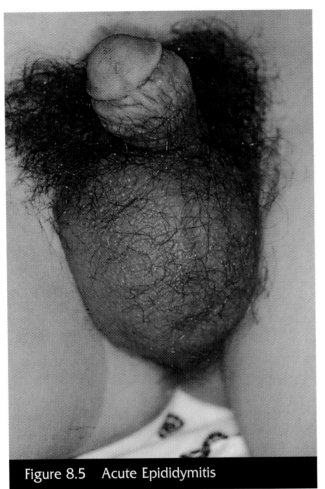

Figure 8.5   Acute Epididymitis

Swelling of the right hemiscrotum shown here is nonspecific. Tenderness was localized to the epididymis in this patient. (Courtesy of Adam R. Saperston, MD, MS.)

Clinical Pearls

1. Elevation of the affected hemiscrotum may provide relief of symptoms (Prehn's sign).
2. Older men should be evaluated for urinary retention, as this is a frequent cause of epididymitis.
3. Testicular tumors are most frequently misdiagnosed as epididymitis.
4. The absence of pyuria or bacteriuria does not exclude the diagnosis.

Associated Clinical Features

Most hydroceles occur in older patients and develop gradually without any significant symptoms. They are generally a soft, pear-shaped, fluid-filled cystic mass anterior to the testicle and epididymis that will transilluminate (Fig. 8.6). However, they can be tense and firm and transilluminate poorly if the tunica vaginalis is thickened. Almost all hydroceles in children are communicating, resulting from the same mechanism that causes inguinal hernia. A persistent narrow processus vaginalis acts like a one-way valve, thus permitting the accumulation of dependent peritoneal fluid in the scrotum. Acute symptomatic hydroceles are more rare, and can occur in association with epididymitis, trauma, or tumor.

Differential Diagnosis

Painless masses that must be differentiated from hydrocele include spermatocele, varicocele, inguinal hernia, and tumor. Painful masses to be differentiated include traumatic hematocele, epididymitis, orchitis, and torsion.

ED Treatment and Disposition

In an acute hydrocele, treatment must be directed at discovering a possible underlying cause. A positive urinalysis may point toward an infectious etiology. Transillumination helps demonstrate whether the mass is cystic or solid. Ultrasound can be very helpful in imaging the scrotal contents and delineating mass composition. Acute hydroceles should not be considered benign and require referral to a urologist to rule out tumor or infection. Chronic accumulations are referred to a urologist on a more routine basis for elective drainage.

Clinical Pearls

1. Ten percent of testicular tumors have a reactive hydrocele as the presenting complaint.
2. An inguinal hernia with a loop of bowel in it will transilluminate.
3. Hydroceles are almost never symptomatic.
4. Acute reactive hydroceles may be caused by infection, trauma, or torsion.

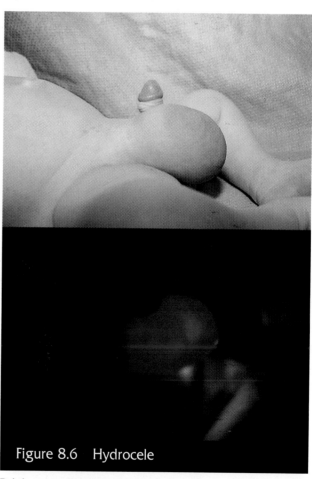

Figure 8.6   Hydrocele

Painless swelling in the scrotum of a young boy (top). Transillumination of the swelling (bottom) identifies the hydrocele. (Courtesy of Michael J. Nowicki, MD.)

Associated Clinical Features

In testicular tumor, a painless, firm testicular mass (Fig. 8.7) is palpated, with the patient often complaining of a "heaviness" of his testicle. If the patient presents early, the mass will be distinct from the testis, whereas later presentations will have generalized testicular or scrotal swelling. It occasionally presents with pain due to infarction of the tumor.

Differential Diagnosis

Epididymitis is the most frequent misdiagnosis, which unfortunately may delay surgical intervention. When the tumor presents with infarction pain, differentiation from epididymitis or torsion can be difficult. In some cases, ultrasound can help differentiate these entities.

ED Treatment and Disposition

Patients should be promptly referred to a urologist for surgical exploration.

Clinical Pearls

1. Acute hydroceles and hematoceles should prompt the physician to consider a tumor as the cause.
2. Pain from tumor infarction is usually not as severe as pain due to torsion or epididymitis.
3. Findings of an unexplained supraclavicular lymph node, abdominal mass, or chronic nonproductive cough resistant to conventional therapy should prompt a testicular examination for tumor.

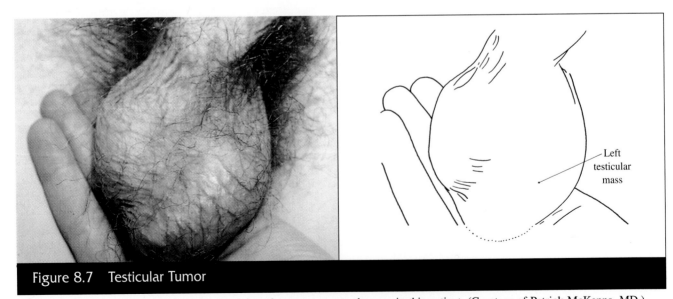

Figure 8.7   Testicular Tumor

This painless left testicular mass is highly suspicious for tumor, as was the case in this patient. (Courtesy of Patrick McKenna, MD.)

Associated Clinical Features

A scrotal abscess is a suppurative mass with surrounding erythema involving the superficial layers of the scrotal wall (Fig. 8.8). The usual history is of progressive swelling of a small pustule or papule followed by increasing pain and induration or fluctuance. Constitutional symptoms and fever are generally absent.

Differential Diagnosis

An apparent superficial scrotal abscess must be distinguished from a deep scrotal abscess or early Fournier's gangrene. In the latter two, patients tend to appear quite ill. The erythema of the skin overlying an abscess should not be mistaken for an urticarial reaction, erythema multiforme, or drug eruption.

ED Treatment and Disposition

Using local anesthesia, simply make a stab incision and drain the abscess. The patient is then instructed to use a sitz bath and to frequently change the dressing. An alternative method of treatment is to unroof the abscess by circumferential excision. This ensures that there is adequate wound drainage. Immunocompromised patients may require intravenous antibiotics and admission.

Clinical Pearl

1. If the patient appears ill out of proportion to the superficial appearance, suspect that this mass is the point of a deep scrotal abscess.

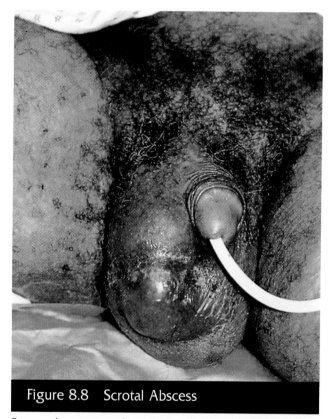

Figure 8.8 Scrotal Abscess

Suppurative mass on the scrotum. (Courtesy of David Effron, MD.)

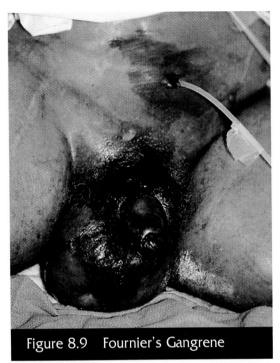

Figure 8.9   Fournier's Gangrene

Markedly swollen, necrotic, tender scrotum, perineum, and adjacent thighs are seen. (Courtesy of David Effron, MD.)

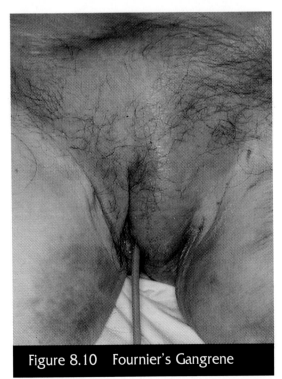

Figure 8.10   Fournier's Gangrene

Swollen, tender, erythematous labia, perineum, and inner thighs in a female patient with Fournier's gangrene. (Courtesy of Daniel L. Savitt, MD.)

Associated Clinical Features

Fournier's gangrene most frequently occurs in a middle-aged diabetic male who presents with swelling, erythema, and severe pain of the entire scrotum (Fig. 8.9), but it is also known to occur in females (Fig. 8.10). In males, the scrotal contents often cannot be palpated because of the marked inflammation. The patient has constitutional symptoms with fever and frequently is in shock. There is often a history of recent urethral instrumentation, an indwelling Foley catheter, or perirectal disease. A localized area of fluctuance cannot be appreciated.

Differential Diagnosis

The differential diagnosis includes cellulitis, superficial scrotal abscess, edema due to heart failure or lymphatic obstruction, allergic reaction, and epididymoorchitis with skin fixation.

ED Treatment and Disposition

These patients require aggressive fluid resuscitation and early surgical consultation for immediate debridement and surgical drainage. Broad spectrum antibiotics effective against gram-positive, gram-negative, and anaerobic organisms should be given as soon as possible in the ED. There is anecdotal experience that treatment is enhanced by hyperbaric oxygen.

Clinical Pearls

1. Pain out of proportion to the clinical findings may represent an early presentation of Fournier's gangrene.
2. A plain pelvic radiograph may reveal subcutaneous air.
3. Fournier's gangrene is usually quite painful, but has been known to present with only a mildly uncomfortable necrosis of the scrotal wall and exposed testis.

Associated Clinical Features

Paraphimosis is the entrapment of a retracted foreskin behind the coronal sulcus that cannot be reduced (Fig. 8.11). Pain, swelling, and erythema are common. If severe, the constriction causes edema and venous engorgement of the glans (Fig. 8.12) that can lead to arterial compromise with subsequent tissue necrosis.

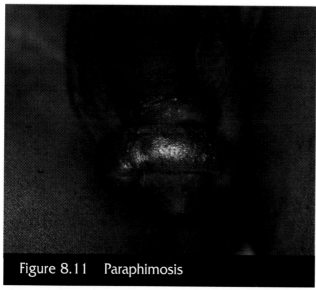

Figure 8.11   Paraphimosis

Moderate edema of the retracted foreskin, which is entrapped behind the coronal sulcus. (Courtesy of Anthony J. Musielewicz, MD.)

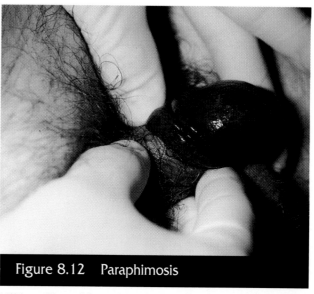

Figure 8.12   Paraphimosis

Mild swelling with erythema of the entrapped foreskin and engorgement of the glans. (Courtesy of Alan B. Storrow, MD.)

Differential Diagnosis

In contrast to paraphimosis, phimosis is the inability to retract the foreskin (Fig. 8.13), usually a chronic condition. Other diagnoses to consider include superficial balanitis, hair tourniquet, contact dermatitis, and urticaria.

ED Treatment and Disposition

Squeezing the glans firmly for 5 min to reduce the swelling can lead to successful reduction of the foreskin. Local infiltration of anesthesia with vertical incision of the constricting band should be performed by a urologist if manual reduction fails.

Clinical Pearls

1. In the presence of arterial compromise, the emergency physician should incise the constricting band if a urologist is not immediately available.
2. The patient should be referred to a urologist for circumcision if successfully reduced.
3. Phimosis is "physiologic" in young males (generally less than 5 to 6 years old).
4. Phimosis, if "reduced" (retracted proximally over the glans), can cause a paraphimosis—a true emergency.

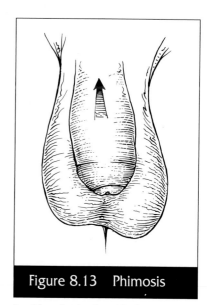

Figure 8.13   Phimosis

In phimosis, the foreskin is not able to be retracted, often due to meatal stenosis and scarring.

Associated Clinical Features

Urethral injury is rarely an isolated event and is associated with the multiple trauma patient. Anterior urethral injuries are most often the result of a straddle injury and may present late (many patients are still able to void) with a local infection or sepsis from extravasated urine. Posterior urethral injuries occur in motor vehicle and motorcycle accidents and are usually the result of pelvic fractures. Patients have blood at the urethral meatus (Fig. 8.14), cannot void, and have perineal bruising. In males, the prostate is often boggy or free floating, or may not be palpable at all if a retroperitoneal hematoma is between the prostate and the rectum.

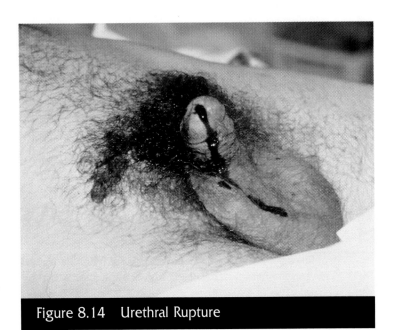

Figure 8.14   Urethral Rupture

Blood at the urethral meatus in a patient with urethral rupture secondary to trauma. (Courtesy of David Effron, MD.)

Differential Diagnosis

Bladder rupture, higher urinary tract injuries, urethritis, and penile fracture may all present with blood at the meatus.

ED Treatment and Disposition

Urethral instrumentation such as Foley catheterization should not occur prior to a retrograde urethrogram with highly concentrated water-soluble contrast. If there is only a partial anterior tear, a gentle attempt at catheterization can be made if it is abandoned at the first sign of resistance. If catheterization is unsuccessful and whenever there is a posterior tear, a suprapubic catheter should be placed in the ED with a trocar if relief of bladder distention is required prior to operative repair.

Clinical Pearls

1. Foley catheter insertion is contraindicated in patients with a suspected urethral injury prior to a retrograde urethrogram.
2. Urethral injury should be suspected in the multiple trauma patient who is unable to void or has blood at the meatus, a high riding prostate, or perineal trauma.
3. Females with vaginal lacerations due to trauma should prompt consideration of a urethral tear.
4. Occasionally urine from an anterior urethral tear will extravasate into the scrotum, causing marked swelling.
5. Posterior injuries are highly associated with other intraabdominal injury.

Associated Clinical Features

Patients usually present complaining of trauma during sexual arousal and often relate experiencing a sudden "snapping" sound or sensation, pain, and deformity which is caused by a tearing of the tunica albuginea. The shaft of the penis is swollen and often angulated at the fracture site (Fig. 8.15).

Differential Diagnosis

Penile fracture can be confused with penile trauma without tear of the tunica albuginea, urethral injury, Peyronie's disease (dorsal contracture), priapism, or foreign bodies.

ED Treatment and Disposition

If the patient cannot urinate, a retrograde urethrogram may be required to rule out urethral injury (Fig. 8.16). These patients require admission and referral to a urologist, who frequently takes them immediately to the operating room for repair.

Clinical Pearls

1. Patients sometimes concoct elaborate, non-sexually-related stories surrounding the circumstances of injury, but penile fracture most commonly occurs during sexual arousal.
2. Penile implants are also subject to injury in a similar fashion.

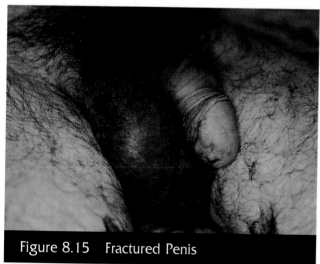

Figure 8.15   Fractured Penis

A swollen, ecchymotic penis is shown. Note the angulation at the midshaft of penis indicating the "fracture" site. Blood at the meatus shown here is further evidence of a urethral injury. (Courtesy of Kevin J. Knoop, MD, MS.)

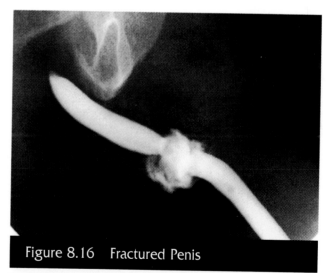

Figure 8.16   Fractured Penis

Retrograde urethrogram showing urethral injury from the fractured penis in Fig. 8.15. (Courtesy of David W. Munter, MD.)

Associated Clinical Features

In straddle injury, the patient has pain, swelling, contusion, and hematoma of the perineum or scrotum following direct blunt trauma (Fig. 8.17 and 8.18). This injury is commonly caused by falls onto bicycle frame cross-tubes, playground equipment, or a toilet seat. Swelling can be severe enough to interfere with urination. Scrotal contents can also be contused or crushed with this injury.

Differential Diagnosis

Fournier's gangrene, cellulitis, and urticaria are similar in appearance, but without the history of trauma. Sexual or physical abuse should be considered.

ED Treatment and Disposition

Treatment is supportive and includes cold packs, elevation, rest, and analgesics. If unable to void, the patient may require catheterization.

Clinical Pearls

1. Laceration of the perineum can be obscured by swelling if a careful examination is not performed.
2. Pelvis radiographs should be obtained in all perineal injuries.
3. Males and females are at high risk for urethral injuries with this type of injury.
4. Straddle injury is differentiated from abuse with a good history from a reliable caregiver that matches the injury.

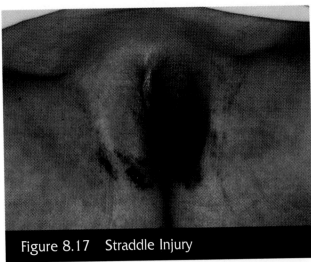

Figure 8.17 Straddle Injury

Ecchymosis, swelling, and contusion of the perineum in a 3-year-old female who tripped and fell on a large plastic toy. (Courtesy of James Mensching, MD.)

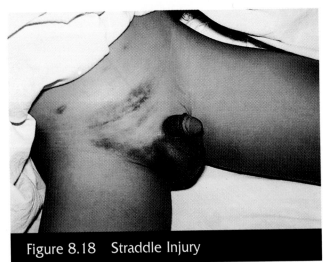

Figure 8.18 Straddle Injury

Contusion of the scrotum and lower abdomen in a young boy consistent with a straddle injury. (Courtesy of David W. Munter, MD.)

Associated Clinical Features

A laceration or avulsion of the scrotum may lead to exposure of the scrotal contents (Fig. 8.19). Other associated injuries may be present, depending on the mechanism of injury (blunt versus penetrating trauma, motor vehicle accident).

Differential Diagnosis

Fournier's gangrene can present with exposed scrotal contents owing to destruction of the scrotal wall.

ED Treatment and Disposition

Every effort should be made to prevent scrotal contents from desiccation by covering them with available scrotal tissue or moist, sterile dressings. A urologist should be consulted immediately for surgical repair.

Clinical Pearls

1. The dramatic presentation of these injuries can divert the examiner's attention and delay the assessment of other, life-threatening injuries.
2. These lacerations can be associated with occult anal sphincter, urethral, intraperitoneal, or retroperitoneal injury.

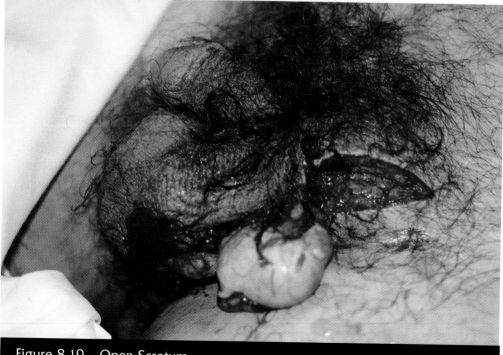

Figure 8.19   Open Scrotum

Laceration of the scrotum with exposed testis. (Courtesy of Kim Feldhaus, MD.)

Associated Clinical Features

Balanoposthitis is an infection and inflammation of the glans penis that also involves the overlying foreskin (prepuce) (Fig. 8.20). *Balanitis* is isolated to the glans, whereas *posthitis* involves only the prepuce. Pain, erythema, and edema of the affected parts of the penis are typically present. Patients may refrain from urination secondary to dysuria, or the edema may induce meatal occlusion, leading to urinary retention or obstruction. Common etiologies include overgrowth of normal bacterial flora secondary to poor hygiene (pediatric), sexually transmitted diseases (adolescents and adults), and candidal infections (elderly or immunocompromised) (Fig. 8.21).

Differential Diagnosis

The diagnosis is usually straightforward; however, the underlying etiology often must also be addressed. Examples are sexually transmitted diseases in healthy adults and diseases associated with immunocompromise (e.g. diabetes mellitus, AIDS, alcoholism). Phimosis occurs when chronic infection due to poor hygiene causes fibrosis and contracture of the preputial opening. Other diagnoses to consider include contact dermatitis, fixed drug eruptions, lichen sclerosus et atrophicus, and squamous cell carcinoma.

ED Treatment and Disposition

Treatment is directed at the suspected etiology. Warm soaks and topical antibiotics (bacitracin) are the mainstay of therapy for infectious etiologies owing to poor hygiene. Parents should be counseled about proper cleansing and handling of the prepuce. Oral or intravenous antibiotics may be indicated if there is an accompanying cellulitis. If urinary obstruction is present, catheterization may be attempted using a small catheter. If catheterization is unsuccessful, urologic consultation for emergent surgical correction of the prepuce is required. Candidal infections are treated with meticulous hygiene and topical antifungal agents. Routine urologic referral is indicated for suspected lichen sclerosus et atrophicus and squamous cell carcinoma.

Clinical Pearls

1. The inability to retract the foreskin completely is normal in young males up to age 4 or 5. Attempting to do so could cause a paraphimosis, a true emergency.
2. Placing the child in a bathtub with warm water will help alleviate difficulty with micturition, assuming no obstruction is present.
3. Candidal balanitis or balanoposthitis may be associated with an undiagnosed immunocompromised state.
4. Suspected sexually transmitted diseases require treatment for the partners as well.

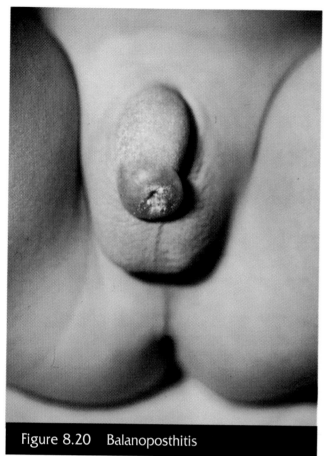

Figure 8.20   Balanoposthitis

Note the erythema, localized edema, and significantly constricted preputial orifice of the distal penis. (Courtesy of Lawrence B. Stack, MD.)

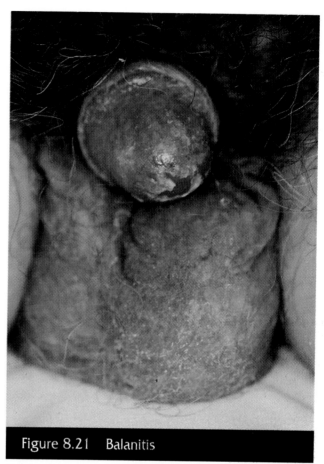

Figure 8.21   Balanitis

Candidal balanitis in an elderly patient with no other complaints. New onset diabetes was diagnosed. (Courtesy of Kevin J. Knoop, MD, MS.)

CHAPTER 9

SEXUALLY TRANSMITTED DISEASE AND ANORECTAL CONDITIONS

Diane M. Birnbaumer
Lynn K. Flowers

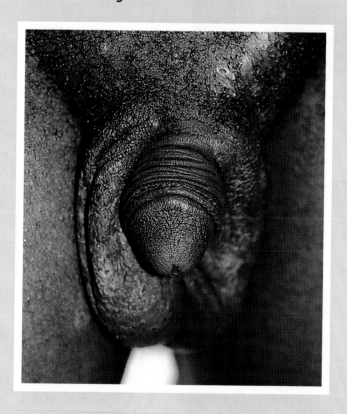

Sexually Transmitted Diseases

PRIMARY SYPHILIS

Associated Clinical Features

Lesions of primary syphilis generally appear after an incubation period of 2 to 6 weeks, but may appear up to 3 months after exposure. The patient usually presents with a solitary, round to oval, painless genital ulcer (Figs. 9.1 and 9.2). However, the ulcer may be slightly painful, and several lesions are sometimes seen. The base of the genital ulcer is dry in males, moist in females; purulent fluid in the base is uncommon. The borders of the ulcer are often indurated. Patients may develop ulcers at any site of inoculation on the body. Bilateral, nontender, nonfluctuant adenopathy is common. Lesions resolve spontaneously in 3 to 12 weeks without treatment as the infection progresses to the secondary stage. Patients with primary syphilis are at risk for concurrent infection with other sexually transmitted diseases.

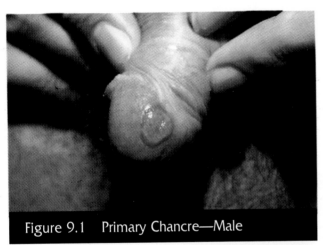

Figure 9.1   Primary Chancre—Male

This dry-based, painless ulcer with indurated borders is typical for a primary chancre in a male patient. (Courtesy of A. Wisdom: *Sexually Transmitted Diseases*. London, Mosby-Wolfe, 1992.)

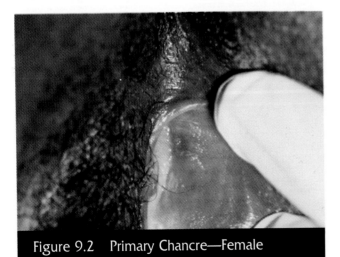

Figure 9.2   Primary Chancre—Female

A solitary, painless genital chancre with a clean base in a patient with primary syphilis. (Courtesy of the Dept. of Dermatology, Naval Medical Center, Portsmouth.)

Differential Diagnosis

Behçet's disease, fixed drug eruption, recurrent genital herpes, chancroid, squamous cell carcinoma, and lesions caused by trauma can have a similar appearance.

ED Treatment and Disposition

Treat with benzathine penicillin G, 2.4 million units IM once. Penicillin-allergic patients should be given doxycycline, 100 mg PO bid for 2 weeks. Other alternatives include tetracycline, 500 mg PO qid for 2 weeks; erythromycin base, 500 mg PO qid for 2 weeks; or ceftriaxone, 250 mg IM once daily for 10 days. An RPR or VDRL should be checked. Partners within the last 90 days should be treated presumptively; partners over the last 90 days should be treated on the basis of their serologic testing results. This is a reportable disease, and appropriate paperwork should be filed.

Clinical Pearls

1. Lesions are usually painless and solitary, but may be slightly painful and two or three lesions may also be seen.
2. Consider dark-field examination of the lesion to rapidly confirm the diagnosis.
3. Chancres of primary syphilis can occur anywhere on the body at the site of inoculation.
4. Evaluate patients with primary syphilis for concurrent sexually transmitted diseases and treat accordingly.

Associated Clinical Features

The rash of secondary syphilis often occurs 2 to 10 weeks after resolution of the primary lesions. It begins as a nonpruritic macular rash that evolves into a papulosquamous rash involving primarily the trunk, palms, and soles (Figs. 9.3, 9.4, 9.5). The rash is often annular in shape. Diffuse, painless lymphadenopathy is also seen at this stage. Mucous patches represent mucous membrane involvement of the tongue and buccal mucosa (Fig. 9.6). Condyloma lata (Fig. 9.7) can be seen during this stage, as can patchy alopecia. The manifestations of this stage resolve without treatment in several months.

Differential Diagnosis

The differential diagnosis depends on the site involved:

Rash: Pityriasis rosea, psoriasis, lichen planus, Reiter's, viral syndrome, allergic rash

Mucous patches: Apthous ulcerations, thrush

Condyloma lata: Condyloma accuminata, squamous cell carcinoma, granuloma inguinale

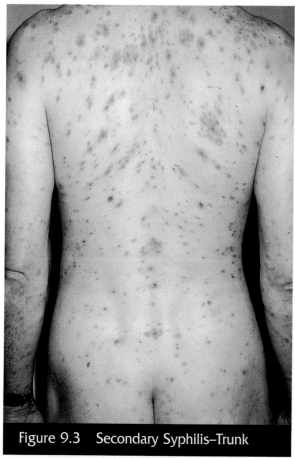

Figure 9.3   Secondary Syphilis–Trunk

Rash on trunk in secondary syphilis. (Courtesy of A. Wisdom: *Sexually Transmitted Diseases*. London, Mosby-Wolfe, 1992.)

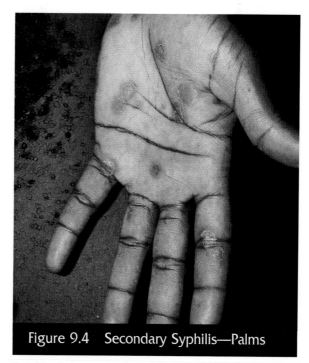

Figure 9.4   Secondary Syphilis—Palms

Papulosquamous rash of secondary syphilis. Note the annular appearance of the palmar rash. (Courtesy of H. Hunter Handsfield: *Atlas of Sexually Transmitted Diseases*. New York, McGraw-Hill, 1992.)

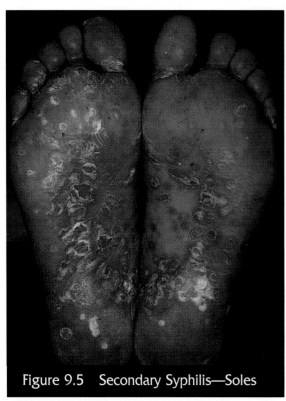

Figure 9.5   Secondary Syphilis—Soles

Hyperkeratotic plantar rash in a patient with secondary syphilis. (Courtesy of H. Hunter Handsfield: *Atlas of Sexually Transmitted Diseases.* New York, McGraw-Hill, 1992.)

ED Treatment and Disposition

Benzathine penicillin G, 2.4 million units IM once; penicillin allergic patients should receive doxycycline, 100 mg PO bid for 2 weeks. RPR or VDRL should be sent and titers followed to determine adequate response to therapy. Suspected and confirmed cases of syphilis must be reported.

Clinical Pearls

1. Lesions of secondary syphilis are very infectious. It is prudent to always wear gloves when examining a patient with a rash that may be due to secondary syphilis.
2. Consider using dark-field examination of scrapings of the rash, mucous patches, and condyloma lata to make a rapid diagnosis.
3. Patients should be warned about the potential development of the Jarish-Herxheimer reaction after they are treated. This syndrome, characterized by fever, headache, malaise, and myalgias, occurs within 24 h of treatment and is caused by massive release of pyrogens by the dying spirochetes.

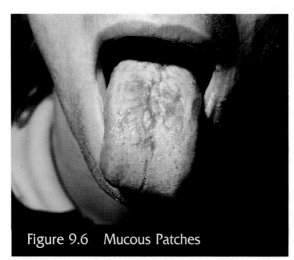

Figure 9.6   Mucous Patches

Oral involvement in secondary syphilis manifested by mucous patches. These lesions are very infectious, and dark-field examination is often positive for spirochetes. (Courtesy of Morse, Moreland, Thompson: *Atlas of Sexually Transmitted Diseases.* London, Mosby-Wolfe, 1990.)

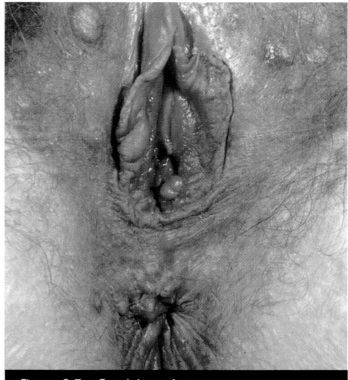

Figure 9.7   Condyloma Lata

Typical appearance of the verrucous, heaped-up lesions of condyloma lata, a manifestation of secondary syphilis. (Courtesy of H. Hunter Handsfield: *Atlas of Sexually Transmitted Diseases.* New York, McGraw-Hill, 1992.)

Associated Clinical Features

Gonorrhea often manifests after a short incubation period of 2 to 5 days. In men, urethritis is characterized by purulent, usually copious urethral discharge (Fig. 9.8) with dysuria; however, up to 10% of men are asymptomatic. Women may also develop urethritis (Fig. 9.9) and complain of dysuria. Cervicitis is often asymptomatic. If symptomatic, women may complain of increased vaginal discharge or vaginal spotting, particularly after intercourse. On speculum examination, the cervix is friable with a mucopurulent endocervical exudate (Fig. 9.10). Patients with gonococcal conjunctivitis have chemosis and copious, purulent exudate (Fig. 9.11); untreated, these patients can develop endophthalmitis and globe perforation. Untreated gonorrhea may disseminate, and more commonly does so in women. Disseminated gonococcal infection (DGI) presents with a monoarticular or oligorticular septic arthritis usually involving the knees, ankles, elbows, or wrists. Skin lesions are necrotic pustules on an erythematous base, may ulcerate, and are more commonly found on the distal extremities (Figs. 9.12, 9.13).

Differential Diagnosis

The differential diagnosis depends on the site involved:

Urethritis and cervicitis: *Chlamydia,* mycoplasma, ureaplasma
Conjunctivitis: Bacterial conjunctivitis, chemical conjunctivitis
Arthritis: Septic arthritis, rheumatic fever, hepatitis B prodrome, immune complex disease, Reiter's syndrome, systemic lupus erythematosus
Skin lesions: Folliculitis, subacute bacterial endocarditis (septic emboli)

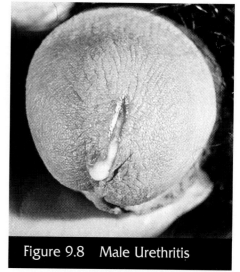

Figure 9.8   Male Urethritis

Purulent, copious urethral discharge in a patient with gonococcal urethritis. (Courtesy of H. Hunter Handsfield: *Atlas of Sexually Transmitted Diseases.* New York, McGraw-Hill, 1992.)

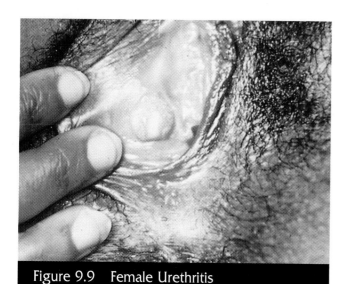

Figure 9.9   Female Urethritis

Gonococcal urethritis in a female patient; note the purulent urethral discharge. (Courtesy of Morse, Moreland, Thompson: *Atlas of Sexually Transmitted Diseases.* London, Mosby-Wolfe, 1990.)

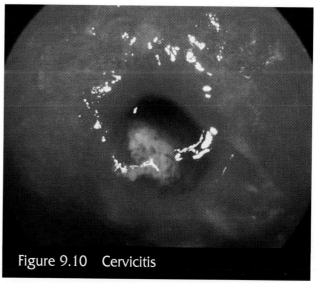

Figure 9.10   Cervicitis

Endocervical purulent exudate in an asymptomatic patient with gonococcal cervicitis. The cervix is very friable. (Courtesy of King K. Holmes, MD from H. Hunter Handsfield: *Atlas of Sexually Transmitted Diseases.* New York, McGraw-Hill, 1992.)

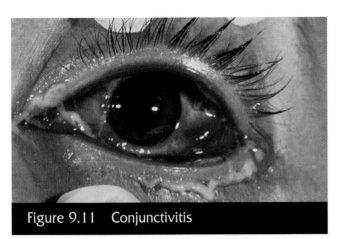

Figure 9.11   Conjunctivitis

Chemotic conjunctiva and copious purulent exudate in a patient with gonococcal conjunctivitis. (Courtesy of H. Hunter Handsfield: *Atlas of Sexually Transmitted Diseases.* New York, McGraw-Hill, 1992.)

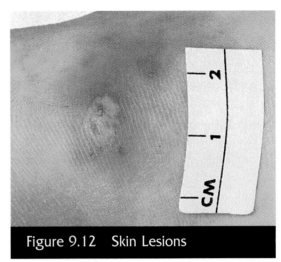

Figure 9.12   Skin Lesions

Small pustules with hemorrhage suggestive of the skin lesions of disseminated gonococcal infection. (Courtesy of H. Hunter Handsfield: *Atlas of Sexually Transmitted Diseases.* New York, McGraw-Hill, 1992.)

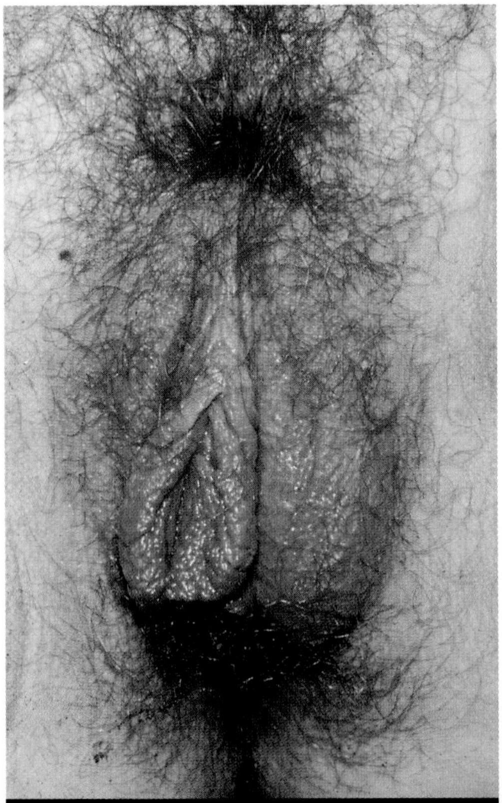

Figure 9.13   Bartholin's Cyst

Enlarged, fluctuant, tender Bartholin's abscess of the labia, usually but not always a result of gonorrhea. (Courtesy of A. Wisdom: *Sexually Transmitted Diseases.* London, Mosby-Wolfe, 1992.)

ED Treatment and Disposition

Treatment is dependent on the site of infection:

Urethritis and cervicitis: Ceftriaxone, 125 mg IM once; cefixime, 400 mg PO once; ciprofloxacin, 500 mg PO once; ofloxacin, 400 mg PO once

Conjunctivitis: Ceftriaxone 1 g IM once; eye irrigation

Disseminated gonococcal infection: Ceftriaxone, 1 g IV or IM daily for 7 to 10 days; may treat with 1 to 2 days of IM ceftriaxone and then change to cefixime, 400 mg PO bid, or ciprofloxacin, 500 mg PO bid, to complete a 7- to 10-day course. Sexual partners should be notified and treated. Gonorrhea is a reportable disease.

Clinical Pearls

1. Patients with gonorrhea need to be treated for concurrent infection with *Chlamydia.* Coinfection with these organisms is seen in 30% of men with urethritis and 50% of women with cervicitis.
2. Gonococcal arthritis is the most common cause of monoarticular arthritis in young, sexually active patients.
3. Suspect gonococcal conjunctivitis in patients with copious eye discharge and chemosis.
4. Cultures are the gold standard for confirming the diagnosis of gonorrhea. Selective media should be used when specimens are obtained from the cervix, pharynx, urethra, or rectum. Nonselective medium (blood agar) should be used when culturing joint fluid, blood, or cerebrospinal fluid.

Associated Clinical Features

After an incubation period of 1 to 3 weeks, males with urethritis may present with a thin, often clear urethral discharge and dysuria (Fig. 9.14). Up to 10% of men may be asymptomatic. Women may also develop urethritis which may only cause dysuria and be misdiagnosed as a urinary tract infection. Cervicitis in women (Fig. 9.15) is almost always asymptomatic. Women may develop pelvic inflammatory disease with upper genital tract infection. Men may develop epididymitis.

Differential Diagnosis

For urethritis and cervicitis, gonorrhea, mycoplasma, and ureaplasma should be considered.

ED Treatment and Disposition

The preferred treatment consists of azithromycin, 1 g PO once, or doxycycline 100 mg PO bid for 7 days. Alternatives include ofloxacin, 500 mg PO bid for 7 days. Pregnant women should receive erythromycin base, 500 mg, or erythromycin ethylsuccinate 800 mg PO qid for 7 days. Partners should be examined and treated appropriately.

Clinical Pearls

1. Chlamydial infection often accompanies gonococcal infection, and patients being treated for gonorrhea should also be treated for chlamydial infection.
2. Women with chlamydial infections may be completely asymptomatic for long periods of time.
3. Consider syphilis serologic testing and HIV testing in patients presenting with sexually transmitted diseases.

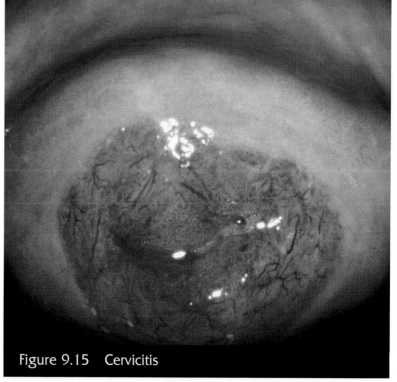

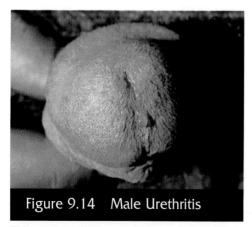

Figure 9.14   Male Urethritis

Thin urethral discharge of chlamydial urethritis. (Courtesy of Walter Stamm, MD, from H. Hunter Handsfield: *Atlas of Sexually Transmitted Diseases.* New York, McGraw-Hill, 1992.)

Figure 9.15   Cervicitis

Mucopurulent cervicitis from chlamydial infection. (Courtesy of H. Hunter Handsfield: *Atlas of Sexually Transmitted Diseases.* New York, McGraw-Hill, 1992.)

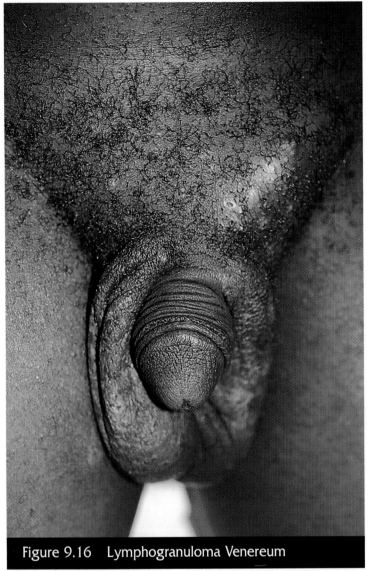

Figure 9.16   Lymphogranuloma Venereum

Unilateral left lymphadenopathy in a patient with lymphogranuloma venereum. (Courtesy of Lawrence B. Stack, MD.)

Associated Clinical Features

Lymphogranuloma venereum (LGV) is caused by a serotype of *chlamydia trachomatous* and is primarily a disease of lymphatic tissue. Initially, LGV is often a painless genital ulceration that is not noticed by the patient more than 90% of the time. Patients often present with painful, non-fluctuant inguinal adenopathy, which is often, but not always, unilateral (Fig. 9.16). Lymphadenopathy may lie above and below the inguinal ligament, causing the "groove sign" suggestive of this diagnosis. Lymphadenopathy may spontaneously open into draining sinus tracts to the skin.

Differential Diagnosis

Chancroid, granuloma inguinale, lymphoma, pyogenic or mycobacterial infection, syphilis, and cat scratch disease may have a similar appearance.

ED Treatment and Disposition

Doxycycline, 100 mg PO bid for 3 weeks. Although rare, patients may need needle aspiration of the lymph nodes if they become fluctuant. Serologic testing is needed to confirm the diagnosis.

Clinical Pearls

1. Patients rarely note the evanescent ulcer associated with LGV.
2. The lymphadenopathy of LGV progresses over several weeks.
3. Treatment for LGV requires 3 weeks of therapy for a cure.

Associated Clinical Features

Herpes genitalis presents in several ways: symptomatic primary infection, first-episode nonprimary infection, and recurrent infection. Symptomatic primary infection occurs when the patient develops symptoms when first acquiring the virus. Some patients may be asymptomatic when primarily infected with the virus, however, and present at a later time with their first symptomatic episode of nonprimary genital herpes. Patients with either symptomatic primary infection or first-episode nonprimary infection may develop recurrences.

Symptomatic primary genital herpes is characterized by multiple vesicles that quickly ulcerate into shallow, painful ulcers (Figs. 9.17, 9.18). The ulcers may coalesce. The lesions are accompanied by a viral syndrome with low-grade fever and myalgias. Up to 10% of patients may develop aseptic meningitis. Women may develop sacral autonomic dysfunction and require urinary catheterization because of urinary retention. The lesions last up to 3 weeks and heal without scarring.

First-episode nonprimary genital herpes and recurrent genital herpes are less dramatic (Fig. 9.19). Patients with first-episode nonprimary genital herpes do not have systemic symptoms, have solitary to several painful lesions, and resolve their symptoms in 1 to 2 weeks. Recurrences of genital herpes are often heralded by a warning prodrome of tingling or numbness in the perineal area. Vesicles and their subsequent ulcers are often solitary. Duration of symptoms is often several days and usually less than a week.

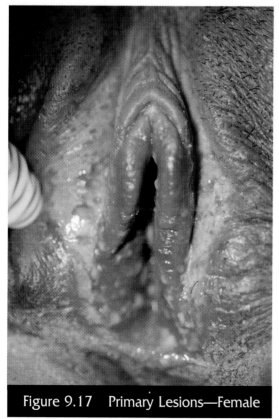

Figure 9.17 Primary Lesions—Female

Multiple, coalescing superficial ulcerations of primary genital herpes. (Courtesy of Lawrence B. Stack, MD.)

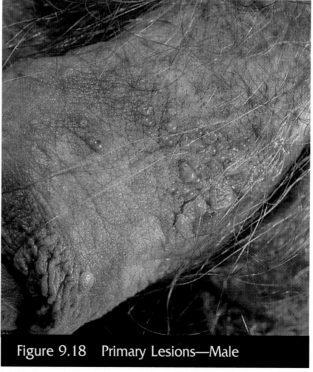

Figure 9.18 Primary Lesions—Male

Multiple genital vesicles of primary genital herpes. (Courtesy of H. Hunter Handsfield: *Atlas of Sexually Transmitted Diseases.* New York, McGraw-Hill, 1992.)

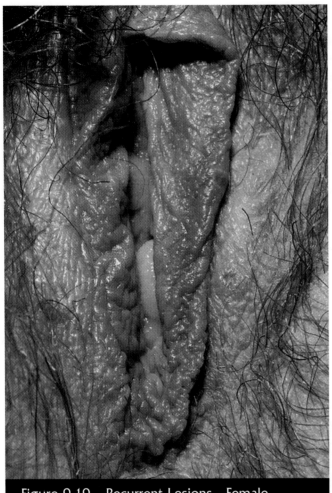

Figure 9.19   Recurrent Lesions—Female

Solitary, minimally painful lesion of recurrent genital herpes. (Courtesy of H. Hunter Handsfield: *Atlas of Sexually Transmitted Diseases.* New York, McGraw-Hill, 1992.)

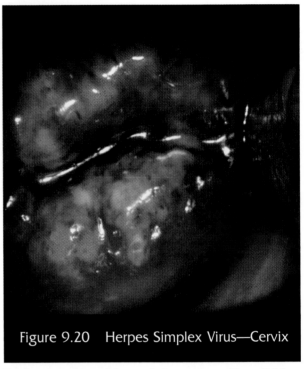

Figure 9.20   Herpes Simplex Virus—Cervix

Erosive ulcerations of the cervix in a patient with genital herpes infection. This patient may be completely asymptomatic and may transmit the disease. (Courtesy of A. Wisdom: *Sexually Transmitted Diseases.* London, Mosby-Wolfe, 1992.)

Differential Diagnosis

Pustular psoriasis, chancroid, erythema multiforme, fixed drug eruption, Behçet's disease, Stevens-Johnson syndrome, pyoderma gangrenosum, syphilis, and pyodermic infection may have a similar appearance.

ED Treatment and Disposition

Primary genital herpes: Acyclovir, 200 mg PO five times daily for 7 to 10 days or until symptoms resolve; 400 mg PO tid may be substituted for patient convenience.

Recurrent genital herpes: Acyclovir, 200 mg PO five times daily; 400 mg PO tid for 5 to 7 days; or Famciclovir, 125 mg PO BID for 5 days.

Clinical Pearls

1. Women with genital herpes must be counseled to inform their obstetrician of this history of herpes when they become pregnant.
2. Genital herpes is the most common cause of ulcerating genital lesions.
3. Patients may initially present with full-blown primary genital herpes symptoms or may have their first clinical presentation as a recurrence of an asymptomatically acquired infection (Fig. 9.20).

Associated Clinical Features

Chancroid is caused by *Haemophilus ducreyi*. After an incubation period of 2 to 10 days, this disease presents with multiple, painful, nonindurated genital ulcerations that are often deep and undermined and may have a purulent base (Fig. 9.21). Inguinal adenopathy may develop and becomes fluctuant, large, and painful (Fig. 9.22). Infected lymph nodes may spontaneously rupture. Systemic symptoms are uncommon.

Differential Diagnosis

Lymphogranuloma venereum, granuloma inguinale, herpes simplex virus, and syphilis should be considered.

ED Treatment and Disposition

Ceftriaxone, 250 mg IM once, or azithromycin, 1 g PO once. Alternatives include amoxicillin and clavulanic acid, 500 mg and 125 mg PO tid for 7 days or ciprofloxacin, 500 mg PO bid for 3 days. Large, fluctuant nodes should be aspirated to prevent rupture; incision and drainage should be avoided to prevent development of chronic draining sinus tracts. Partners should be notified of exposure to the disease.

Clinical Pearls

1. Chancroid is usually found in high-risk populations: drug-abusing, inner city.
2. Chancroid is a diagnosis of exclusion, as culturing *H. ducreyi* requires special medium not readily available. Genital herpes and syphilis must be ruled out.
3. The lymphadenopathy of chancroid is often very tender and fluctuant.
4. Chancroid lesions are very tender and usually multiple.

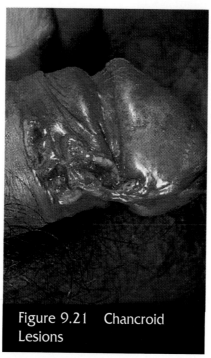

Figure 9.21 Chancroid Lesions

Multiple painful, deep ulcerations of chancroid. (Courtesy of H. Hunter Handsfield: *Atlas of Sexually Transmitted Diseases.* New York, McGraw-Hill, 1992.)

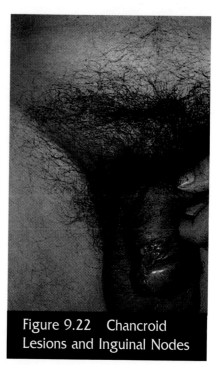

Figure 9.22 Chancroid Lesions and Inguinal Nodes

Chancroid lesions with an enlarged lymph node; on examination this node is tender and fluctuant. (Courtesy of H. Hunter Handsfield: *Atlas of Sexually Transmitted Diseases.* New York, McGraw-Hill, 1992.)

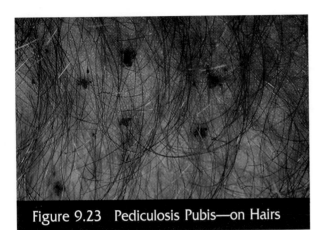

Figure 9.23 Pediculosis Pubis—on Hairs

Phthirus pubis, or the crab louse, in the pubic hair of a patient complaining of itching. Note also the nits attached to the hairs. (Courtesy of Morse, Moreland, Thompson: *Atlas of Sexually Transmitted Diseases.* London, Mosby-Wolfe, 1990.)

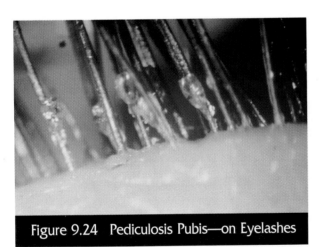

Figure 9.24 Pediculosis Pubis—on Eyelashes

Phthirus pubis lice noted in the eyelashes. (Courtesy of Spalton, Hitchings, Hunter: *Atlas of Clinical Ophthalmology,* 2d ed. London, Mosby-Year Book Europe, 1994.)

Associated Clinical Features

Pediculosis can be caused by either the body louse or the crab louse. Body lice (Fig. 17.21) are not sexually transmitted and tend to cluster around the waist, shoulders, axillae, neck, and head. Extremely itchy, patients may present with excoriations and intense pruritus. The lice are very small and may not be easily seen. The larval form of the louse, the nit, may be mistaken for dandruff in the hair. Unlike dandruff, however, the nits are extremely adherent to the hair shaft and cannot be brushed out of the hair. The adult lice and their eggs are often found in the seams of clothing.

Pubic infestation is caused by *Phthirus pubis,* the crab louse (Fig. 9.23, 17.20). Patients may present with intense itching in the pubic area; however, as many as half of patients with this infestation may be asymptomatic. Patients may notice the lice or may note tiny rust-colored spots on their underwear, which represent bleeding from the sites of louse bites. Nits may be found at the base of pubic hairs and hatch in 5 to 10 days.

Differential Diagnosis

Tinea, contact dermatitis, scabies, and heat rash may have a similar appearance.

ED Treatment and Disposition

Lindane shampoo (Kevell™) should be lathered into the pubic, perineal, and perianal hair, or lindane lotion applied in the affected areas and left on for 10 min and rinsed off. Synergized pyrethrins (RID™), or synthetic pyrethrins (NIX™, Elmite™), may also be used. Since lindane may be toxic, pyrethrins are preferred in pregnant women and children. Treatment should be repeated in 1 week to treat any nits that may have hatched. Clothing worn or linen used in the preceding 24 h should be washed. Mechanical removal of nits attached to hairs should be attempted. Petrolatum jelly or any bland ophthalmic ointment can be applied to the eyelashes twice daily for a week to treat infestation of the eyelashes (Fig. 9.24). Sexual contacts should be examined.

Clinical Pearls

1. Nits are easier to find on examination than are mature lice; the average number of lice in an infestation is only 10.
2. Patients with pediculosis pubis should be considered at risk for other sexually transmitted diseases and examined.
3. Lindane shampoo or lotion should not be used in infants under 1 year of age or in pregnant women.

Associated Clinical Features

Caused by human papilloma virus (HPV), these flesh-colored lesions may be flat, sessile, or pedunculated (Figs. 9.25, 9.26). They often have a cauliflowerlike appearance and are usually asymptomatic, but may be seen or felt by patients or their sexual partners. They range in size from 1 to 4 mm to masses that may be several centimeters large (giant warts, Figs. 9.27 to 9.28).

Differential Diagnosis

Condyloma lata due to secondary syphilis is the primary alternative diagnosis (Fig. 9.7). Bowen's disease, molluscum contagiosum, and carcinoma may have a similar appearance.

ED Treatment and Disposition

Local caustic agents (e.g., podophyllin) are used to treat the lesions; multiple treatment is often needed, and recurrence is common. Other therapies include cryotherapy, electrocautery, and trichloracetic acid. Laser therapy or surgery may be needed in cases of giant warts.

Clinical Pearls

1. Evidence suggests that HPV is linked with increased risk of cervical cancer.
2. Women with genital warts need to have a Pap smear to rule out coexisting carcinoma in situ.
3. Large lesions should be biopsied to rule out cancer.
4. Patients should be advised that it may take several to many visits to completely eradicate the condyloma.
5. In cases where the diagnosis is not obvious, rule out condyloma lata (secondary syphilis) by sending serologic studies.

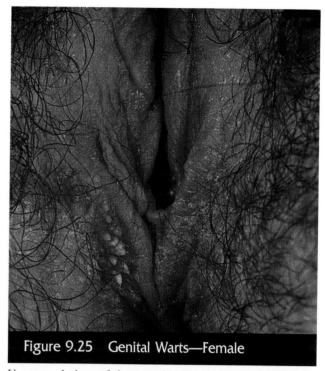

Figure 9.25   Genital Warts—Female

Verrucous lesions of the posterior fourchette in a patient with condyloma acuminata. (Used with permission from H. Hunter Handsfield: *Atlas of Sexually Transmitted Diseases.* New York, McGraw-Hill, 1992.)

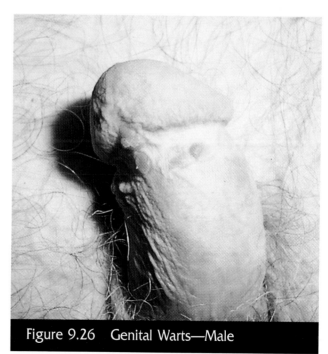

Figure 9.26   Genital Warts—Male

Typical appearance of condyloma acuminata of the glans penis. (Courtesy of Morse, Moreland, Thompson: *Atlas of Sexually Transmitted Diseases.* London, Mosby-Wolfe, 1990.)

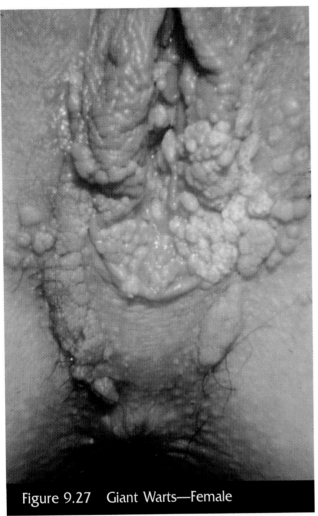

Figure 9.27   Giant Warts—Female

Giant warts of a female patient with extensive condyloma acuminata. (Courtesy of Morse, Moreland, Thompson: *Atlas of Sexually Transmitted Diseases.* London, Mosby-Wolfe, 1990.)

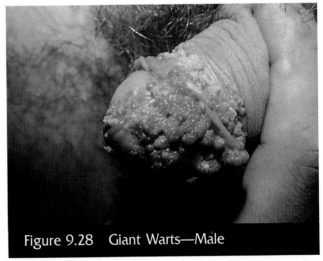

Figure 9.28   Giant Warts—Male

Giant warts in a male patient with extensive condyloma acuminata. (Courtesy of A. Wisdom: *Sexually Transmitted Diseases.* London, Mosby-Wolfe, 1992.)

ANORECTAL CONDITIONS

Associated Clinical Features

An anal fissure is a longitudinal tear in the skin of the anal canal and usually extends from the dentate line to the anal verge. Fissures are thought to be caused by the passage of hard or large stools with constipation, but may also be seen with diarrhea. The fissures are typically a few millimeters wide and occur in the posterior midline (Fig. 9.29), but can occur elsewhere. An anal fissure that is off the midline may have a secondary cause such as inflammatory bowel disease or sexually transmitted infection. Although often seen in infants, this condition is found mostly in young and middle-aged adults. Patients present with the complaint of intense sharp, burning pain during and after bowel movements. They may also note bright red blood at the time or shortly after the passage of stool. Gentle examination with separation of the buttocks usually provides good visualization (Fig. 9.29). Anoscopy should be performed, if possible.

Differential Diagnosis

The diagnosis of inflammatory bowel disease, ulcerative colitis or Crohn's disease, should be considered, particularly if the fissure is atypical. Anal fissures may be the result of a sexually transmitted disease such as *Chlamydia*, gonorrhea, herpes, and syphilis. Tuberculosis, anal neoplasms, and sickle cell disease can also present as an anal fissure. An anal abscess and thrombosed hemorrhoids may cause similar symptoms, but can usually be ruled out on physical examination.

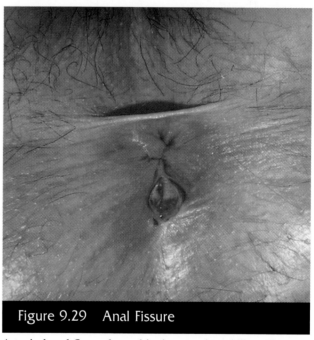

Figure 9.29   Anal Fissure

A typical anal fissure located in the posterior midline. (Courtesy of Paul J. Kovalcik, MD.)

ED Treatment and Disposition

Acute treatment of anal fissures consists of anal hygiene, bulk fiber diet supplements to soften stools, warm sitz baths, and topical anesthetics. Oral pain medication and muscle relaxants such as diazepam may be required in certain patients.

Clinical Pearls

1. Pain and involuntary sphincter spasm may preclude a routine digital or anoscopic examination and require an examination under anesthesia.
2. A proctoscopic examination should be done at some point to rule out secondary causes.
3. Most anal fissures heal spontaneously, but refractory cases may require surgical repair.

Associated Clinical Features

The perianal abscess is the most common anorectal abscess. It is associated with pain in the anal area that is exacerbated by bowel movements, straining, coughing, or palpation. On examination, a fluctuant and possibly erythematous mass is found at the perianal region (Fig. 9.30). Perianal abscesses are usually fairly superficial and easy to drain with local anesthesia. The patient may notice swelling or a pressure sensation. Perirectal abscesses tend to be more complex and are named according to the involved space: ischiorectal, intersphincteric, or supralevator (Fig. 9.31). These are fluctuant masses that are usually palpable along the rectal wall. Patients may complain of pain, fever, and mucous or bloody discharge with bowel movement.

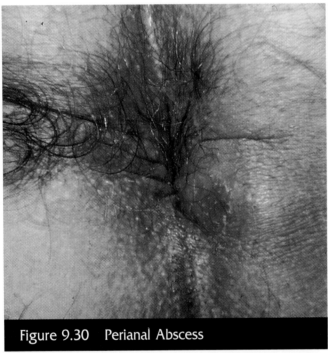

Figure 9.30 Perianal Abscess

Swelling and erythema around the anus consistent with a perianal abscess. (Courtesy of the American Society of Colon and Rectal Surgeons.)

Differential Diagnosis

Crohn's disease should be considered because 36% of Crohn's patients have a perianal abscess at the presentation of their disease. An underlying process may exist such as diabetes mellitus, leukemia, or other malignancy.

ED Treatment and Disposition

Incision and drainage of perianal abscesses should be performed with a small radial or cruciate incision lateral to the external sphincter. For an uncomplicated abscess this can be accomplished under local anesthesia. The cavity should be cleared of loculations and then loosely packed with iodoform gauze, which should be removed in 24 to 48 h. All patients require outpatient follow-up. Antibiotic therapy is not indicated unless there is underlying disease affecting the patient's immunologic function, or the patient appears septic. Surgical consultation should be obtained for treatment of perirectal abscesses under anesthesia.

Clinical Pearls

1. Surgical consultation and treatment may be required in the patient with a large or complicated perianal abscess or where adequate analgesia cannot be obtained.
2. Consider admission for debilitated, elderly, febrile, obese, or otherwise ill-appearing patients.
3. All patients warrant follow-up referral due to the high incidence of fistulae with anorectal abscesses.

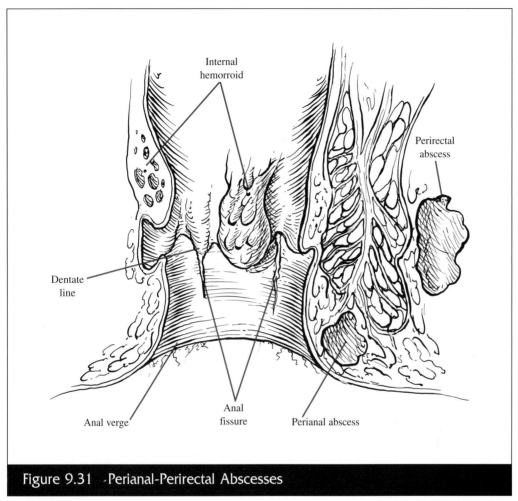

Figure 9.31 · Perianal-Perirectal Abscesses

The anatomy of perianal and perirectal abscesses is illustrated. Also shown are anal fissure and internal and external hemorrhoids.

Associated Clinical Features

External hemorrhoids result from the dilatation of the venules of the inferior hemorrhoidal plexus below the dentate line. They have a covering of skin, or anoderm, versus internal hemorrhoids that have a mucosal covering. Hemorrhoids commonly present with an episode of rectal bleeding of bright red blood after defecation. This results from the passage of the fecal mass over the thin-walled venules causing abrasions and bleeding. Symptoms from external hemorrhoids include complaints of swelling and burning rectal pain. Numerous associated factors exist, such as constipation, family history, pregnancy, portal hypertension, or increased intraabdominal pressure. Hemorrhoids are commonly found at three anatomic locations: right anterior, right posterior, and left lateral positions (Fig. 9.32). A thrombosed external hemorrhoid contains intravascular clots and causes exquisite pain the first 48 h.

Internal hemorrhoids (Figs. 9.31, 9.33) present with painless rectal bleeding or possibly the sensation of prolapse. They are graded according to the degree of prolapse where the first degree is identifiable at the dentate line and the fourth degree shows irreducible prolapse through the anus. Internal hemorrhoids are not typically painful, whereas external hemorrhoids do cause pain.

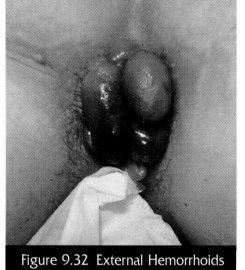

Figure 9.32 External Hemorrhoids

Multiple engorged external hemorrhoids are seen in all quadrants. (Courtesy of the American Society of Colon and Rectal Surgeons.)

Differential Diagnosis

Other diagnoses to consider include infection, perianal or perirectal abscess, inflammatory bowel disease, malignancy, local trauma, herpes or other sexually transmitted infection, rectal polyp, or rectal prolapse.

ED Treatment and Disposition

In the case of severe bleeding, fluid resuscitation would need to be instituted and the bleeding vessel located, clamped, and ligated. The treatment for less severe cases warrants more conservative therapy, including increased dietary fiber, increased fluid intake, hot sitz baths, bedrest, and nonnarcotic pain medication. Advanced cases may require surgical consultation and treatment. ED treatment of thrombosed external hemorrhoids includes an elliptical excision and extrusion of the clot under local anesthesia.

Clinical Pearls

1. Many patients with any anorectal problem complain of hemorrhoids. Therefore, careful examination and consideration of the differential diagnosis should be undertaken with each patient.
2. Having the patient strain during the examination may reveal bleeding or prolapse that may otherwise go unnoticed.
3. Hemorrhoids are a rare cause of anorectal pruritus.

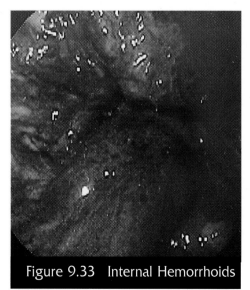

Figure 9.33 Internal Hemorrhoids

Internal hemorrhoids are seen in this endoscopic view of the rectum. (Courtesy of Virender K. Sharman, MD.)

Associated Clinical Features

Rectal prolapse occurs when anorectal tissue slides through the anal orifice and can include mucosa or a full-thickness layer. This is due to several anatomic features including laxity of the pelvic floor, weak anal sphincters, and lack of mesorectal fixation. Patients complain of bleeding, mucous discharge, rectal pressure, or a mass (Fig. 9.34). Problems with fecal incontinence, constipation, and rectal ulceration are common as well. Prolapse may be associated with an increased familial incidence, chronic cough, dysentery, or parasitic infection.

Differential Diagnosis

Usually reduction is possible with gentle manual pressure. However, if this cannot be accomplished, surgical consultation and admission is needed. Surgical treatment is also indicated with a complete prolapse. All patients should undergo an anoscopic and sigmoidoscopic examination at some point and, if rectal bleeding is a problem, full colonic evaluation should be completed.

Clinical Pearls

1. This is commonly seen in children with cystic fibrosis (22%); therefore, all children with rectal prolapse should have a sweat chloride test.
2. Examination of rectal prolapse reveals concentric mucosal rings and a sulcus between the anal canal and the rectum, whereas prolapsed hemorrhoids are separated by radial grooves and the sulcus is absent.
3. To confirm the diagnosis, prolapse may be reproduced by having the patient bear down.

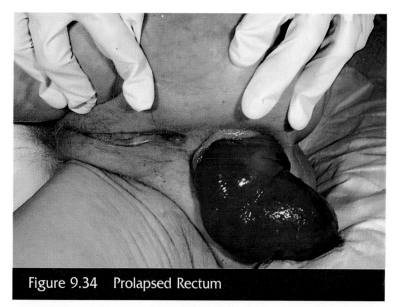

Figure 9.34   Prolapsed Rectum

The rectum is completely prolapsed in this elderly patient. (Courtesy of Alan B. Storrow, MD.)

Associated Clinical Features

Pilonidal abscesses are typically seen at or just superior to the gluteal fold (Fig. 9.35) and are more common in teenage and young adult males. Patients complain of localized pain, swelling, and drainage, but usually do not have systemic symptoms. The abscess begins with the formation of a small opening in the skin that develops into a cystic structure involving surrounding hairs. This opening is occluded by hair or keratin, creating a closed space that does not allow drainage. The acute abscess contains mixed organisms including *Staphylococcus aureus* and *Streptococcus,* but anaerobes and gram-negative organisms may also be present.

Differential Diagnosis

Evidence of cellulitis in the sacrococcygeal area may result from a simple abscess or furuncle. However, other causes should be considered such as anal fistulae, hidradenitis, inflammatory bowel disease, or tuberculosis.

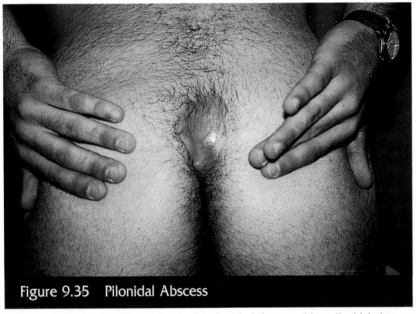

Figure 9.35   Pilonidal Abscess

Redness, fluctuance, and tenderness in the gluteal cleft seen with a pilonidal abscess. (Courtesy of Louis La Vopa, MD.)

ED Disposition and Treatment

An acutely fluctuant abscess requires incision and drainage under local anesthesia with removal of pus and debris. The patient should be instructed on meticulous wound care and sitz baths. Antibiotic therapy is not indicated unless the patient is immunocompromised. Surgical referral is given, particularly with a chronic or recurrent cyst that may require surgical excision and closure.

Clinical Pearls

1. Pilonidal abscesses almost always occur in the midline, but can have sinus tracts extending off the midline.
2. Pilonidal disease is three times more common in men than in women.

Associated Clinical Features

The diagnosis of rectal foreign body is usually made by history and confirmed by digital examination. Most often the foreign body is inserted (Fig. 9.36), but it is possible to have an ingested foreign body trapped in the rectum. The most serious complication of a rectal foreign body is perforation of the rectum or distal colon. The patient must be carefully evaluated for evidence of perforation with x-rays demonstrating free air and clinically for the presentation of an acute abdomen. Perforation above the peritoneal reflection is associated with free air in the abdominal cavity and peritoneal signs. Perforation below the peritoneal reflection presents with more insidious signs of pain and infection in the perianal or perineal region. It is important to determine the size, shape, and number of objects to assess the risk of perforation. In children rectal foreign bodies usually present as rectal bleeding.

Differential Diagnosis

Depending on the clinical scenario, the diagnoses of sexual assault or child abuse should be considered.

ED Disposition and Treatment

Removal can often take place in the ED with sedation of the patient and local anesthesia of the anal sphincter. If the risk of perforation appears high or adequate relaxation and anesthesia cannot be obtained, then the patient is prepared for emergency surgery. After removal, proctoscopic or sigmoidoscopic examination is recommended to rule out perforation or laceration.

Clinical Pearls

1. A Foley catheter or an endotracheal tube may be used to release the vacuum effect of some foreign bodies, and the balloon can be inflated and aid in the removal.
2. A rectal foreign body in a child should raise the suspicion of abuse.

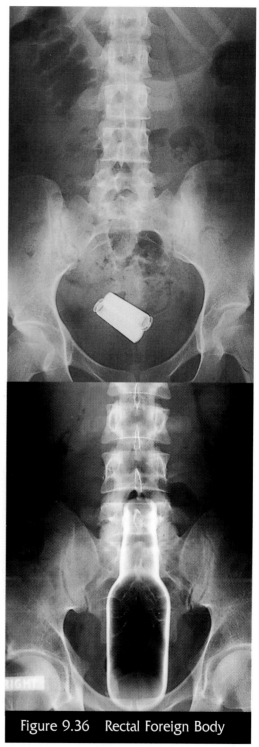

Figure 9.36 Rectal Foreign Body

Top The metallic outline of two batteries is seen in this x-ray. *Bottom* This foreign body (a 7-oz beer bottle) required removal in the operating room. (Courtesy of David W. Munter, MD. [*Top*] and Kevin J. Knoop, MD, MS. [*Bottom*].)

Associated Clinical Features

Gastrointestinal bleeding commonly presents with the alteration of stool color. By definition, melena is the passage of dark, pitchlike stools stained with blood pigments (Fig. 9.37). Generally, but not always, melena results from bleeding into the upper gastrointestinal tract proximal to the ligament of Treitz. Black stools have been seen with as little as 60 mL of blood in the upper gastrointestinal tract, but melena typically does not develop until 100 to 200 mL is present. Melena can be found in lower bleeds with decreased transit time, as with an obstruction distal to the site of bleeding.

Differential Diagnosis

Melenic stools may occur from swallowed blood such as from epistaxis or other oropharyngeal bleeding. Dark or black stools can also be seen with the ingestion of bismuth salicylate, food coloring, and iron supplements.

ED Disposition and Treatment

Patients with melenic stools should be evaluated in a monitored setting and undergo assessment for signs and symptoms of hypovolemia and treated accordingly. At least one large-bore IV should be placed and saline infused. Depending on the patient's stability, type-specific packed red blood cells or other blood products may be required. Abdominal radiographs are done to look for free air in the peritoneum, and gastric aspiration should be done to assess for active gastric bleeding. Stable patients who present with melena may be admitted to the ward. Evidence of unstable vital signs, continued bleeding, severe anemia, or co-morbid disease warrants admission to the intensive care unit. Consultation with a gastroenterologist should be sought unless patients require more than two units of blood for resuscitation, which would call for surgical intervention.

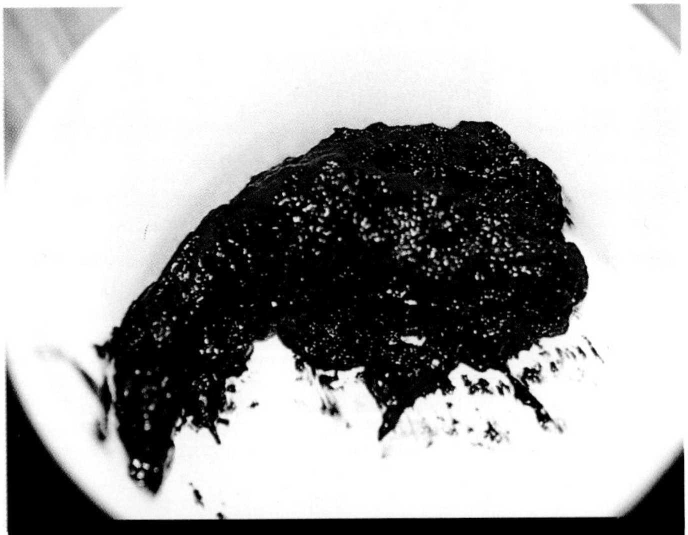

Figure 9.37   Melena

The black, tarry appearance of melena in a patient with a duodenal ulcer. (Courtesy of Alan B. Storrow, MD.)

Clinical Pearls

1. Melena is the most common presenting symptom of bleeding from peptic ulcer disease.
2. Melena represents approximately 200 mL of blood loss in the gastrointestinal tract.

CHAPTER 10

GYNECOLOGIC AND OBSTETRIC CONDITIONS

Robert G. Buckley
Kevin J. Knoop

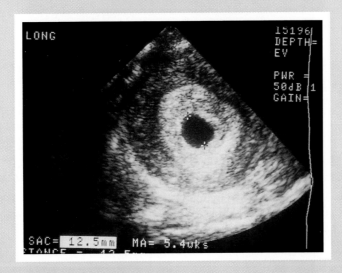

Gynecologic Conditions

VAGINITIS

Associated Clinical Features

Candidal vaginitis is characterized by a thick curdy white discharge, (Fig. 10.1) and vulvar discomfort. Intense vulvar erythema, pruritus, or burning are often present. A microscopic slide prepared with 10% potassium hydroxide yielding characteristic branch chain hyphae and spores establishes the diagnosis (Fig. 17.13). The pH of the discharge is less than 4.5. Predisposing factors which should be considered include oral contraceptive, antibiotic, or corticosteroid use; pregnancy; and diabetes. Sexually transmitted diseases are not usually associated with isolated candidal vaginitis.

Trichomonas vaginitis presents as a persistent, thin, copious discharge that is often frothy (Fig. 10.2), green, or foul smelling. The pH of these secretions is greater than 4.5. The amount of vaginal and cervical erythema and inflammation varies considerably; thus the diagnosis depends on the presence of motile flagellates on normal saline wet mount microscopy. Occasionally, multiple petechiae on the vaginal wall (strawberry spots) or cervix (strawberry cervix) are seen.

Bacterial vaginosis (previously termed *Haemophilus,* or *Gardnerella* vaginitis) is characterized by a malodorous, homogeneous discharge (Fig. 10.3) with a pH greater than 4.5 and a transient amine (fishy) odor when mixed with a drop of KOH solution (positive sniff test). Clue cells present on normal saline wet mount establish the diagnosis (Fig. 17.14). Other associated vaginal or abdominal complaints are minimal and, if significant, may represent another disease process.

Differential Diagnosis

Vaginal foreign bodies, especially in prepubescent girls, may present with a heavy white discharge, but would be unaccompanied by vulvar erythema or the microscopic appearance of hyphae. Atrophic vaginitis is commonly found in postmenopausal women and is discriminated from candidal vaginitis by mucosal dryness, atrophy, dyspareunia, and minimal discharge, and itching. Other considerations include contact dermatitis, local irritation secondary to tight fitting underwear, and contact dermatitis from toiletry items.

ED Treatment and Disposition

For *candidal vaginitis,* various regimens of topical antifungal agents are the mainstay of treatment (clotrimazole 1% cream, one applicatorful inserted high into the vaginal vault for 7 nights, clotrimazole, two 100-mg vaginal tablets for 3 nights or one 500-mg vaginal tablet for single-dose treatment). Oral fluconazole (Diflucan, 150 mg as a single dose) is also effective. Nystatin vaginal tablets (100,000 U daily for 2 weeks) are generally considered safe for use in the first trimester of pregnancy.

For *Trichomonas vaginitis* a single, one-time dose of metronidazole (2 g) is generally curative. Alternatively, 250 mg given three times daily can be used for recurrent or refractory cases. Metronidazole is contraindicted in pregnancy and is associated with an Antabuse-like reaction when taken with alcohol. For the pregnant patient, clotrimazole (100-mg vaginal suppositories daily for 7 to 14 days) may provide symptomatic relief.

For *Bacterial vaginosis,* metronidazole (500 mg twice daily for 7 days) is recommended in the nonpregnant patient. Amoxicillin (500 mg tid for 7 days) or clindamycin (300 mg bid) for 7 days is a safe, but less effective, alternative during pregnancy. Treatment for asymptomatic infection or for male sexual partners is not generally recommended.

Clinical Pearls

1. Diabetes mellitus or immunosuppression should be considered in refractory or recurrent cases of candidal vaginitis.
2. A history of balanitis in the sexual partner should be sought and, if present, treated.
3. *Trichomonas* should be considered a sexually transmitted disease. It is generally recommended, therefore, that concomitant culturing for gonorrhea and *Chlamydia* be performed. Serologic testing for syphilis, HIV, and hepatitis B should be considered.
4. Patients treated with metronidazole should abstain from alcohol for the duration of treatment and for at least 24 h after their last dose.

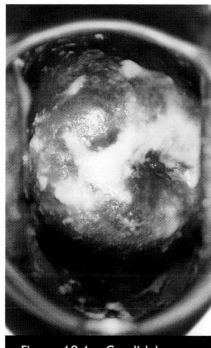

Figure 10.1   Candidal Vaginitis

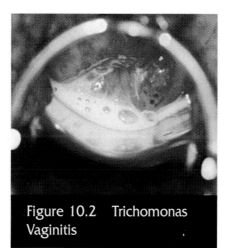

Figure 10.2   Trichomonas Vaginitis

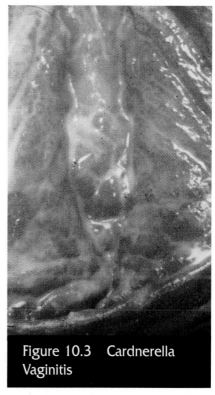

Figure 10.3   Cardnerella Vaginitis

Thick, curdy white discharge secondary to candidal vaginitis. (Courtesy of Kevin J. Knoop, MS, MD.)

Thin vaginal discharge suggestive of *Trichomonas* vaginitis. (Courtesy of H. Hunter Handsfield: *Atlas of Sexually Transmitted Diseases.* New York, McGraw-Hill, 1992.)

Thin milky white discharge suggestive of *Cardnerella* vaginitis. (Courtesy of Curatek Pharmaceuticals.)

Associated Clinical Features

The patient's chief complaint is often a purulent vaginal discharge. Speculum examination reveals a purulent, viscous discharge emanating from the cervical os (Fig. 10.4). Otherwise, a purulent discharge may be seen on a cervical swab. A Gram's stain may reveal either gram-negative intracellular diplococci consistent with *Neisseria* gonorrhoeae (Fig. 17.11) or be nonspecific, consistent with *Chlamydia trachomatis,* a coinfectant with *Gonococcus* about 50% of the time. When accompanied by symptoms of lower abdominal pain and signs of pelvic peritonitis such as cervical motion and adnexal tenderness, the diagnosis of pelvic inflammatory disease should be considered.

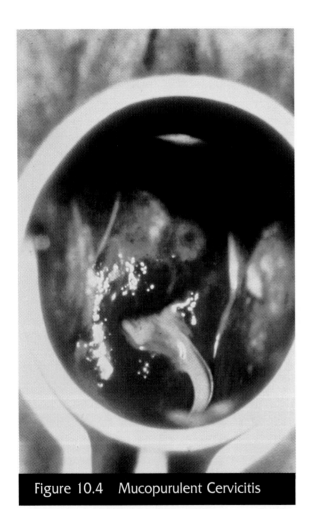

Figure 10.4   Mucopurulent Cervicitis

Viscous, opaque discharge emanating from the cervical os, consistent with mucopurulent cervicitis. The string from an intrauterine device is seen descending through the os in this patient. (Courtesy of Sue Rist FNP.)

Differential Diagnosis

Physiologic cervical mucous discharge at the time of ovulation may occur, but is generally clear, with few white blood cells on Gram's stain.

ED Treatment and Disposition

Cultures for *Chlamydia trachomatis* and *Neisseria gonorrhoeae* should be obtained prior to initiation of therapy. Ceftriaxone (125 mg as a single intramuscular dose) provides coverage for *Neisseria gonorrhoeae*. Single-dose oral quinolones (ciprofloxacin, 500 mg, or ofloxacin, 400 mg) can be used in penicillin-allergic patients. Doxycycline (100 mg) or ofloxacin (300 mg bid for 7 days or a single 1-g dose of azithromycin) provides coverage for *Chlamydia*. Erythromycin (base 500 mg qid for 7 days) is the alternative for pregnant patients.

Clinical Pearls

1. The discharge of candidal, trichomonal or *Gardnerella* vaginitis is almost never limited solely to the cervix.
2. Mucopurulent cervicitis is almost always secondary to a sexually transmitted disease; thus sexual partners should be treated as well.
3. Refer all patients for formal gynecologic follow-up after culture and treatment, since early cervical neoplasia may have a similar appearance.

Associated Clinical Features

Bartholin's glands and ducts are located over the lower third of the introitus near the labia minora. A cyst or abscess can result from an obstructed duct which usually occurs secondary to scarring from trauma, delivery, or episiotomy. Infection of the cyst is usually with mixed vaginal or fecal flora (*Escherichia coli*), but may also contain *Neisseria gonorrhoeae* and *Chlamydia trachomatis*. Progressive enlargement and infection leads to increasing pain, swelling, and dyspareunia. A tender, fluctuant cystic mass with surrounding labial edema is easily appreciated on examination (Fig. 10.5).

Differential Diagnosis

Epidermal inclusion cysts and sebaceous cysts of the labia majora may look similar, but are generally smaller. When inflamed or infected, maximal fluctuance generally points toward the external aspect of the labium, as opposed to Bartholin's gland cysts, which point medially. Occlusion and infection of apocrine sweat glands can lead to subcutaneous abscess formation—known as hidradenitis suppurativa. Vulvar hematoma, leiomyoma, lipoma, and fibromas may occasionally be confused with a noninfected Bartholin's cyst. Vulvar cancer usually arises in postmenopausal women and is generally either ulcerated, excoriated, or exophytic.

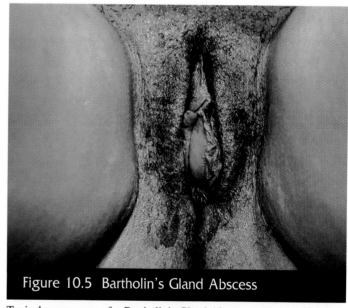

Figure 10.5 Bartholin's Gland Abscess

Typical appearance of a Bartholin's Gland Abscess with the labial fluctuance pointing medially. (Courtesy of the Medical Photography Department, Naval Medical Center, San Diego.)

ED Treatment and Disposition

Simple incision and drainage (Fig. 10.6) followed by sitz baths provide the most effective and expeditious relief on an emergency basis. Unfortunately, reocclusion and reaccumulation of cystic swelling are common. Definitive therapy of recurrent Bartholin's gland cysts involves marsupialization by suturing the introital mucosa to the inner cyst wall.

Clinical Pearls

1. Antibiotics, although commonly used, are usually not required.
2. Placement of a Word catheter into the cyst cavity (Fig. 10.7) decreases the incidence of reocclusion, but must be allowed to remain in place for up to 6 weeks to ensure epithelialization of the drainage tract.

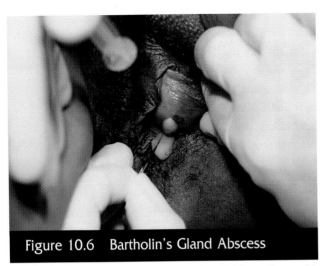

Figure 10.6   Bartholin's Gland Abscess

Medial incision of the cyst yielding purulent fluid, consistent with a Bartholin's gland abscess. (Courtesy of the Medical Photography Department, Naval Medical Center, San Diego.)

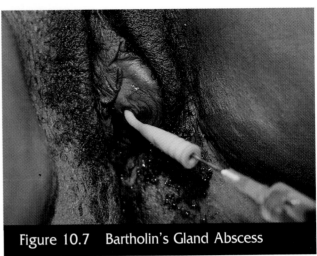

Figure 10.7   Bartholin's Gland Abscess

Insertion and inflation of a Word catheter into the cyst cavity. The free end of the catheter can be tucked into the vagina for long-term placement, allowing for the epithelialization of the incision site. (Courtesy of the Medical Photography Department, Naval Medical Center, San Diego.)

DIAGNOSIS   SPONTANEOUS ABORTION

Associated Clinical Features

Spontaneous abortion is associated with vaginal bleeding and abdominal discomfort. Severe pain, heavy bleeding with the passage of clots or tissue (Fig. 10.8), fever, and hypotension may also be present. *Threatened abortion* is diagnosed when mild cramping and vaginal bleeding are not accompanied by the complete or partial extrusion of tissue, cervical dilation, or ectopic pregnancy. Uterine cramping with progressive dilation of the cervix, with or without partial extrusion of the products of conception, indicates the presence of an *inevitable abortion* (Fig. 10.9). In an *incomplete abortion,* some elements of the conceptus have passed (Fig. 10.10), yet retained intrauterine tissue leads to ongoing uterine cramping, cervical dilation, and persistent bleeding.

Differential Diagnosis

Ectopic pregnancy should be considered in all first-trimester females with lower abdominal pain or vaginal bleeding. The presence of frank tissue passage or cervical dilation essentially excludes this diagnosis. Large blood clots or an intrauterine decidual cast (Fig. 10.11), however, may occasionally be mistaken for products of conception.

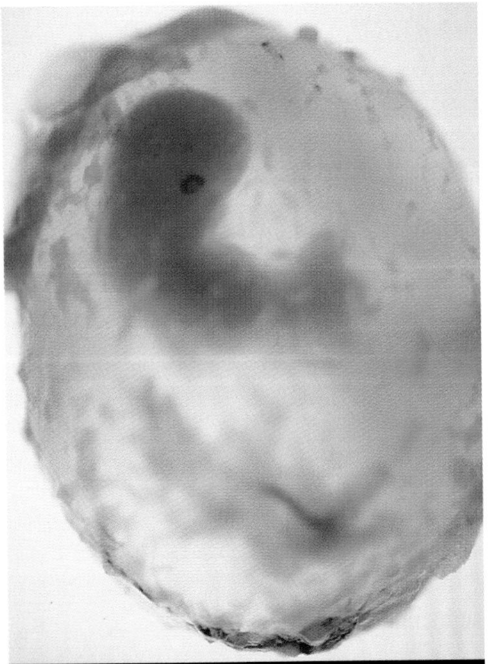

Figure 10.8   Spontaneous Abortion

Passage of tissue in a spontaneous abortion at 4 weeks. (Courtesy of Lawrence B. Stack, MD.)

ED Treatment and Disposition

Intravenous access, fluid resuscitation, cross-matching of blood, and urgent gynecologic consultation should be made in the presence of severe pain, heavy bleeding, or hypovolemia. All tissue should be sent to pathology for definitive identification. Occasionally, patients who initially have an open cervical os will rapidly expel the remaining products of conception, with subsequent resolution of all pain and bleeding. These patients may be discharged from the emergency department with the diagnosis of completed abortion if otherwise clinically stable. Anti-Rh immunoglobulin (RhoGAM) should be administered in all cases of vaginal bleeding in the pregnant patient where the mother is Rh negative and the father is not Rh negative.

Clinical Pearls

1. The passage of large clots usually indicates rapid heavy bleeding.
2. *Completed abortion* is characterized by the passage of tissue, followed by resolution of bleeding and closure of the cervical os.
3. Fever, leukocytosis, pelvic tenderness, and malodorous cervical discharge should suggest *septic abortion*.

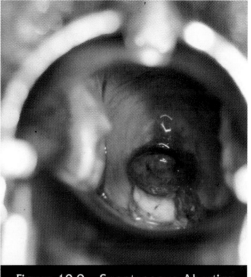

Figure 10.9   Spontaneous Abortion

Dilation of the cervical os with partial extrusion of tissue in the setting of an inevitable abortion. (Courtesy of Robert Buckley, MD.)

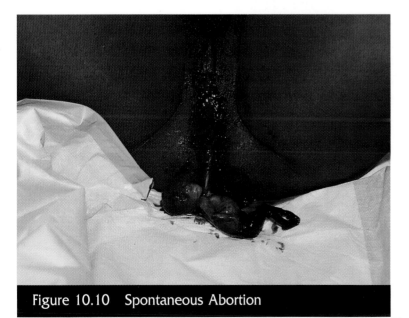

Figure 10.10   Spontaneous Abortion

Expulsion of fetal tissue in a second-trimester spontaneous abortion. (Courtesy of Robert Buckley, MD.)

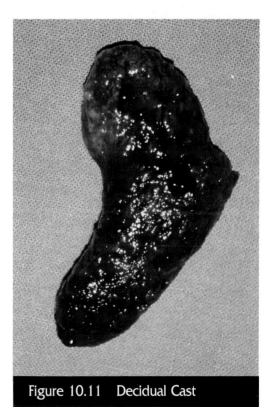

Figure 10.11   Decidual Cast

A decidual cast or organized clot may occasionally be mistaken for products of conception. (Courtesy of the Medical Photography Department, Naval Medical Center, San Diego.)

Associated Clinical Features

Patients who present for examination and treatment following an incident of sexual assault are ideally cared for by a multidisciplinary team capable of addressing the immediate medical and psychosocial needs of the patient in concert with forensic and legal requirements. A thorough general examination may reveal associated contusions and other soft-tissue injuries. A meticulous inspection of the perineum, rectum, vaginal fornices, vagina, and cervix is required to identify inflicted injuries. Toluidine staining and colposcopy are often useful in enhancing less apparent injuries such as those to the posterior fourchette following sexual assault (Fig. 10.12). These are most commonly found between the 3 and 9 o'clock distribution when the patient is examined in the dorsal lithotomy position. Perianal lacerations (Fig. 10.13) may also be seen as toluidine-enhanced linear tears (Fig. 10.14). Examination of the cervix and posterior vaginal vault may reveal injuries to those structures (Fig. 10.15).

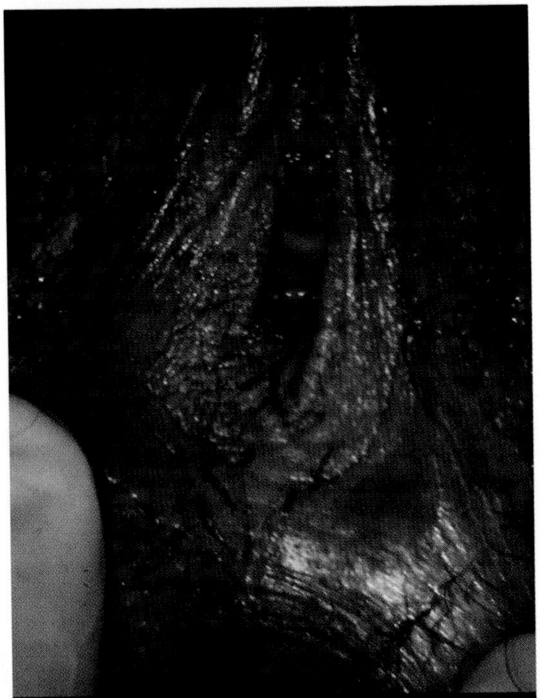

Figure 10.12   Genital Trauma (Posterior Fourchette)

Linear tears to the posterior fourchette due to sexual assault enhanced by toluidine staining. (Courtesy of Hillary J. Larkin, PA-C and Lauri A. Paolinetti, PA-C.)

Differential Diagnosis

Perineal injuries from accidental trauma may be indistinguishable from those of sexual assault and should be interpreted in the context of the history. The assessment of assault or rape is technically a legal one; therefore, the examiner should be careful to document the medical appearance of the wounds, rather than speculate as to the specific mechanism by which each injury occurred.

ED Treatment and Disposition

Treatment is preceded by forensic evidence gathering, consisting of a Wood's lamp examination to identify semen for collection, pubic hair sampling and combing, vaginal and cervical smears (air-dried), a cervical and vaginal wet mount to identify sperm, vaginal aspirate to test for acid phosphatase, and rectal or buccal swabs for sperm. A prepackaged kit with directions may be available to facilitate evidence collection.

Cervical cultures for *Chlamydia* and gonorrhea should be obtained as well as serum testing for syphilis, hepatitis, and HIV. Empiric antibiotic coverage against sexually transmitted diseases should be provided and an oral contraceptive offered (after confirming a nonpregnant state) to prevent unwanted pregnancy.

Clinical Pearls

1. The medical care of the patient who has been sexually assaulted should ideally be performed by experienced supportive staff familiar with the details of forensic evidence gathering and colposcopic photography.
2. Normal findings on physical examination and no sperm on wet preparation do *not* exclude the possibility of assault.

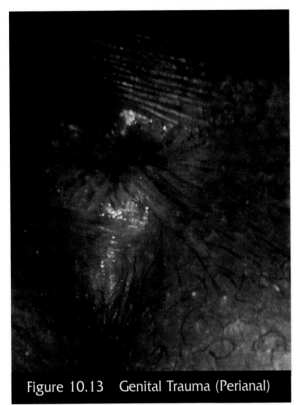

Figure 10.13   Genital Trauma (Perianal)

Perianal lacerations following sexual assault. (Courtesy of Hillary J. Larkin, PA-C and Lauri A. Paolinetti, PA-C.)

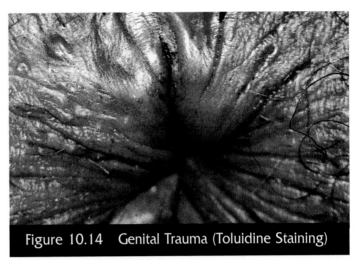

Figure 10.14   Genital Trauma (Toluidine Staining)

Toluidine staining showing subtle perianal lacerations following forceful anal penetration. (Courtesy of Aurora Mendez RN.)

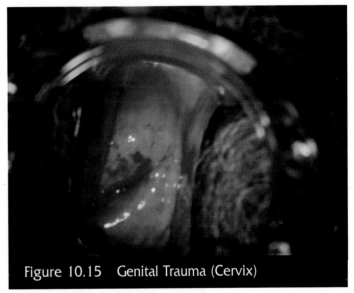

Figure 10.15   Genital Trauma (Cervix)

Cervical trauma in an elderly victim of sexual assault. Petechiae and freshly bleeding abrasions are noted from 10 to 3 o'clock. (Courtesy of Hillary J. Larkin, PA-C and Lauri A. Paolinetti, PA-C.)

Associated Clinical Features

Uterine prolapse is defined as the propulsion of the uterus through the pelvic floor or vaginal introitus. In first-degree prolapse, the cervix descends into the lower third of the vagina. In second-degree prolapse, the cervix usually protrudes through the introitus, whereas in third-degree prolapse, or procidentia, the entire uterus is externalized with inversion of the vagina. (Fig. 10.16) Symptoms include a sensation of inguinal traction, low back pain, urinary incontinence, and the presence of a vaginal mass.

Differential Diagnosis

Uterine prolapse can occasionally be confused with a cystocele, enterocele, or a soft-tissue tumor. These disorders, which may all be accompanied by introital bulging, are easily distinguished by the absence of cervicouterine descent.

ED Treatment and Disposition

Patients with first- or second-degree prolapse should be referred to a gynecologist for pessary placement or surgical correction. With procidentia, the uterus should be manually reduced into the vaginal vault and the patient placed at bedrest until evaluated by a gynecologic consultant.

Clinical Pearl

1. With procidentia, the exposed uterus is prone to abrasion and possible secondary infection.

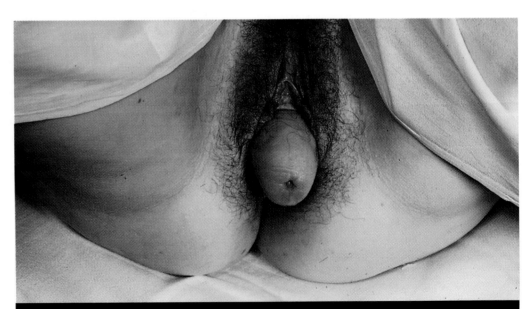

Figure 10.16   Third-Degree Uterine Prolapse

Note the protrusion of the entire uterus with cervix visable through the vaginal introitus. (Courtesy of Matthew Backer, Jr., MD.)

Associated Clinical Features

A cystocele occurs when there is relaxation and bulging of the posterior bladder wall and trigone into the vagina (Fig. 10.17) and is usually due to birth trauma. Patients complain of bulging or fullness over the introitus that is worsened with Valsalva (Fig. 10.18) and relieved with recumbency. It is often associated with urinary incontinence or symptoms of incomplete emptying. Most cystoceles, however, are asymptomatic. Examination reveals a thin-walled bulging of the anterior vaginal wall, which, in severe cases, may pass through the introitus with Valsalva.

Differential Diagnosis

An enterocele may lead to a similar bulging of the anterior vaginal wall but is much less common and is generally limited to those patients who have had a hysterectomy. Rectocele, uterine prolapse, and soft-tissue tumors should also be considered.

ED Treatment and Disposition

Larger cystoceles or those associated with urinary symptomatology, pain, or bothersome bulging should be referred to a gynecologist for further evaluation.

Clinical Pearl

1. Most cystoceles are asymptomatic and are detected incidentally at the time of pelvic examination.

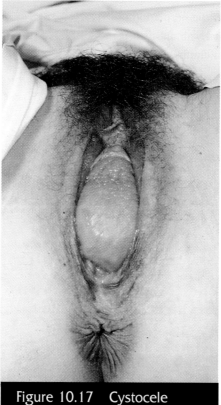

Figure 10.17 Cystocele

Cystocele with bulging of the posterior bladder wall into the vagina. (Courtesy of Matthew Backer, Jr., MD.)

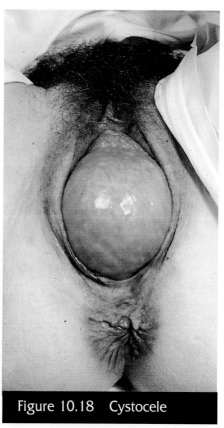

Figure 10.18 Cystocele

Cystocele worsening with Valsalva. (Courtesy of Matthew Backer, Jr., MD.)

Associated Clinical Features

Most small rectoceles are completely asymptomatic, though symptoms of introital bulging, constipation, and incomplete rectal evacuation may occur. Bulging of the introitus can be seen grossly on physical examination (Fig. 10.19) and can become worse with Valsalva (Fig. 10.20). Rectovaginal examination reveals a thin-walled protrusion of the rectovaginal septum into the lower part of the vagina.

Differential Diagnosis

Cystocele, enterocele, uterine prolapse, and soft-tissue tumors should all be easily distinguished by careful inspection.

ED Treatment and Disposition

Supportive measures with hydration, laxatives, and stool softeners are generally all that is needed to relieve the patient's symptoms. Those patients with large symptomatic rectoceles, who do not desire further childbearing, are candidates for posterior colpoperineorrhaphy.

Clinical Pearl

1. A rectocele is the herniation of the rectovaginal wall and is usually due to childbirth.

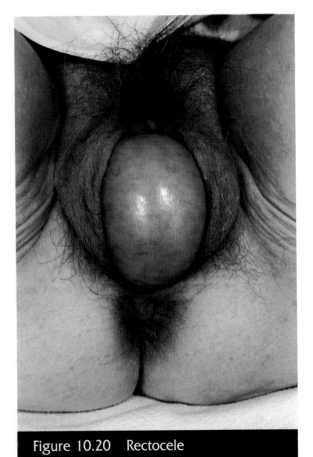

Figure 10.20   Rectocele

Worsening of the rectocele with Valsalva. (Courtesy of Matthew Backer, Jr., MD.)

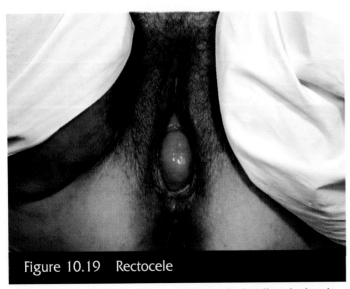

Figure 10.19   Rectocele

Characterized by bulging of the posterior vaginal wall at the introitus. (Courtesy of Matthew Backer, Jr., MD.)

Associated Clinical Features

Ectopic pregnancy is the leading cause of maternal obstetric morbidity in the first trimester of pregnancy. Presentations commonly include mild vaginal bleeding and lower abdominal pain, but patients can present in shock secondary to massive hemorrhage. The menstrual history, although often unreliable, may reveal a missed or recent abnormal menses. The presence of early signs of pregnancy (breast changes, morning sickness, fatigue) is variable. On examination, the uterus may be slightly enlarged, and adnexal tenderness is not always present. The visualization of an intrauterine pregnancy (IUP) by ultrasound (US) essentially excludes the diagnosis of ectopic pregnancy, the exception being a rare dual pregnancy (IUP and ectopic). The appearance of a gestational sac at about 5 weeks (Fig. 10.21) is the first significant finding on US *suggestive* of an IUP; however, definitive diagnosis of IUP should be deferred until a yolk sac is present (Fig. 10.22). A fetal pole develops next and can be seen on part of the yolk sac (Fig. 10.23). The double decidual sac sign is evidence of a true gestational sac and should be differentiated from the pseudogestational sac formed from a decidual cast in ectopic pregnancy (Fig. 10.24). When no gestational sac is visualized ("empty uterus") (Fig. 10.25), ectopic pregnancy cannot be distinguished from an early IUP too small to be seen on US.

Differential Diagnosis

Ectopic pregnancy should be considered in all first-trimester females presenting to the emergency department with either lower abdominal pain or tenderness, or vaginal bleeding. A spontaneously completed abortion with an empty uterine cavity may lead to confusion if the beta human chorionic gonadotropin (βhCG) level is elevated above the institution's or sonographer's discriminatory zone (generally above 2000 mIU/mL) and clinical evidence for the passage of products of con-

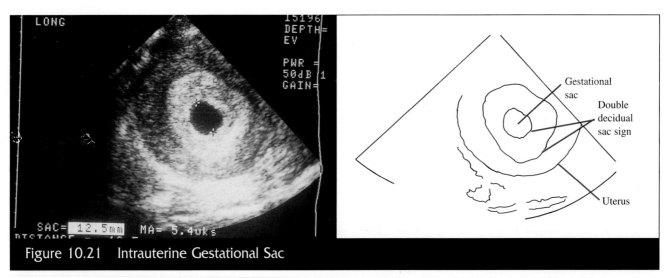

Figure 10.21   Intrauterine Gestational Sac

Discrete ring of an intrauterine gestational sac seen on transvaginal ultrasound. No yolk sac is visualized. A double decidual sac sign is seen, however, lending evidence of a true gestational sac versus a pseudogestational sac formed from a decidual cast in ectopic pregnancy. A thorough look in the adnexa is important in diagnosing ectopic pregnancy when a gestational sac is the only finding. (Courtesy of Janice Underwood.)

ception is lacking. Alternative causes of first-trimester lower abdominal pain or vaginal bleeding include threatened or incomplete abortion, molar pregnancy, ruptured corpus luteum cyst, adnexal torsion, urinary tract infection, appendicitis, pelvic inflammatory disease, and ureteral calculi.

ED Treatment and Disposition

Unstable patients require aggressive resuscitation with fluid and blood followed by surgery. Stable patients with an ultrasound diagnosis consistent with ectopic pregnancy (Fig. 10.24) warrant immediate gynecologic consultation. Definitive therapeutic options range from observation in asymptomatic patients with declining hCG levels, traditional or laparoscopic surgery, to pharmacologic therapy with methotrexate. Despite the diminished diagnostic accuracy of ultrasound at lower levels (up to half of all ectopic pregnancies have a serum hCG level less than 2000 mIU/mL), if there is a strong clinical suspicion for ectopic pregnancy, gynecologic consultation should be considered. Those patients in whom a normal intrauterine pregnancy is visualized can be safely discharged with early outpatient follow-up.

Clinical Pearls

1. Ectopic pregnancy should be considered in all women of reproductive age presenting with vaginal bleeding, abdominal pain or tenderness, or a missed menstrual period.

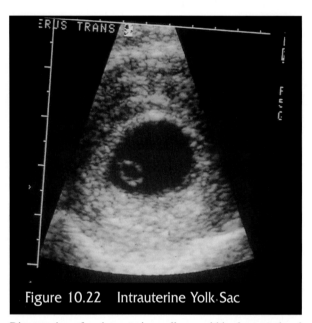

Figure 10.22   Intrauterine Yolk Sac

Discrete ring of an intrauterine yolk sac within the gestational sac seen on transvaginal ultrasound. Definitive diagnosis of IUP should be deferred until a fetal pole is present in the sac. (Courtesy of Janice Underwood.)

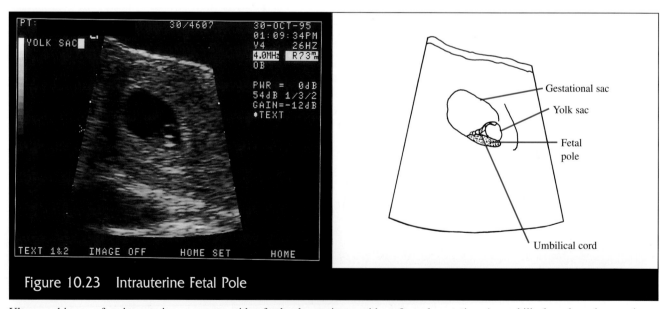

Figure 10.23   Intrauterine Fetal Pole

Ultrasound image of an intrauterine pregnancy with a fetal pole consistent with an 8-week gestation. An umbilical cord can be seen interposed between the yolk sac and the fetal pole. (Courtesy of Robert Buckley, MD.)

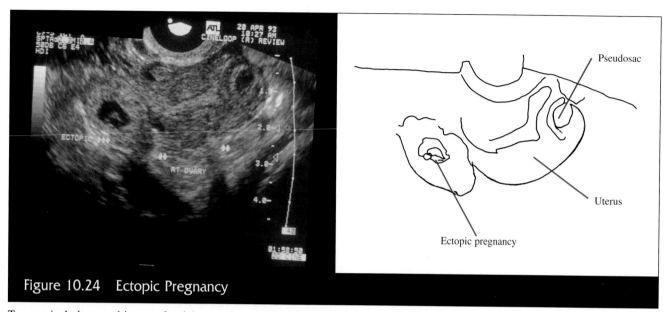

Figure 10.24   Ectopic Pregnancy

Transvaginal ultrasound image of a right ectopic pregnancy with a decidual reaction in the uterus resembling a gestational sac, or "pseudosac." Visualization of a pseudogestational, or "single," sac sign could be consistent with an early gestational sac or an ectopic pregnancy with a uterine decidual cast. (Courtesy of Janice Underwood.)

2. Failure to visualize an intrauterine pregnancy by transvaginal ultrasonography by the time the serum hCG level has reached approximately 2000 mIU/mL or by abdominal ultrasound once it has reached a level of approximately 6000 mIU/mL is highly suggestive of the diagnosis of ectopic pregnancy.

3. The ability of ultrasound and quantitative βhCG to diagnose ectopic pregnancy is highly dependent on the resolution of the machine, the skill of the examiner, and the βhCG assay used. Thus, every institution and examiner must develop a specific "discriminatory zone," the level of βhCG on which to base diagnostic decisions.

4. A decidual cast in the uterus of an ectopic pregnancy may resemble a gestational sac of an intrauterine pregnancy on ultrasound.

5. Consider ectopic pregnancy in any female of reproductive age presenting with syncope.

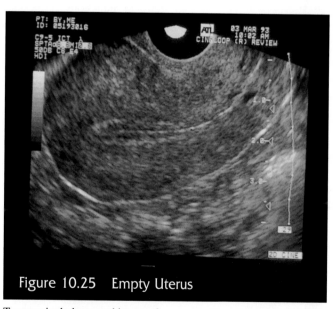

Figure 10.25   Empty Uterus

Transvaginal ultrasound image of an apparently empty uterus. Ectopic pregnancy should be strongly suspected if a transvaginal ultrasound reveals an empty uterus in the setting of a serum quantitative hCG level above the institution's discriminatory zone. (Courtesy of Janice Underwood.)

Obstetric Conditions

Associated Clinical Features

Trauma is a major cause of maternal and fetal mortality. In addition to the common solid organ and hollow viscous injuries associated with blunt abdominal trauma, special consideration should be given to the possibility of preterm labor, fetal-maternal hemorrhage, uterine rupture, and most importantly, abruptio placentae. Abruptio placentae is defined as the premature separation of the placenta from the site of uterine implantation. It is found in up to 50% of major blunt trauma patients and up to 5% of those with apparent minor injuries. There are generally signs of uterine hyperactivity and fetal distress when significant placental detachment occurs. Most patients have vaginal bleeding, although in up to 20%, the margins of detachment are above the cervical os and therefore have little or no vaginal bleeding. Laboratory evidence of a consumptive coagulopathy is occasionally seen with significant abruption. Electronic fetal monitoring is of paramount importance in all cases of significant trauma in patients beyond 20 weeks' gestation. As the pregnancy progresses toward term, a normal heart rate averages between 120 and 160 bpm. Rapid frequent fluctuations in the baseline are characteristic of normal "reactivity" (Fig. 10.26). The loss of this reactivity can occur during a normal sleep cycle, following narcotic administration, or most importantly, in the setting of fetal hypoxia or distress (Fig. 10.27). Decelerations are transient reductions in the fetal heart rate. Late decelerations begin after the contraction begins and return to baseline well after it ends, with the nadir of the deceleration occurring after the peak of the uterine contraction. Late decelerations should suggest fetal hypoxia, especially when accompanied by a loss of normal baseline variability (Fig. 10.28). Variable decelerations are characterized by deep, broad decreases in fetal heart rate, often falling below 100 bpm (Fig. 10.29). They can occur slightly before, during, or after the onset of a uterine contraction, hence the term *variable*. Variable decelerations are caused by the transient compression of the umbili-

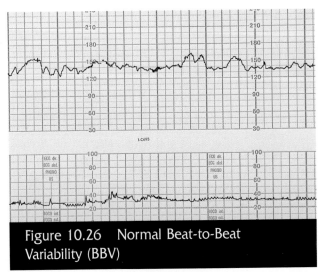

Figure 10.26   Normal Beat-to-Beat Variability (BBV)

A normal reactive fetal monitor strip showing a baseline heart rate between 120 and 160 with fluctuations in the short- and long-term heart rate. (Courtesy of Timothy Jahn, MD.)

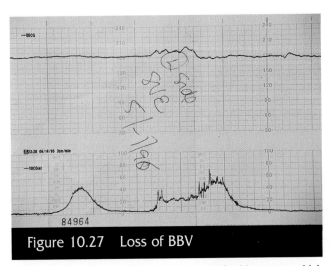

Figure 10.27   Loss of BBV

Loss of beat-to-beat variability (BBV) in the fetal heart rate, which may forewarn of fetal distress. This same pattern may also be seen during a normal sleep cycle or following maternal narcotic administration. (Courtesy of Gerard Van Houdt, MD.)

cal cord during a contraction and are rarely associated with significant hypoxia or acidosis, unless they are frequent or prolonged. They are most commonly appreciated during the second stage of labor, when forceful uterine compression transiently occludes the umbilical cord as the infant is propelled through the birth canal.

Differential Diagnosis

Another alternative cause of bright red vaginal bleeding in the third trimester of pregnancy is placenta previa. This can generally be differentiated from abruption by the visualization of a low-lying placenta on ultrasound.

ED Treatment and Disposition

An obstetrician should be consulted immediately in all trauma patients beyond 20 weeks' gestation. Blood for type- and cross-matching, complete blood count, prothrombin time (PT), partial

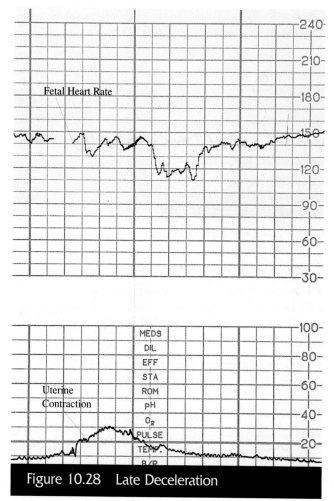

Figure 10.28   Late Deceleration

The nadir of a late deceleration always follows the peak of the uterine contraction with the heart rate approaching the baseline after the completion of the uterine contraction, suggestive of hypoxia. (Courtesy of James Palombaro, MD.)

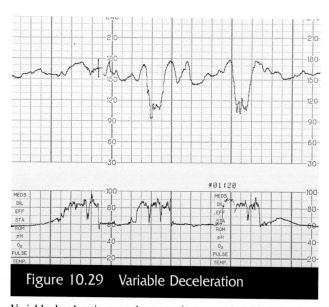

Figure 10.29   Variable Deceleration

Variable decelerations are due to cord compression. They are characterized by a rapid onset and recovery and may occur slightly before, during, or after the onset of the contraction. (Courtesy of John O. Boyle, MD.)

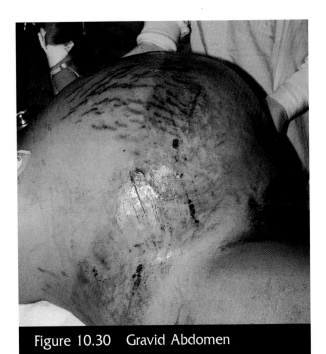

Figure 10.30 Gravid Abdomen

A third-trimester gravid abdomen with ecchymotic markings imparted by a significant blunt force. Fetal assessment should occur simultaneously with maternal resuscitation. (Courtesy of John Fildes, MD.)

thromboplastin time (PTT), fibrinogen, and fibrin degradation products or D-dimer should be obtained. It is generally recommended that patients undergo continuous tocofetal monitoring for a minimum of 4 h to rule out preterm labor or fetal distress. Ultrasound is essential in visualizing placental abruption. Indications for emergency cesarean section include placental abruption, signs of ongoing fetal distress, or uncontrolled maternal hemorrhage.

Clinical Pearls

1. A gravid abdomen with ecchymotic markings imparted by a significant blunt force (Fig. 10.30) are not always present; thus, a careful history of the mechanism of trauma and associated complaints is essential.
2. Anti-Rh immunoglobulin should be administered for all cases of significant third-trimester blunt abdominal trauma if the mother is Rh-negative and the father is not Rh-negative as well.

DIAGNOSIS   FERNING PATTERN OF AMNIOTIC FLUID

Associated Clinical Features

Patients beyond the 20th week of pregnancy presenting with a history of uncontrolled leakage of fluid should undergo sterile speculum examination to determine the presence of amniotic fluid. The diagnosis of membrane rupture can be made by observing the passage of fluid from the cervix or pooling in the vaginal vault. Without gross evidence of rupture, secretions from the vaginal vault can be placed on a slide and allowed to air dry. The characteristic arborization, or ferning pattern (Fig. 10.31), is diagnostic of amniotic fluid, thus rupture of the membranes. In addition, the secretions can be applied to nitrazine paper. The pH of normal vaginal secretions generally falls between 4.5 and 5.5, whereas amniotic fluid generally ranges between 7.0 and 7.5, yielding a dark blue tint.

Differential Diagnosis

Urinary incontinence is the most common alternative diagnosis in a third-trimester patient who presents with a history of possible membrane rupture. The passage of the cervical mucous plug, known as bloody show, may rarely be confused with the passage of amniotic fluid. Although a small, subclinical amniotic fluid leak can never be completely excluded, the presence of an acid pH, the absence of gross fluid in the vaginal vault and ferning, all point against the diagnosis of membrane rupture.

ED Treatment and Disposition

All patients with confirmed ruptured fetal membranes should be admitted to the labor and delivery area and the obstetrical consultant notified, irrespective of the presence or absence of uterine contractions. The greatest risk to the fetus before 37 weeks is that of preterm delivery. The fetus at term is at risk for infection, secondary to chorioamnionitis, if the time from membrane rupture to vaginal delivery exceeds 24 h.

Clinical Pearls

1. With a strong suspicion of membrane rupture by history and no objective evidence of amniotic fluid on examination, a large sterile pad may be placed on the perineum and the patient reexamined after brief ambulation. This assumes the absence of uterine contractions and the presence of a reactive fetal monitor strip.

2. Umbilical cord prolapse should be excluded in all cases of membrane rupture with a speculum examination.

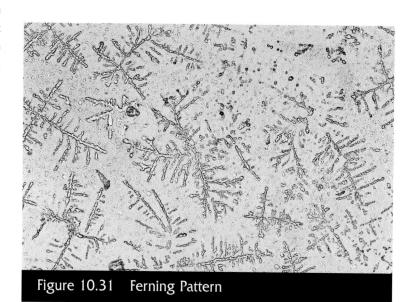

Figure 10.31   Ferning Pattern

The arborization pattern found when a drop of amniotic fluid is allowed to air dry on a microscope slide, known as ferning. (Courtesy of Robert Buckley, MD.)

EMERGENCY DELIVERY:
IMMINENT VERTEX DELIVERY—CROWNING

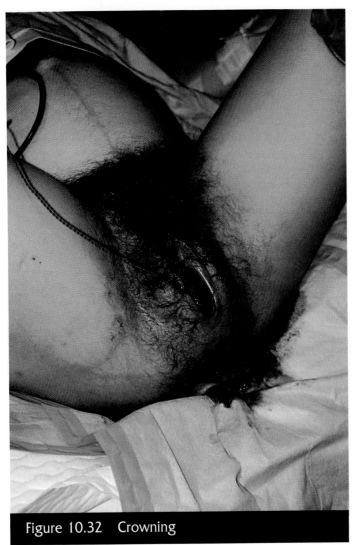

Figure 10.32   Crowning

Descent of the fetal head with separation of the labia is known as crowning and heralds imminent vertex delivery. (Courtesy of William Leninger, MD.)

Associated Clinical Features

The second stage of labor begins when the cervix is fully dilated, allowing for the gradual descent of the head toward the vaginal outlet. As the head approaches the perineum, the labia begin to separate with each contraction, then recede, once the contraction subsides. Crowning is the term applied when the head separates the labial margins without receding at the end of the contraction. (Fig. 10.32)

ED Treatment and Disposition

The appearance of crowning heralds imminent vaginal delivery. Equipment for delivery and neonatal resuscitation should be brought to the bedside. Both the on-call obstetric consultant and pediatrician should be notified while preparations are being made for emergency department delivery.

Clinical Pearls

1. Primigravida patients may still require multiple sets of contractions and pushing to fully expel the head through the vaginal outlet.
2. If meconium secretions are detected well before delivery, continuous electronic tocofetal monitoring should be begun and the obstetric and pediatric consultants notified.

Associated Clinical Features

A gravid female with regular forceful contractions and the urge to strain (push) can present without warning. Crowning may be present and heralds imminent vaginal delivery. Important historical questions include the number of previous pregnancies, a diagnosis of twin gestations, and whether there has been prenatal care or complications. The presence of greenish brown fetal stool, known as meconium, is associated with fetal hypoxia and is a clinical indicator of fetal distress. Fetal bradycardia or late decelerations (Fig. 10.28) may be present and are also evidence of fetal distress.

Differential Diagnosis

Complications (discussed below) should be considered when the progress of delivery is altered or when the presenting part is something other than the occiput. Twin gestations should be considered in all emergency deliveries and asked about early in the history.

ED Treatment and Disposition

Intravenous access, oxygen, and equipment for delivery and neonatal resuscitation (suction, oxygen, warming light, etc) are immediately obtained as preparation for the impending delivery.

Delivery of the Head

As the vertex passes through the vaginal outlet, extension of the head occurs, followed by the appearance of the forehead and chin. Extension and delivery of the fetal head can be facilitated by applying gentle pressure upward on the chin through the perineum—known as the modified Ritgen maneuver (Fig. 10.33). Simultaneously, the fingers of the other hand can be used to elevate the scalp to help extend the head. Once the head has been delivered, the occiput promptly rotates toward a left or right lateral position. At this stage, the nuchal region should be swept to detect the presence of a nuchal umbilical cord. Before the delivery of the shoulders, the nasopharynx should be gently suctioned with a bulb syringe to clear away any blood or amniotic debris. If thick meconium is present, deeper and more thorough suctioning of the posterior pharynx and glottic region should be accomplished with a mechanical suction trap, since aspiration of thick meconium by the newborn can lead to pneumonitis and hypoxia.

Delivery of the Shoulders

Delivery of the shoulders generally occurs spontaneously with little manipulation. Occasionally, gentle downward traction applied by grasping the sides of the head with two hands eases the delivery of the anterior shoulder (Fig. 10.34). The head can then be directed upward to permit the delivery of the posterior shoulder (Fig. 10.35). Following delivery of both shoulders, the body and legs are easily delivered. Attention is then directed toward the immediate care of the newborn. The cord is doubly clamped and ligated (Fig. 10.36) and inspected for three vessels: two umbilical arteries and one umbilical vein (Fig. 10.37). The child's pediatrician should be notified if a two-vessel umbilical cord is found at delivery. The newborn is immediately placed under a warming lamp for drying and gentle stimulation while being observed for signs of distress (heart rate <100, limp muscle tone, poor color, weak cry).

Delivery of the Placenta

Following delivery, gentle traction can be placed on the cord while the opposite hand is used to massage the uterine fundus (Fig. 10.38). The placenta will generally be delivered within 15 to 20 min (Fig. 10.39) and should be grossly inspected. Retention of small fragments should be suspected when inspection of the placenta reveals evidence of a missing segment or cotyledon (Fig. 10.40). The attending obstetric consultant should be notified, since retained placental fragments often warrant manual exploration of the uterus, especially in the context of persistent postpartum bleeding.

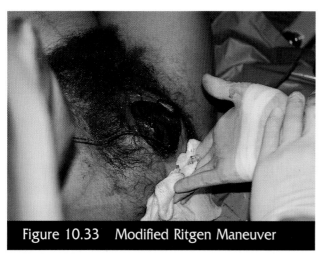

Figure 10.33   Modified Ritgen Maneuver

Modified Ritgen maneuver: upward pressure is applied on the fetal chin through the perineum. (Courtesy of William Leninger, MD.)

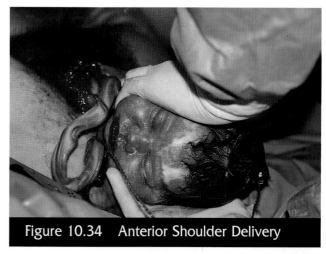

Figure 10.34   Anterior Shoulder Delivery

Delivery of the anterior shoulder is facilitated with downward traction. (Courtesy of William Leninger, MD.)

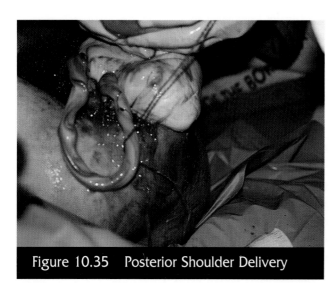

Figure 10.35   Posterior Shoulder Delivery

Delivery of the posterior shoulder with upward traction. (Courtesy of William Leninger, MD.)

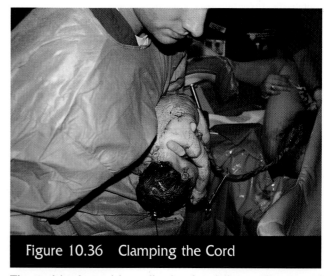

Figure 10.36   Clamping the Cord

The cord is clamped immediately after delivery. (Courtesy of William Leninger, MD.)

Clinical Pearls

1. Both obstetric and pediatric consultants should be alerted that preparations are being made for emergency department delivery.
2. A two-vessel cord may be found in about 1 in 500 singleton deliveries and is associated with an increased incidence of congenital defects.
3. Retained placental fragments should be considered in the setting of postpartum hemorrhage or endometritis.

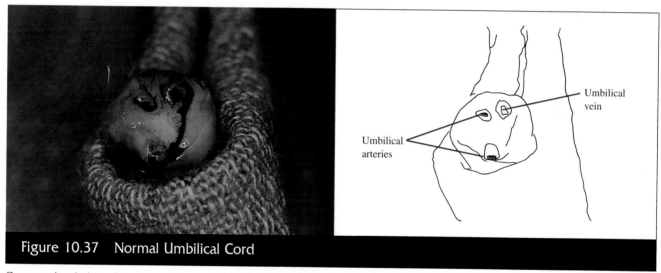

Figure 10.37 Normal Umbilical Cord

Cross-sectional view of the two arteries and single vein of a normal three-vessel umbilical cord. (Courtesy of Jennifer Jagoe, MD.)

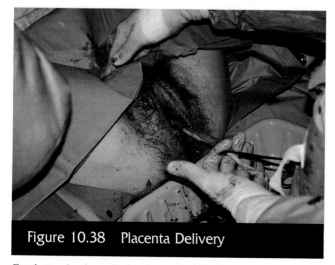

Figure 10.38 Placenta Delivery

Gentle traction is applied to the cord while the opposite hand massages the uterus. (Courtesy of William Leninger, MD.)

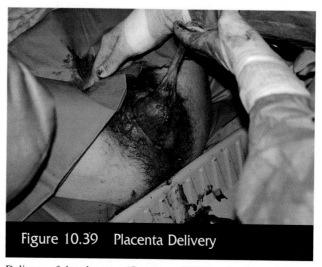

Figure 10.39 Placenta Delivery

Delivery of the placenta. (Courtesy of William Leninger, MD.)

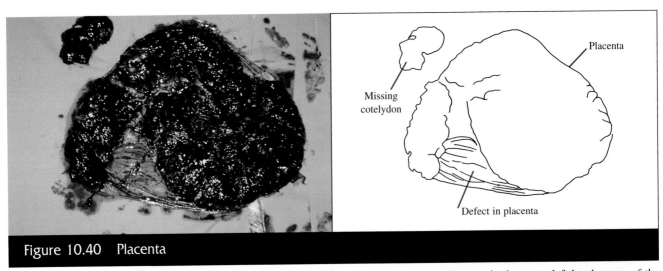

Figure 10.40   Placenta

Placenta with evidence of a missing segment or cotyledon. The missing placental tissue can be seen in the upper left-hand corner of the photograph. (Courtesy of John O. Boyle, MD.)

DIAGNOSIS

UMBILICAL CORD PROLAPSE IN EMERGENCY DELIVERY

Associated Clinical Features

In an overt cord prolapse, a loop of umbilical cord is visualized either at the introitus (Fig. 10.41) or on speculum examination following membrane rupture (Fig. 10.42). Alternatively, a small loop of cord may be palpated at the cervical os. In a funic cord prolapse, a loop of umbilical cord is palpated directly through intact fetal membranes. Occult prolapse occurs when the umbilical cord descends between the presenting part and the lower uterine segment, but is not visible or directly palpable on examination. Intermittent compression of the umbilical cord with each uterine contraction may be detected by the presence of variable decelerations of the fetal monitor (Fig. 10.29). The new onset of variable decelerations should always prompt immediate cervical examination to rule out an overt cord prolapse. Severe persistent bradycardia may ensue if cord compression is sustained beyond the duration of the contraction, which is often the case in an overt prolapse.

Differential Diagnosis

Rarely, an inexperienced examiner may mistake a presenting hand or foot for a prolapsed cord. This may be clarified by careful digital or speculum examination.

ED Treatment and Disposition

Prolapse of the umbilical cord presents an immediate threat to the fetal circulation and constitutes an obstetric emergency. If an overt prolapse is detected in the emergency department, the

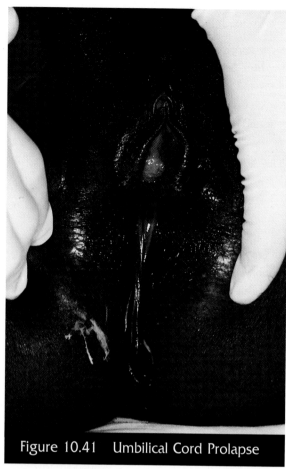

Figure 10.41   Umbilical Cord Prolapse

Prolapsed umbilical cord visible at the vaginal introitus in a patient with twin gestations. (Courtesy of Kevin J. Knoop, MD., MS.)

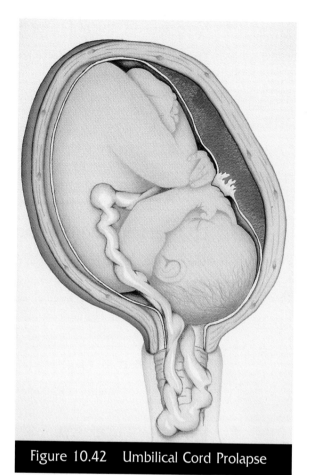

Figure 10.42   Umbilical Cord Prolapse

Schematic drawing of an overt prolapse of the umbilical cord through partially dilated cervical os. (Courtesy of Judy Christianson.)

patient should immediately be placed in a knee-chest position and continuous upward pressure applied by the examining hand to relieve the pressure of the presenting part on the lower uterine segment. An obstetrician should be summoned immediately and the patient taken directly to the operating room for cesarean delivery. Continuous upward pressure should be applied to the presenting part of the fetus at all times during transport. Occasionally, precipitous vaginal delivery may ensue in the emergency department shortly after detecting a cord prolapse. Resuscitative equipment should be available in anticipation of a physiologically compromised infant. If a funic prolapse is appreciated in the emergency department, an obstetrician should be notified and the patient prepared for cesarean delivery. Under no circumstance should the membranes be broken. Occult prolapse is rarely appreciated in the emergency department.

Clinical Pearl

1. Pelvic examination to exclude umbilical cord prolapse should be performed immediately following rupture of membranes, the appearance of variable decelerations, or the detection of bradycardia.

Associated Clinical Features

The incidence of singleton breech presentation is approximately 3%, but rises to higher than 20% in preterm infants weighing less than 2000 g. In a frank breech, both hips are flexed and both knees extended. In a complete breech, both hips and knees are flexed, whereas a footling breech has one or both legs extended below the buttocks. Frank breech is most common in full-term deliveries, whereas footling presentation can be found in up to half of all preterm deliveries. Breech deliveries carry a much higher mortality rate than cephalic deliveries. Complications of breech delivery include umbilical cord prolapse, nuchal arm obstruction, and difficulty in delivery of the following head (Fig. 10.43).

ED Treatment and Disposition

The specific maneuvers for breech extraction are beyond the scope of this text. If breech delivery appears imminent, support and gentle traction should be applied as the various parts spontaneously pass through the vaginal outlet, keeping in mind that the biparietal diameter is greater than either the bitrochanteric or bisacromial diameter.

Clinical Pearl

1. Immediate obstetric consultation should be obtained in all breech deliveries.

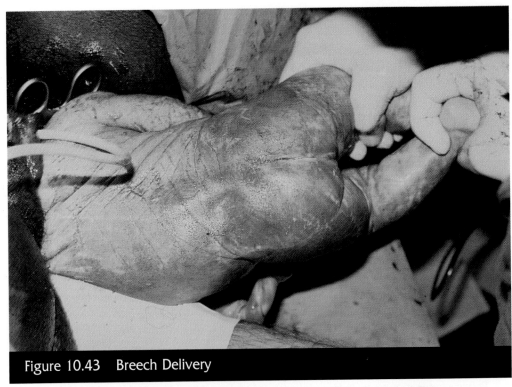

Figure 10.43 Breech Delivery

Footling breech vaginal delivery of the following head. (Courtesy of John O. Boyle, MD.)

Associated Clinical Features

The circumferential wrapping of the umbilical cord around the child's neck occurs in about 20% of all deliveries. (Fig. 10.44) Tight approximation of the cord around the infant's neck can lead to transient disruption of uterine blood flow during contractions leading to variable decelerations of the fetal heart rate monitor (Fig. 10.29), as well as impede delivery once the head passes through the introitus.

ED Treatment and Disposition

Once a cord is identified around the neck, it is readily slipped over the head. Occasionally two coils are identified.

Clinical Pearl

1. A loosely applied cord should be pulled over the child's head. If the cord is wrapped too tightly, it can be clamped and ligated on the perineum, followed by the immediate delivery of the shoulders and body.

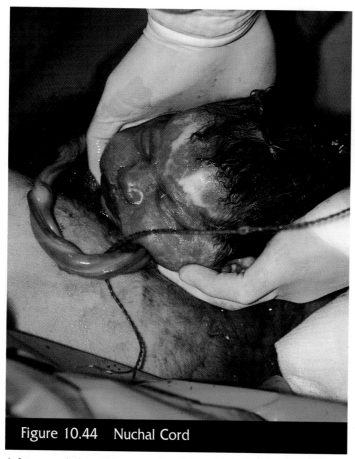

Figure 10.44   Nuchal Cord

A loose nuchal cord is seen around the neck. (Courtesy of William Leninger, MD.)

Associated Clinical Features

Shoulder dystocia is defined as failure to deliver the shoulders, following delivery of the head, because of impaction of the fetal shoulders against the pelvic outlet (Fig. 10.45). Risk factors include gestational diabetes, prior delivery of large infants, and postterm delivery.

ED Treatment and Disposition

Shoulder dystocia is an acute obstetric emergency, with the immediate life threat being asphyxia from prolonged delivery. Every effort should be made to provide for immediate obstetric consultation. Equipment for neonatal resuscitation should be set up and, ideally, a pediatric consultant should be summoned. In the absence of an obstetric consultant, a wide episiotomy should be performed. The least invasive maneuver is to forcefully flex the mother's knees toward her chest (McRobert's maneuver). This extreme dorsal lithotomy position occasionally allows for the appropriate engagement of the fetal shoulders. If this is unsuccessful, a Wood's maneuver can be attempted, by hooking two fingers behind the infant's posterior scapula and rotating the entire body in a screwlike manner. As the posterior shoulder rotates upward, it can generally be delivered past the symphysis pubis. If the Wood's maneuver fails to deliver the anterior shoulder, delivery of the posterior arm may be attempted by inserting two fingers into the sacral fossa and bringing down the entire posterior arm by flexing it at the elbow. The remaining anterior shoulder should then deliver, either spontaneously or else following rotation into the oblique position to facilitate its delivery.

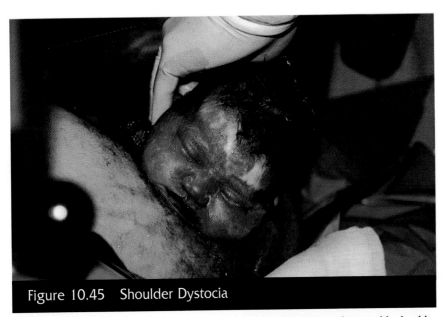

Figure 10.45   Shoulder Dystocia

Firm approximation of the fetal head against the vaginal outlet consistent with shoulder dystocia. (Courtesy of William Leninger, MD.)

Clinical Pearls

1. Shoulder dystocia is an acute obstetric emergency that requires quick action:
   Call for help.
   Cut a wide episiotomy.
   Perform McRobert's maneuver.
   Rotate the posterior shoulder.
2. After delivery, look for fracture of the clavicles or humerus and possible brachial plexus injury.

Associated Clinical Features

Lacerations to the perineum occur commonly following a rapid, uncontrolled expulsion of the fetal head. Postpartum perineal lacerations range from minor to severe.

Differential Diagnosis

Perineal lacerations due to birth trauma are categorized into four groups. First-degree lacerations are limited to the mucosa, skin, and superficial subcutaneous and submucosal tissues (Fig. 10.46). Second-degree lacerations penetrate deeper into the superficial fascia and transverse perineal musculature (Fig. 10.47). In addition to these structures, a third-degree laceration disrupts the anal sphincter, whereas a fourth-degree laceration extends into the rectal lumen (Fig. 10.48).

ED Treatment and Disposition

In most precipitous emergency department deliveries, the repair of the episiotomy and/or perineal lacerations can often be performed by the obstetric consultant, the details of repair being beyond the scope of this book.

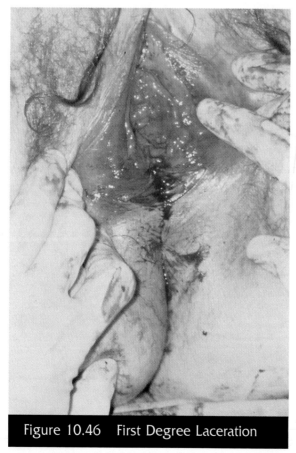

Figure 10.46   First Degree Laceration

First-degree laceration limited to the mucosa, skin, and superficial subcutaneous and submucosal tissues. There is no involvement of the underlying fascia and muscle. (Courtesy of Jerry Van Houdt, MD.)

Clinical Pearl

1. Perineal laceration repair fundamentally involves the sequential anatomic reapproximation, using absorbable suture material, of the rectal mucosa, anal sphincter, transverse perineal musculature, vaginal mucosa, and skin.

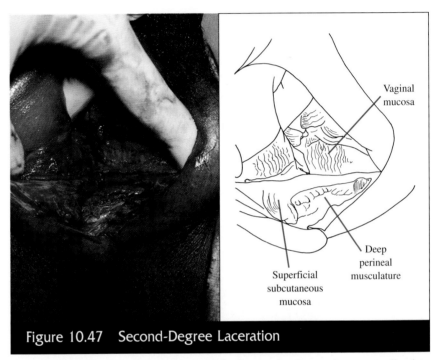

Figure 10.47   Second-Degree Laceration

There is disruption of the hymenal ring and the deep perineal musculature extending into the vaginal mucosa and transversalis fascia, but no involvement of the anal sphincter or mucosa. (Courtesy of Pamela Ambroz, MD.)

Fourth-degree perineal laceration revealing wide separation of the perineal fascia and anal sphincter. The examiner's small finger is in the rectal lumen, showing extension of the tear proximally. (Courtesy of Timothy Jahn, MD.)

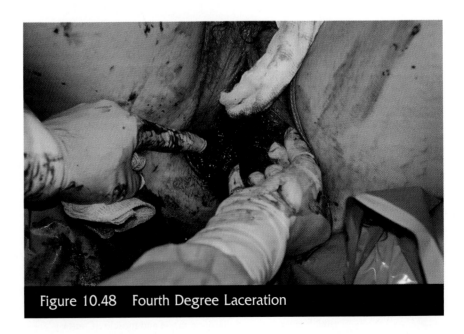

Figure 10.48   Fourth Degree Laceration

CHAPTER 11

EXTREMITY TRAUMA

Cathleen M. Vossler
Daniel L. Savitt
Alan B. Storrow

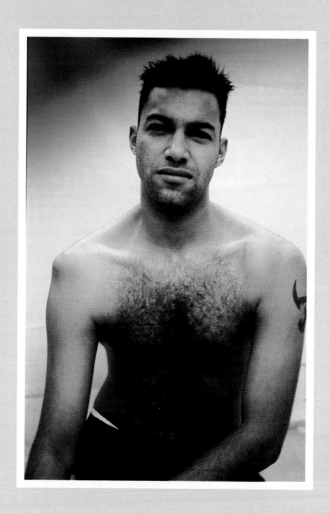

Upper Extremity

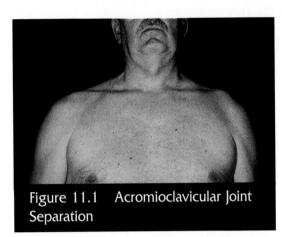

Figure 11.1   Acromioclavicular Joint Separation

Subtle prominence of the left distal clavicle. The upward displacement of the clavicle is due to stretching or disruption of the suspending ligaments. (Courtesy of Frank Birinyi, MD.)

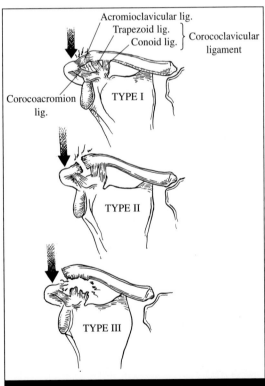

Figure 11.2   Acromioclavicular Joint Injuries

Classification of acromioclavicular joint injuries. (Adapted with permission from Rockwood CA, Green DP, Bucholz RW: *Rockwood and Green's Fractures in Adults,* 3d ed. Philadelphia, JB Lippincott, 1991.)

Associated Clinical Features

Injury to the acromioclavicular (AC) joint is a common finding in the ED resulting from direct trauma with an adducted arm, or indirectly from a fall on an outstretched arm with pressure directed to the joint (Fig. 11.1). There are three degrees of injury (Fig. 11.2). A first-degree injury is equivalent to a sprain. There is an incomplete tear of the ligament. Radiographs are negative. A second-degree injury consists of subluxation of the AC joint and disruption of the ligament. Subluxation of the clavicle from the acromion of less than 50% is only evident on stress radiographs. Complete disruption of the AC, coracoacromial, and coracoclavicular ligaments is a third-degree injury. Stress radiographs reveal more than 50% displacement of the clavicle from the acromion. All patients complain of pain at the joint site with moderate to severe amounts of swelling. Stress radiographs are obtained by suspending 5 to 10 lb of weight from each arm and taking a bilateral anteroposterior (AP) shoulder film. The joint space and any subluxation is easily visualized.

Differential Diagnosis

Clavicular fracture, scapular fracture, rotator cuff injury, shoulder dislocation, contusion, or isolated coracoclavicular ligament damage can be confused with AC joint separation.

ED Treatment and Disposition

First- and second-degree injuries are treated with rest, ice, analgesics, and a simple sling, until acute pain with movement is relieved. Third-degree injury treatment is controversial. Many experts advocate immobilization with a sling for 3 weeks, whereas others advocate operative repair. Orthopedic referral is essential for all third-degree injuries.

Clinical Pearls

1. The AC joint stress test is an accurate means of testing for AC joint separation. The patient is instructed to bring the arm across the chest and try to align the opposite shoulder with the elbow. The production of pain over the AC joint confirms the diagnosis.
2. The classic AP stress film indicating a second-degree injury shows distal clavicle-acromion separation of less than one-half the diameter of the clavicle.

Associated Clinical Features

Anterior shoulder dislocations are the most common dislocation seen in the ED. They are caused by external rotation and abduction that disrupts the capsule and glenohumeral ligaments. The affected extremity is held in slight abduction and external rotation. Often, the patient supports the dislocated shoulder with the other arm. The acromion becomes prominent and there is a squared off boxlike appearance to the top of the shoulder. The rounded contour of the deltoid is lost (Fig. 11.3). These patients complain of shoulder pain and refuse to move the shoulder on the affected side. Many patients will appear diaphoretic and pale. A neurologic examination of the upper extremity should be performed to rule out associated injury, most commonly of the axillary nerve (sensation over the deltoid). Radiographic examination is necessary to evaluate for associated fracture (Fig. 11.4). Posterior shoulder dislocations are commonly missed because of subtle radiographic findings (Figs. 11.5 and 11.6). The arm is held internally rotated and adducted. There is no external rotation. On examination, a posterior prominence exists. Posterior dislocations commonly occur during seizures. The Hill-Sachs deformity (an impaction of the humeral head) can occur in a significant percentage (11 to 50%) of these patients.

Differential Diagnosis

Acromioclavicular separation, fracture of the greater tuberosity, humeral fracture, and fracture of the humeral head are commonly mistaken for a shoulder dislocation prior to radiographic examination.

ED Treatment and Disposition

Closed reduction is the treatment of choice and may require conscious sedation. There are many methods to reduce shoulder dislocations, including Stimson, traction-countertraction, and external rotation. Neurovascular and radiographic examination should occur before and after reduction. The patient should be placed in a sling and swathe after reduction. The shoulder should remain immobilized for 2 to 5 weeks (shorter periods for older patients owing to their greater ability to develop shoulder stiffness).

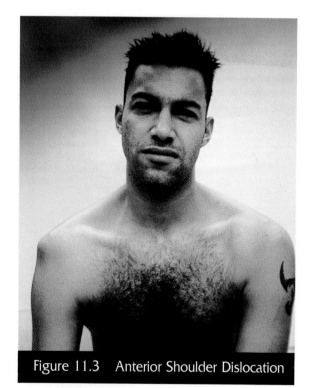

Figure 11.3   Anterior Shoulder Dislocation

This right anterior shoulder dislocation occurred when the patient fell while playing basketball. There is an obvious contour deformity as well as prominence of the acromion. (Courtesy of Kevin J. Knoop, MD, MS.)

Clinical Pearls

1. Patients with dislocated shoulders usually cannot touch the contralateral shoulder with the hand of the affected side.
2. Relaxation of the pectoral musculature is an excellent aid in shoulder reduction. This can be accomplished by manual massage of the muscle. Some patients can voluntarily relax this muscle when asked to do so (e.g., weightlifters).
3. Luxatio erecta is inferior glenohumeral dislocation. The humeral head is forced below the inferior aspect of the glenoid fossa. These patients present with the arm locked 180 deg overhead.

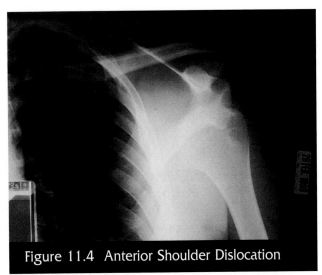

Figure 11.4   Anterior Shoulder Dislocation

Radiographic evaluation of this anterior shoulder dislocation demonstrates that the humeral head is not in the glenoid fossa, but is located anterior and inferior to it. (Courtesy of Kevin J. Knoop, MD, MS.)

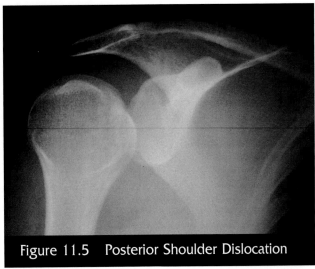

Figure 11.5   Posterior Shoulder Dislocation

AP radiograph of this rare type of shoulder dislocation. Because of internal rotation of the greater tuberosity, the humeral head appears like a dip of ice cream on a cone, thus called the "ice cream cone sign." (Courtesy of Alan B. Storrow, MD.)

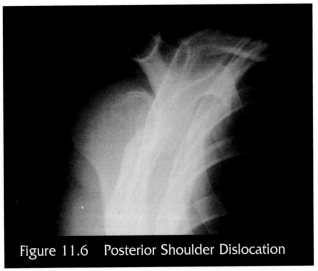

Figure 11.6   Posterior Shoulder Dislocation

A scapular Y view of the same patient confirms the diagnosis. (Courtesy of Alan B. Storrow, MD.)

Associated Clinical Features

Dislocations of the elbow can be anterior, posterior, medial, or lateral. All dislocations require immediate reduction to relieve pain and prevent circulatory compromise. Elbow dislocations require a considerable amount of force, and approximately 40% have an associated fracture. Posterior dislocation is the most common (Fig. 11.7), occurring after a fall on an outstretched hand. The arm is extended and abducted. The elbow is held in a flexed position and is swollen, tender, and deformed. The olecranon is very prominent. Neurovascular status must be evaluated immediately because of associated injury. Anterior dislocations are rare. They occur if the elbow is in a flexed position and is hit from behind on the olecranon. The elbow is extended with the forearm supinated and elongated. The upper arm appears shortened. Injury to nerves and vessels is more common with anterior dislocation.

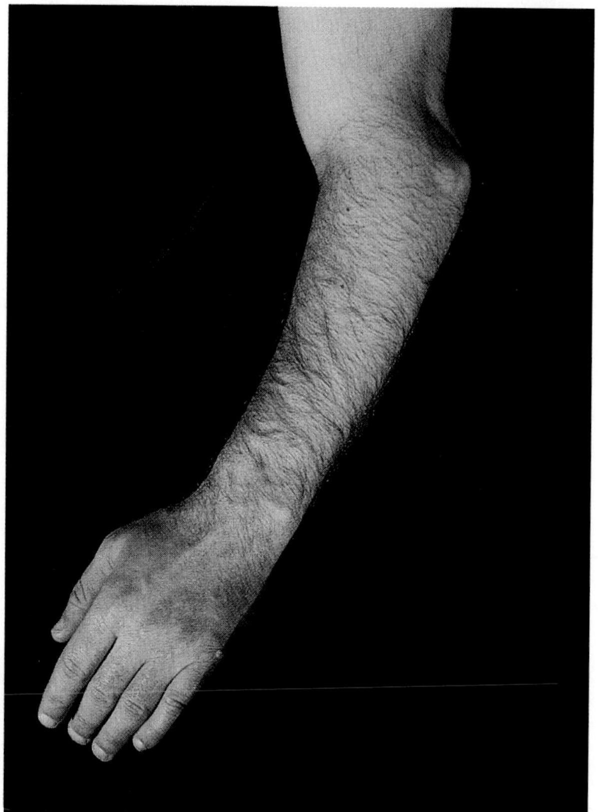

Differential Diagnosis

Contusion, radial or ulnar fracture, or supracondylar fracture of the humerus are commonly confused with an elbow dislocation until radiographic examination.

ED Treatment and Disposition

Most patients require analgesia and muscle relaxants prior to reduction. After reduction, the elbow should be immobilized in 90 to 120 deg of flexion in a posterior splint and sling.

Figure 11.7 Posterior Elbow Dislocation

This patient dislocated his elbow while playing basketball. Note the flexed position of the elbow and the prominence of the olecranon. (Courtesy of Frank Birinyi, MD.)

Neurologic and radiographic examination should occur after any attempt at reduction. The patient should be observed in the ED for vascular compromise. Elbow dislocations with associated fractures may make closed reduction difficult, as well as leave the joint unstable. In these cases, consultation with an orthopedic surgeon is recommended prior to reduction attempts.

Clinical Pearls

1. Patients should not be placed in a circular cast because of the necessity for re-examination.
2. Factors which increase the index of suspicion for arterial injury include pulselessness prior to reduction, open dislocations, and concurrent serious traumatic injury.
3. The ulnar nerve is the most common nerve injured.
4. For posterior dislocations, palpate the two epicondyles and the tip of the olecranon. If they are in the same place, a supracondylar fracture is likely. If the olecranon is displaced, a dislocation is likely.

Associated Clinical Features

Colles' fracture (Fig. 11.8) occurs most commonly from a fall on an outstretched hand. This results in dorsiflexion of the wrist and a transverse fracture of the metaphysis of the radius. There is no intraarticular involvement, and the fracture fragment is displaced dorsally. The original description by Colles was for an isolated radial fracture as described above, though the term is frequently applied to a radial fracture in combination with an ulnar styloid fracture. Patients complain of pain, swelling, tenderness, and decreased range of motion. Associated injuries include carpal fractures, distal radioulnar subluxation, flexor tendon injuries, and median or ulnar nerve injuries.

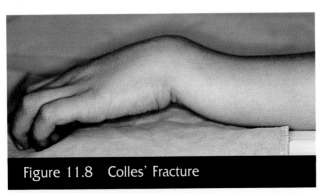

Figure 11.8   Colles' Fracture

The classic dinner fork deformity is demonstrated in this photograph. The distal forearm is displaced dorsally. (Courtesy of Cathleen M. Vossler, MD.)

Differential Diagnosis

Barton's fracture (dorsal rim fracture of the distal radius), Smith's fracture (fracture of the distal radius with volar angulation), Hutchinson's fracture (radial styloid fracture), wrist sprain, Galeazzi's fracture (displaced distal radial fracture with radioulnar subluxation), carpal bone dislocation, radial dislocation, Chauffeur's fracture (a transverse nondisplaced fracture of the radial styloid), and ulnar dislocation can all be confused with a Colles' fracture (Fig. 11.9). Classically, a Colles' fracture results from extension, a Smith's fracture from flexion, and both Hutchinson's and Barton's fractures from a push-off.

ED Treatment and Disposition

Nondisplaced fractures require no manipulation and can be casted. Displaced fractures may be reduced by using finger traps for distraction while applying dorsal pressure to the distal fragment. Optimal anesthesia is a regional block. A regional block is accomplished by axillary block of the brachial plexus. Alternative methods of anesthesia include hematoma and Bier blocks. Initial immobilization with a double sugar tong splint with the forearm in 20 deg of supination is adequate. The goals of reduction include restoration of volar tilt and radial inclination, as well as maintaining radial length. Long-term complications include stiffness, malunion, nonunion, and chronic pain. Therefore, all Colles' fractures should be followed by an orthopedic surgeon.

Clinical Pearls

1. Median nerve function must be evaluated before and after any reduction because of associated paresthesias which occur secondary to tension or pressure on the nerve.
2. Some Colles' fractures are unstable and require more aggressive treatment including external or internal fixation. Colles' fractures with intraarticular involvement, comminution, more than 20 deg of angulation, and more than 1 cm of shortening may be unstable and require fixation. These fractures are more likely to lead to complications such as loss of reduction, joint instability, and arthritis.

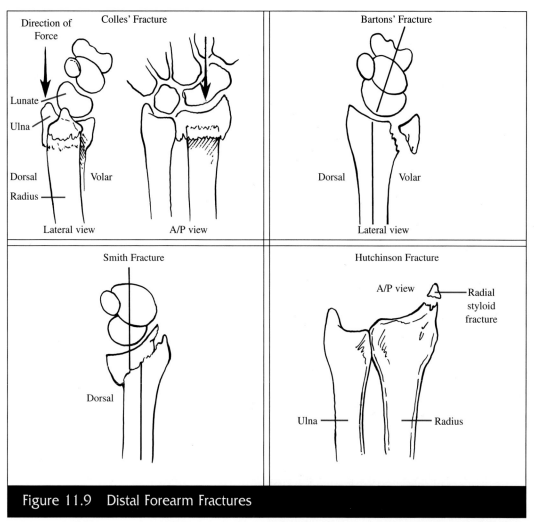

Figure 11.9   Distal Forearm Fractures

These illustrations depict the different types of distal forearm fractures: Colles', Smith's, Barton's, and Hutchinson's. (Adapted from Simon R: *Emergency Orthopedics: The Extremities.* Norwalk, CT, Appleton and Lange, 1987, pp 118–119.)

Associated Clinical Features

Flexor and extensor tendon injury occur from lacerations or wounds to the hand. Tendon rupture can also occur secondary to forces applied to the hand causing avulsion of the bone or rupture of the tendon. Many patients state that they are unable to flex or extend the digit (Fig. 11.10). Tendon function must be checked with any injury to the hand. Accurate assessment of a tendon can be misleading, since a 90% lacerated tendon can still retain function. Partial tendon lacerations can often be identified by testing strength against resistance. Strength against resistance is decreased if a partial tendon laceration exists. It is helpful to evaluate the resting hand. Note the flexor cascade of the fingers. An abnormal resting posture is suspicious for tendon injury. Flexor digitorum profundus and superficialis as well as all individual flexor and extensor tendons should be tested. Ask the patient to extend each digit individually while the other digits are held in place. Suspicion for an extensor tendon laceration should arise if this cannot be done.

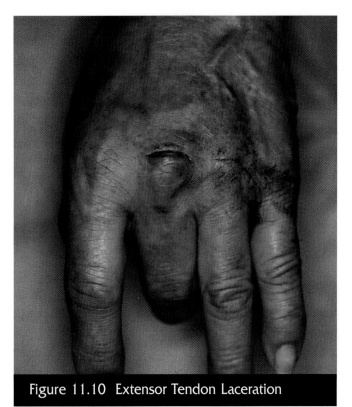

Figure 11.10 Extensor Tendon Laceration

Note the laceration over the third metacarpal head. The inability to extend the long finger is strong clinical evidence of complete extensor tendon disruption. (Courtesy of Kevin J. Knoop, MD, MS.)

Differential Diagnosis

Partial tendon laceration, tendon sheath laceration, tenosynovitis, or acute arthritis may be confused with tendon injury.

ED Treatment and Disposition

Initial wound care should include irrigation, exploration for foreign bodies, debridement, antibiotics, and tetanus prophylaxis if needed. Treatment of a partial tendon laceration requires no repair and is treated with a protective splint. Extensor tendon repair can be performed in the ED after careful irrigation, inspection, and debridement or later by the consultant. Flexor tendon repair requires immediate orthopedic consultation for operative repair.

Clinical Pearls

1. Wounds should be examined through a full range of motion. A tendon laceration sustained with the finger in flexion will be missed if the finger is examined only in extension secondary to retraction of the tendon.
2. Excellent hemostasis is required for a complete tendon examination. The brief use of a blood pressure cuff or other tourniquet may be necessary.

Associated Clinical Features

The clenched fist injury classically occurs during a fight when the metacarpophalangeal (MCP) joint contacts human teeth resulting in a laceration in the skin (Fig. 11.11). Many patients will not divulge the true circumstances surrounding the injury; therefore all wounds at the MCP joint are considered a clenched fist injury until proven otherwise. Once these wounds occur, the inoculated organisms are sealed in a warm closed environment allowing rapid spread and destruction. Serious complications can result, including infection, loss of function, and amputation. Most wounds are polymicrobial. Patients who present initially may have little on physical examination, whereas those who present more than 18 h after injury are more likely to have evidence of infection including pain, swelling, erythema, and purulent drainage.

Differential Diagnosis

Abrasions or lacerations secondary to a source other than human teeth can be mistaken for a clenched fist injury.

ED Treatment and Disposition

All wounds should be irrigated, debrided, explored, elevated, and immobilized. Patients should receive antibiotics directed at both oral and skin flora. Tetanus prophylaxis is given if needed. Radiographs should be obtained to evaluate for fractures and any foreign bodies remaining in the wound. These wounds should never be closed initially. All patients require careful follow-up with a hand specialist. Reliable patients who present early, without evidence of infection or significant medical history (e.g., diabetes), and have no involvement of bone, joint, or tendon may be treated on an outpatient basis. They must return in 24 h for a wound check, sooner if any signs of infection develop. Any patient that does not meet these requirements must be hospitalized for IV antibiotics and wound care.

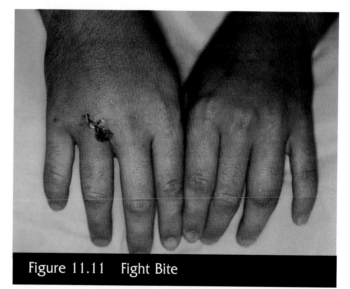

Figure 11.11   Fight Bite

The small lacerations seen in this photograph were sustained from human teeth during a fight. (Courtesy of Lawrence B. Stack, MD.)

Clinical Pearls

1. Complications include cellulitis, lymphangitis, septic arthritis, abscess formation, osteomyelitis, and tenosynovitis.
2. All wounds need to be examined in full flexion and extension so tendon injuries are not missed. A tendon injury sustained with the fingers flexed will be missed if the hand is only examined in extension due to the retraction of the tendon with extension.

Associated Clinical Features

A boxer's fracture is a metacarpal neck fracture of the fifth, and sometimes fourth digit, which commonly occurs after a direct blow to the metacarpophalangeal joints of the clenched fist. The proximal metacarpal bone is angulated dorsally and the metacarpal head is angulated volarly. On physical examination, the "knuckle" is missing and can be palpated on the volar surface (Figs. 11.12 and 11.13). Any associated laceration should be considered secondary to human teeth ("fight bite," see "Clenched Fist Injury" Fig. 11.11).

Differential Diagnosis

Metacarpal head fracture, metacarpal shaft fracture, hematoma, sprain, clenched fist injury, and metacarpophalangeal dislocation are often mistaken for a boxer's fracture until radiographic evaluation is performed.

ED Treatment and Disposition

Prior to reduction, the injury must be evaluated for rotational malalignment. This is easily done by having the patient place all fingers in the palm; all fingers should point to the scaphoid bone (Fig. 11.14). Rotational deformities of greater than 15% require reduction. An ulnar nerve block provides sufficient anesthesia for the fifth metacarpal, but median and radial nerve blocks can be used for the other metacarpals. Hematoma block can be used as an alternative. Once adequate anesthesia is achieved, reduction can be attempted. A nondisplaced nonangulated fracture requires no reduction. Treatment includes ice, elevation, and immobilization in a gutter splint. For reduction, the distal interphalangeal (DIP), proximal interphalangeal (PIP), and metacarpophalangeal (MCP) joints are all held in flexion at 90 deg. Pressure is exerted on the proximal phalanx directed upward to push the metacarpal head dorsally back into position. At the same time, the metacarpal shaft is stabilized with pressure on the dorsum over the shaft. The patient should be splinted with the MCP at 90 deg of flexion. Postreduction radiographs are necessary to ensure adequate reduction. Early follow-up (within 7 days) with a hand specialist is essential, since simple splinting may not adequately maintain proper reduction and fractures with higher degrees of angulation and instability may require fixation.

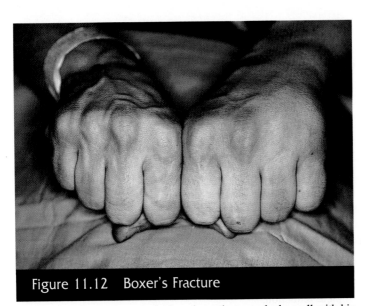

Figure 11.12   Boxer's Fracture

This boxer's fracture occurred when the patient punched a wall with his hand. There is loss of the "knuckle" when the dorsum of the hand is examined, especially noticeable when the patient makes a fist. (Courtesy of Cathleen M. Vossler, MD.)

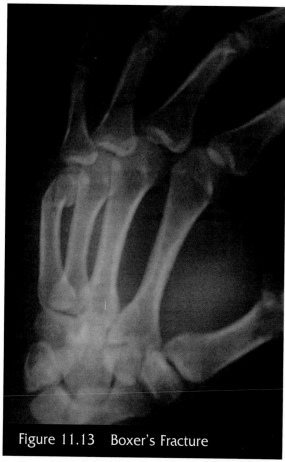

Figure 11.13   Boxer's Fracture

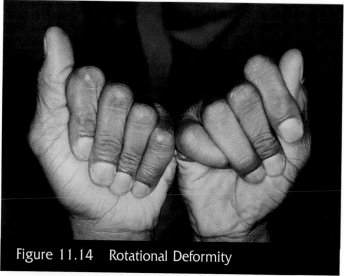

Figure 11.14   Rotational Deformity

Radiographic examination reveals a fracture through the neck of the metacarpal and volar displacement of the fractured segment. (Courtesy of Cathleen M. Vossler, MD.)

Malpositioning of the right fifth digit due to a boxer's fracture. Normally, all the digits point toward a single spot on the scaphoid. (Courtesy of Alexander T. Trott, MD.)

Clinical Pearls

1. Second and third metacarpal neck fractures will not tolerate any angulation and require orthopedic referral for anatomic reduction. Fourth and fifth metacarpal neck fractures can tolerate up to 30 and 50 deg of angulation, respectively, before function is impaired.

2. Subtle malrotation can be recognized by looking at the alignment of the nail beds with the digits flexed. Complications include collateral ligament damage, extensor injury damage, and malposition or clawing of the fingers secondary to incomplete reduction.

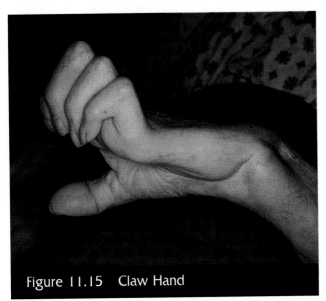

Figure 11.15   Claw Hand

This photograph demonstrates the claw hand appearance resulting from median and ulnar nerve injury. Note metacarpophalangeal joint hyperextension. (Courtesy of Daniel L. Savitt, MD.)

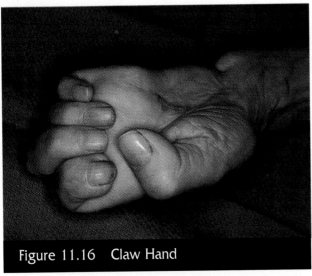

Figure 11.16   Claw Hand

Atrophy of the thenar and hypothenar eminences also occurs as a result of damage to the median and ulnar nerve respectively. Note the concavity to the hypothenar eminence. (Courtesy of Cathleen M. Vossler, MD.)

Associated Clinical Features

Ulnar nerve injury results in the classic claw hand deformity (Fig. 11.15) because of the wasting of small hand muscles. The deformity is formed by hyperextension of the metacarpophalangeal joint and flexion at the proximal and distal interphalangeal joints of the fourth and fifth digits. There is wasting of the interosseous and hypothenar muscles, as well as the hypothenar eminence (Fig. 11.16). The patient is unable to abduct or adduct the digits.

Median nerve damage results in the claw hand deformity but to the second and third digits. Damage to the proximal portion of the nerve results in weakness of wrist flexion, forearm pronation, thumb apposition, and flexion of the first three digits. Atrophy of the thenar eminence also occurs. There is a sensory loss over the area of distribution for each nerve. These findings are not seen acutely, but are chronic signs from an old injury.

Wrist drop is the most common symptom seen with *radial nerve* damage occurring in situations of acute compression. It is frequently referred to as Saturday night palsy (a person who has been drinking alcohol, falls asleep on an arm or with the arm over a chair and there is temporary damage to the nerve).

Differential Diagnosis

Rheumatoid arthritis, osteoarthritis, and undiagnosed proximal (cervical osteophyte) or distal (carpal tunnel syndrome) entrapment syndromes can be mistaken for peripheral nerve injury.

ED Treatment and Disposition

Treatment is aimed at recognizing the underlying cause of the nerve damage. These include laceration of the nerve, compression from swelling, or hematoma formation. In the ED, splinting and appropriate referral is the treatment.

Clinical Pearl

1. Long-term nerve injury results in muscle wasting. Prior to any nerve damage, the thenar and hypothenar eminences have a full appearance. This is lost in patients with nerve damage. Initially, there is flattening of each eminence followed by a concave or hollow appearance.

Associated Clinical Features

These patients complain of pain, swelling, and decreased range of motion at the base of the thumb (Fig. 11.17). Bennett's fracture is an intraarticular fracture at the ulnar aspect of the base of the first metacarpal with disruption of the carpometacarpal joint (Fig. 11.18). The first metacarpal is displaced radially and proximally, with subluxation or complete dislocation (Fig. 11.19). Rolando's fracture is an intraarticular comminuted fracture at the base of the first metacarpal with dorsal and volar fragments resulting in a Y- or T-shaped intraarticular fragment (Fig. 11.20).

Differential Diagnosis

Sprain, first metacarpal shaft fracture, or a gamekeeper's thumb (disruption of the ulnar collateral ligament of the metacarpophalangeal joint) are commonly mistaken for Bennett's or Rolando's fracture prior to radiographic evaluation.

ED Treatment and Disposition

The treatment of these fractures in the ED consists of ice, elevation, and immobilization in a thumb spica splint and early referral to a hand specialist. These fractures generally require operative reduction and fixation.

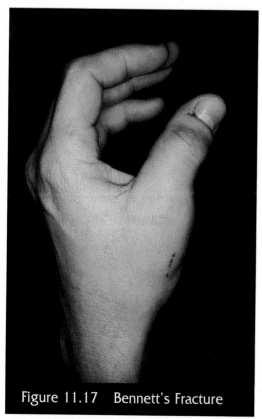

Figure 11.17   Bennett's Fracture

Bennett's fracture involves the base of the first metacarpal. The digit is swollen and ecchymotic over the affected area. (Courtesy of Daniel L. Savitt, MD.)

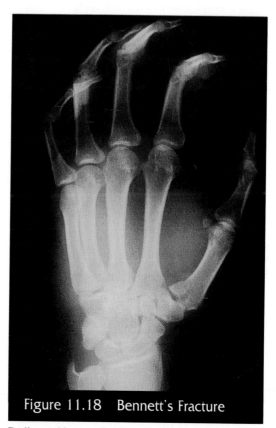

Figure 11.18   Bennett's Fracture

Radiographic examination of a Bennett's fracture illustrates an intraarticular fracture at the base of the first metacarpal with the metacarpal displaced radially and proximally. (Courtesy of Cathleen M. Vossler, MD.)

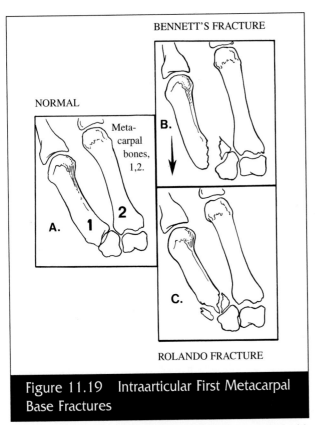

NORMAL

BENNETT'S FRACTURE

Meta-carpal bones, 1,2.

A. 1 2

B.

C.

ROLANDO FRACTURE

Figure 11.19   Intraarticular First Metacarpal Base Fractures

An intraarticular fracture at the base of the first metacarpal with radial and proximal displacement is a Bennett's fracture. A comminuted intraarticular fracture at the base of the first matacarpal is a Rolando's fracture.

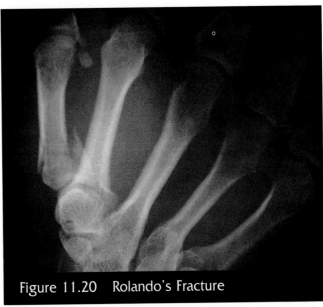

Figure 11.20   Rolando's Fracture

Note the comminuted intraarticular fracture at the base of the first metacarpal. (Courtesy of Cathleen M. Vossler, MD.)

Clinical Pearls

1. Carpometacarpal dislocations are frequently difficult to reduce and require open reduction and fixation approximately 50% of the time.
2. Osteoarthritis is a common long-term complication, even after optimal management.

DIAGNOSIS   BOUTONNIÈRE AND SWAN NECK DEFORMITIES

Associated Clinical Features

The boutonnière deformity is a result of injury or disruption to the insertion of the extensor tendon on the dorsal base of the middle phalanx. Common causes of this problem are proximal interphalangeal (PIP) joint contusion, forceful flexion of the PIP joint against resistance, and palmar dislocation of the PIP joint. Initially, a deformity may be absent, but will develop over the course of time if the injury remains untreated. The lateral bands sublux and exert a proximal pull on the middle phalanx. The result is flexion of the PIP joint and extension of the DIP joint (Figs. 11.21 and 11.22). Radiographically, a small fragment of bone may be visualized at the proximal portion of the dorsal aspect of the middle phalanx.

Swan neck deformity occurs as a result of the shortening of interosseous muscles secondary to systemic diseases such as rheumatoid arthritis. The digit is contorted with hyperextension of the PIP and flexion of the distal interphalangeal (DIP) and metacarpophalangeal (MCP) joints (Fig. 11.23).

Differential Diagnosis

Fracture, dislocation, or tendon damage can be mistaken for a boutonnière or swan neck deformity.

ED Treatment and Disposition

When dealing with a closed injury resulting in a boutonnière deformity, immobilization of the PIP joint in extension is adequate. Splinting the MCP and DIP joints is not necessary. The splint should be used for 4 weeks, at which point active range of motion can start. Open injuries must be carefully explored and repaired. Swan neck deformities are treated by splinting the digit to prevent further deformity. Both deformities require referral to a hand specialist.

Clinical Pearls

1. Boutonnière deformity generally develops weeks after the initial injury as the lateral bands contract; therefore, it is frequently missed in the emergency department. Early diagnosis can be made with the proper examina-

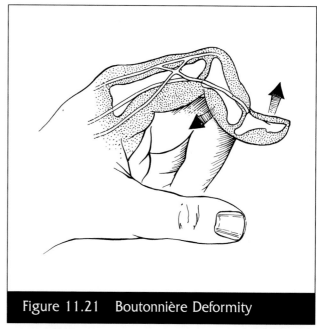

Figure 11.21   Boutonnière Deformity

This depiction of a boutonnière deformity illustrates the rupture of the central slip and the resultant subluxation of the lateral bands. The subluxation exerts a pull on the middle phalanx resulting in the deformity.

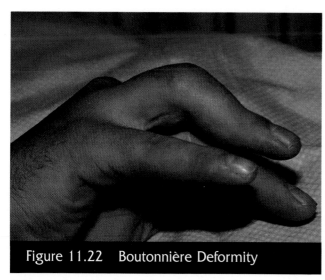

Figure 11.22   Boutonnière Deformity

A boutonnière deformity of the fourth digit. Note the flexion of the PIP joint and the extension of the DIP joint. (Courtesy of E. Lee Edstrom, MD.)

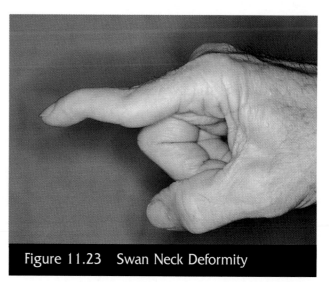

Figure 11.23   Swan Neck Deformity

A swan neck deformity of the index finger. Note the hyperextension of the PIP joint and the flexion of the DIP joint. (Courtesy of Cathleen M. Vossler, MD.)

tion of the finger. The digit should be adequately anesthetized, then examined for range of motion and joint stability.

2.   Any injury involving the dorsal PIP surface should be reexamined for development of a boutonnière deformity after 7 to 10 days.

3.   Surgical repair may be required for cases where conservative therapy yields inadequate results.

DIAGNOSIS   HIGH-PRESSURE INJECTION INJURY

Associated Clinical Features

A large number of commercial devices are able to deliver liquids and gases at high pressures. Occasionally, substances from these devices are injected into the body, especially the upper extremities. The most common devices include spray guns, diesel injectors, and hydraulic lines. The injury occurs when the device accidentally fires during cleaning or mishandling. The injury can be very misleading if seen soon after the event. On early examination, a small puncture wound or no apparent break in the skin may be found with minimal swelling. Swelling and pain increase over time (Fig. 11.24). Vascular compromise can occur directly from compression secondary to swelling or from the inflammatory response that the body produces to the materials injected. The injected material tends to spread along fascial planes, so the extent of injury can be quite misleading and is often subtle on initial presentation.

Differential Diagnosis

Puncture wound, hematoma, or tenosynovitis can be confused with a hydraulic pressure injury.

ED Treatment and Disposition

Immediate operative debridement is the treatment of choice. Therefore, early consultation with a hand specialist is necessary. Radiographic examination evaluates for fracture and may outline spread of injected material. Tetanus and broad spectrum antibiotics should be administered. The affected extremity should be elevated and splinted.

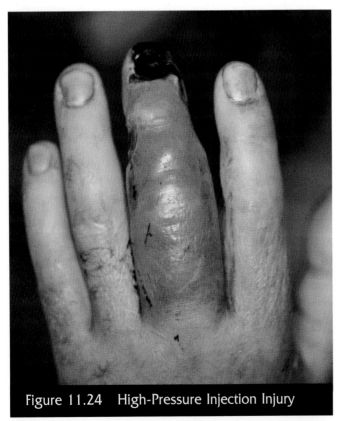

Figure 11.24   High-Pressure Injection Injury

This photograph illustrates injury incurred by a grease gun. The patient was cleaning the device and the gun accidently discharged into his hand. Note the swelling and erythema. The patient was taken to the operating room for initial debridement. (Courtesy of Richard Zienowicz, MD.)

Clinical Pearls

1. Do not be misled by the "benign" appearance of the initial injury.
2. Delays in treatment can lead to compartment syndrome.
3. Digital blocks are contraindicated because of the potential for increased tissue pressure and compromise of tissue perfusion.

PHALANGEAL DISLOCATIONS   DIAGNOSIS

Associated Clinical Features

Phalangeal dislocations are common and can occur at all three finger joints. Distal interphalangeal (DIP) dislocations are the rarest, but can occur when a force is applied to the distal phalanx. Gross deformity is noted on examination with the distal phalanx generally displaced dorsally. Proximal interphalangeal (PIP) dislocations (Figs. 11.25 and 11.26) are common and easily reducible. These are generally dorsally dislocated, caused by hyperextension, and may have associated volar plate damage (Fig. 11.27). PIP volar dislocations can be irreducible secondary to rupture of the extensor tendon or herniation of the proximal phalanx through the extensor mechanism, both requiring operative repair. Metacarpophalangeal (MCP) joint dorsal dislocations are often due to hyperextension.

Differential Diagnosis

Phalangeal fracture, metacarpal fracture, tendon damage, ligamentous injury, or boutonnière deformity can be confused with a phalangeal dislocation.

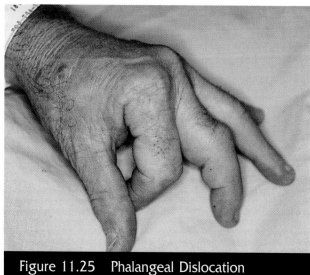

Figure 11.25   Phalangeal Dislocation

This patient dislocated the long finger PIP joint during an altercation. The PIP joint is displaced dorsally with an obvious deformity. (Courtesy of Cathleen M. Vossler, MD.)

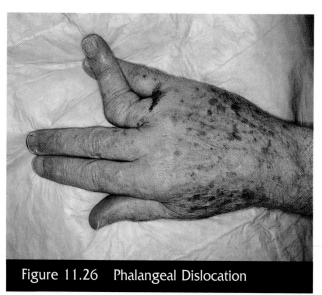

Figure 11.26   Phalangeal Dislocation

This photograph illustrates lateral angulation of the ring finger suggesting PIP dislocation. (Courtesy of Daniel L. Savitt, MD.)

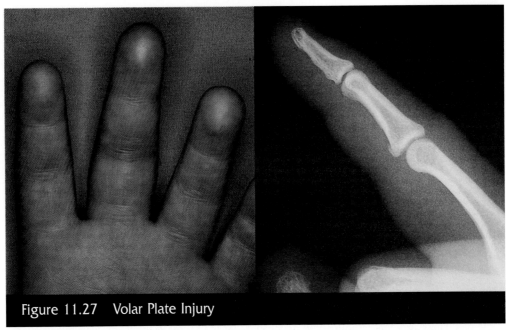

Figure 11.27   Volar Plate Injury

This photograph demonstrates subtle PIP swelling and ecchymosis of the second digit often seen with a volar plate injury. Hyperextension injuries cause disruption of the volar plate and result in swelling, ecchymosis, and tenderness along the volar aspect of the joint. These injuries are initially treated conservatively with splinting, but if they are unstable, operative repair is required. (Courtesy of Daniel L. Savitt, M.D.) Right: Radiographic examination of the digit reveals a small fragment on the proximal volar surface of the PIP joint. (Courtesy of Cathleen M. Vossler, MD.)

ED Treatment and Disposition

Digital nerve block is appropriate anesthesia for the PIP and DIP joints. Ulnar, median, or radial nerve blocks are necessary for the MCP joints. Reduction with splinting is the treatment of choice. Reduction is accomplished via hyperextension of the joint with concurrent application of horizontal traction. Flexion at the MCP joint will facilitate reduction of distal joints. Postreduction radiographs are necessary to ensure adequate reduction. The DIP joint should be splinted in slight flexion and the PIP joint in 20 deg of flexion for 3 to 5 weeks depending on the degree of ligament damage. Hand specialist follow-up is mandatory.

Clinical Pearls

1. All joints should be tested for instability after reduction, using a digital nerve block to facilitate testing.
2. PIP joint volar dislocation can be unstable, requiring open reduction and internal fixation.
3. Joint dislocations that have volar plate entrapment may be impossible to reduce and require surgical repair for successful reduction.

Associated Clinical Features

Mallet finger commonly occurs after the distal finger, specifically the distal interphalangeal (DIP) joint, is forcibly flexed such as from a sudden blow to the tip of the extended finger. This injury represents complete avulsion or laxity of the extensor tendon from the proximal dorsum of the distal phalanx (Fig. 11.28). The patient presents with an inability to extend the distal phalanx, and it remains in a flexed position (Fig. 11.29). On radiograph, a small chip fragment on the dorsum at the DIP joint may be visualized.

Differential Diagnosis

Intraarticular fracture of the distal phalanx, distal tuft fracture, or extensor tendon laceration can be confused with a mallet finger.

ED Treatment and Disposition

A closed mallet finger without involvement of the joint can be treated by splinting the DIP joint in extension to *mild* hyperextension. True hyperextension is to be avoided. This should be worn for 6 to 8 weeks, at which point active range of motion begins. There is no need to splint the other joints. Motion of the PIP joint should not be blocked with the splint. Hand surgery follow-up is required.

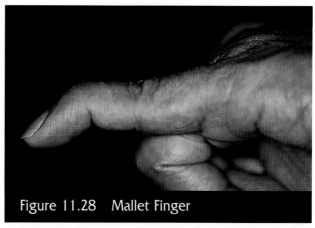

Figure 11.28   Mallet Finger

This photograph depicts a mallet finger. The distal phalanx is held in flexion and the patient is unable to extend it. (Courtesy of Kevin J. Knoop, MD, MS.)

Clinical Pearls

1. During follow-up, some patients exhibit hyperextension of the distal phalanx while out of the splint. This is due to a weakness in the volar plate. These patients should be splinted with the DIP joint in flexion and followed closely.
2. Avulsion of a significant portion of the articular surface (more than one-third) may require open reduction with internal fixation by a hand surgeon.

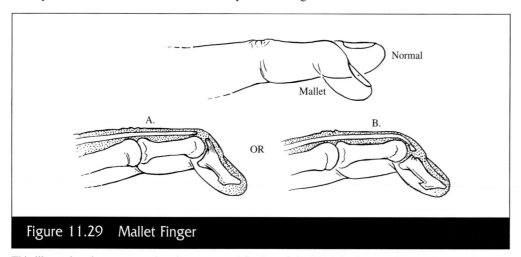

Figure 11.29   Mallet Finger

This illustration demonstrates that the unopposed flexion of the DIP joint is secondary to the complete tear (A) or avulsion (B) of the tendon.

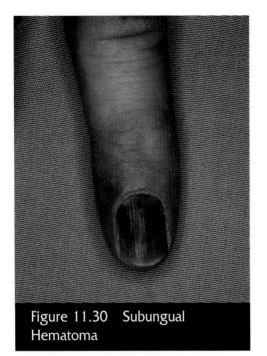

Figure 11.30   Subungual Hematoma

This subungual hematoma occurred after the patient hit his finger with a hammer. The hematoma covers approximately 50% of the subungual area. (Courtesy of Margaret P. Mueller, MD.)

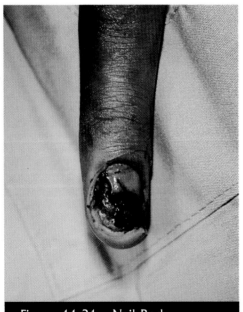

Figure 11.31   Nail Bed Laceration

Bleeding from a nail bed laceration causes a subungual hematoma. This image depicts a nail bed laceration seen after removal of the nail. (Courtesy of Alan B. Storrow, MD.)

Associated Clinical Features

A subungual hematoma is a collection of blood found underneath the nail, usually occurring secondary to trauma to the distal fingers (Fig. 11.30). They can be quite painful because of pressure beneath the nail. There also can be swelling, tenderness, and a decreased range of motion of the associated finger. Associated injuries include nail bed trauma (Fig. 11.31) and distal tuft fractures.

Differential Diagnosis

A nail bed melanoma may resemble a subungual hematoma and is differentiated from a hematoma by lack of a history of recent trauma and subsequent appearance of the "lesion."

ED Treatment and Disposition

A radiograph should be done to evaluate for possible fracture. If there is no associated nail bed injury and the subungual hematoma covers less than 25%, trephining the nail with a sterile needle is adequate to relieve pain by allowing drainage. Management of larger hematomas is somewhat controversial. Some authors advocate removal of the nail if the hematoma covers more than 50% of the nail or there is an associated fracture. A more recent conservative approach states that removal of the nail is best reserved for those injuries which damage the nail plate and surrounding tissues, regardless of the size of the hematoma or presence of a tuft fracture. In many cases, trephination of the nail is sufficient to relieve pain.

Clinical Pearls

1. Subungual hematomas are a sign of nail bed injury.
2. Subungual hematomas with surrounding nail bed and nail fold injuries require nail removal and evaluation of the nail bed for injury and careful repair if needed.
3. A hand-held, high-temperature, portable cautery device is a good tool for drainage of a subungual hematoma.

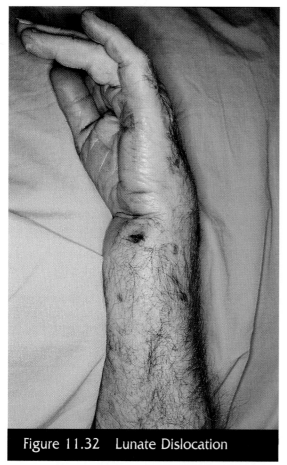

Figure 11.32   Lunate Dislocation

This photograph demonstrates swelling associated with a volar lunate dislocation. (Courtesy of Cathleen M. Vossler, MD.)

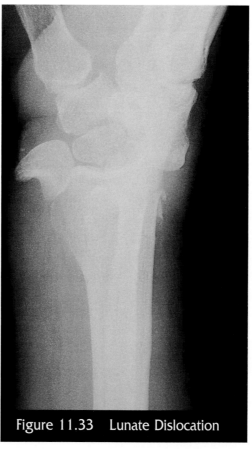

Figure 11.33   Lunate Dislocation

Radiographic examination of a dorsal lunate dislocation. (Courtesy of Cathleen M. Vossler, MD.)

Associated Clinical Features

Carpal and carpometacarpal dislocations are serious wrist injuries usually occurring from hyperextension. Their diagnosis requires careful physical and radiographic examination. Patients complain of decreased range of motion, pain, swelling, and ecchymosis.

Lunate dislocation (Fig. 11.32) can occur in a volar or dorsal position with the lunate displaced relative to the other carpal bones (Fig. 11.33). The normal lunoradial relationship is disrupted. The median nerve is most commonly involved and should be evaluated.

If the lunoradial articulation is intact, and the other carpal bones are dislocated relative to the lunate, it is termed a perilunate dislocation.

Another potentially serious injury is scapholunate dislocation, often mistakenly diagnosed as a sprained wrist. Although the physical examination may be unremarkable except for wrist pain, an anteroposterior (AP) radiograph reveals a widening of the scapholunate joint space

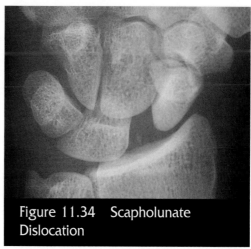

Figure 11.34   Scapholunate Dislocation

Radiographic evidence of a scapholunate dislocation. Note the widened scapholunate joint space. This injury is often misdiagnosed as simple wrist sprain. (Courtesy of Alan B. Storrow, MD.)

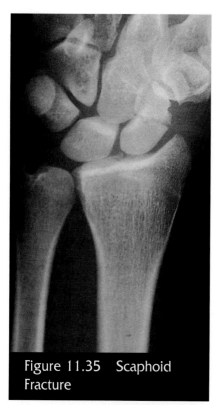

Figure 11.35   Scaphoid Fracture

Fracture of the waist, or middle third, of the scaphoid. These injuries can be associated with delayed healing and avascular necrosis. (Courtesy of Alan B. Storrow, MD.)

(Fig. 11.34). This space is normally less than 3 mm. A space of 4 mm or greater should prompt suspicion of this problem. In addition, the lateral radiograph may reveal an increase of the scapholunate angle to greater than 60 to 65 deg (normal 45 to 50 deg).

All these dislocations may present with concomitant fractures of the carpal bones or distal forearm. A scaphoid fracture is particularly troublesome, since misdiagnosis of this problem can result in later delayed healing or avascular necrosis (Fig. 11.35). This potentially serious problem is due to lack of a direct blood supply to the proximal portion of the bone. Tenderness on palpation of the anatomic snuffbox, or with axial loading, is a common finding. Unfortunately, negative radiographs do not rule out an occult scaphoid fracture.

Carpometacarpal dislocations are fortunately rare, since they are often devastating injuries requiring extensive repair (Fig. 11.36). Functional loss is marked and common.

Differential Diagnosis

Arthritis, carpal tunnel syndrome, and joint infections should be considered in patients with wrist pain.

ED Treatment and Disposition

Initial management includes adequate radiographic evaluation followed by ice, elevation, and splinting. Referral to a hand specialist is essential for adequate reduction and long-term care.

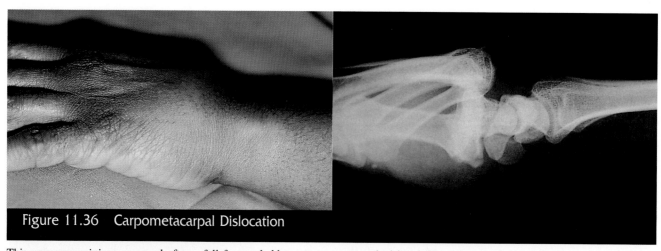

Figure 11.36   Carpometacarpal Dislocation

This uncommon injury occurred after a fall from a ladder onto an outstretched hand. Note the prominent deformity of the proximal metacarpals, II to IV, on the dorsal hand. Also note the normal prominence of the ulnar styloid, which helps the examiner in anatomic location of the dislocation. Right: Radiographic examination of the patient depicted above. (Courtesy of Alan B. Storrow, MD.)

Clinical Pearls

1. A true lateral wrist radiograph best demonstrates a lunate dislocation by exhibiting the usual cup-shaped lunate bone as lying on its side and displaced either dorsally or volarly.
2. On lateral wrist radiographs, the metacarpal, capitate, lunate, and radius should all be aligned so that a line drawn through the long axis will bisect all four bones including the lunate. If this is not found, then some element of dislocation, subluxation, or ligament instability exists.
3. Patients in whom there is a clinical suspicion of an occult scaphoid fracture (anatomic snuffbox tenderness or axial load tenderness of the thumb without radiologic evidence of fracture) should receive a thumb spica splint and a repeat examination in 7 to 10 days.

COMPARTMENT SYNDROME

DIAGNOSIS

Associated Clinical Features

Compartment syndrome develops when the pressure in a closed or inelastic fascial space increases to a point where it causes compression and dysfunction of vascular and neural structures. The five "Ps" that characterize compartment syndrome are pain, pallor, paresthesias, increased pressure, and pulselessness.

The earliest symptom is severe pain out of proportion to the injury. The pain is worsened with passive stretching of muscle within the compartment. Anesthesia-paresthesia is an early sign of nerve compromise. Motor weakness and pulselessness are late signs. Causes include compression, exercise, circumferential burns, constrictive dressings, arterial bleeding, soft-tissue injury, and fracture. Locations where compartment syndrome can occur include interossei of the hand, volar and dorsal compartments of the forearm (Fig. 11.37), gluteus medius, and anterior, peroneal, and deep posterior compartments of the leg. A creatine phosphokinase (CPK) of 1000 to 5000 units per milliliter may add to suspicion of the diagnosis. Myonecrosis can cause myoglobinuria and renal failure.

Differential Diagnosis

Soft-tissue swelling, deep vein thrombosis (DVT), neuropraxia, cellulitis, arterial intimal damage, inflammation, or hematoma formation can be mistaken for a compartment syndrome.

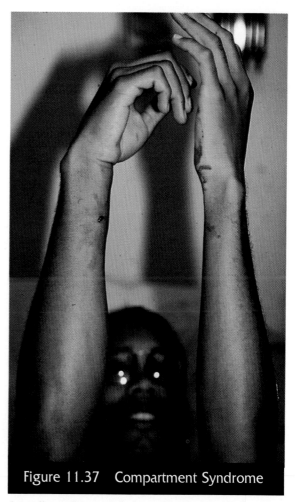

Figure 11.37 Compartment Syndrome

A swollen and tense right forearm typical for the presentation of compartment syndrome. (Courtesy of Lawrence B. Stack, MD.)

ED Treatment and Disposition

The initial treatment is removal of any constrictive dressing and frequent evaluation. If there is no improvement or there are no constrictive dressings in place, then decompression via a fasciotomy should be considered. Intracompartmental pressure monitoring should be performed to assess the need for immediate decompression. Pressures greater than 30 mmHg with signs and symptoms are suggestive of compartment syndrome, whereas pressures greater than 40 are diagnostic.

Clinical Pearls

1. The diagnosis of compartment syndrome should be made early and based on clinical evaluation and the mechanism of injury. Crush or compression injuries should heighten suspicion.
2. The most common areas of the extremities affected by compartment syndrome are anterior compartment of the lower leg due to proximal tibial fractures and the volar compartment of the forearm secondary to fracture of the ulna or radius and supracondylar fracture.
3. If a compartment syndrome is suspected, the compartment pressure should be measured.

Pelvis and Hip

DIAGNOSIS   **HIP DISLOCATION**

Associated Clinical Features

Hip dislocations can be anterior, posterior, or central. Posterior hip dislocations are the most common, resulting from forces exerted on a flexed knee (e.g., a passenger in a motor vehicle accident whose knees hit the dashboard). The extremity is found shortened, internally rotated, and adducted (Fig. 11.38). Associated fractures occur commonly. Anterior hip dislocations occur

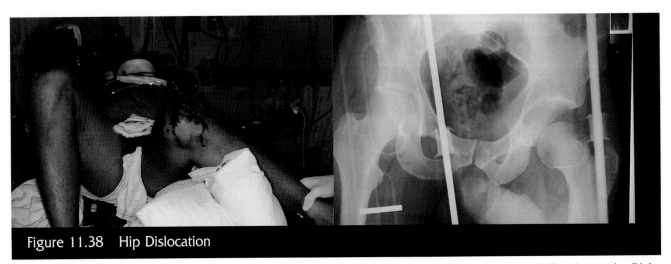

Figure 11.38   Hip Dislocation

Typical clinical appearance and patient position of a left posterior hip dislocation. Note internal rotation of the affected extremity. Right: Radiograph of patient on the left. (Courtesy of Cathleen M. Vossler, MD.)

when there is forced abduction to the femoral head, which forces the head out through an anterior capsule tear. Anterior dislocations can be superior (pubic) or inferior (obturator). The leg is abducted, externally rotated, and flexed with an inferior anterior hip dislocation. A superior anterior hip dislocation has the leg positioned in extension, slight abduction, and external rotation. Patients complain of severe hip pain and decreased range of motion.

Differential Diagnosis

Femoral head fracture, pelvic fracture, femoral neck fracture, acetabular fracture, and femoral shaft fracture are sometimes mistaken for hip dislocations on initial examination.

ED Treatment and Disposition

Treatment for dislocations is early closed reduction using sedation, analgesia, and muscle relaxants. Anterior dislocations are reduced using strong in-line traction with the hip flexed and internally rotated, followed by abduction. Posterior dislocations are reduced using in-line traction with the hip flexed to 90 deg, followed by gentle internal to external rotation. A neurovascular examination and radiographic evaluation should occur before and after any attempts at reduction. Orthopedic consultation should be obtained as early as possible. These patients require admission with frequent neurovascular evaluation.

Clinical Pearls

1. Complications of posterior hip dislocations include sciatic nerve injury and avascular necrosis.
2. Immediate reduction is imperative. The longer the delay in reduction, the greater the incidence of avascular necrosis.
3. Patients with prosthetic joints are at greater risk for dislocation and often require only slight trauma.

HIP FRACTURE

DIAGNOSIS

Associated Clinical Features

Fractures of the femoral head, femoral neck, and intertrochanteric fractures are termed *hip fractures*. For classification, hip fractures are generally divided into intracapsular (femoral head and neck fractures) and extracapsular (trochanteric, intertrochanteric, and subtrochanteric fractures) (Fig. 11.39). Accurate classification is important because of the different prognosis associated with each group. Intracapsular fractures are more likely to have disruption of the vascular supply and resultant avascular necrosis. On the other hand, extracapsular fractures rarely impair the vascular supply.

All patients have complete immobility at the hip joint. Complaints include hip and groin pain, tenderness, and an inability to walk or place pressure on the affected side. There is shortening of the affected leg, as well as abduction and external rotation (Fig. 11.40). Intertrochanteric fractures are associated with significant pain, a shortened extremity, marked external rotation, swelling, and ecchymosis around the hip (Fig. 11.41). Femoral neck fractures are suggested when the extremity is held in slight external rotation, abduction, and shortening. Dislocation of the hip is commonly associated with femoral head fractures. Patients with anterior dislocation and a femoral head fracture hold the lower extremity in abduction and external rotation. Patients with a posterior dislocation hold the extremity in adduction, internal rotation, and display notable shortening.

The femoral head has a tenuous vascular supply which includes three sources: artery of the ligamentum teres, the metaphyseal arteries, and the capsular vessels. Any injury that disturbs the anatomy of the hip can lead to compromise of this vascular supply.

Shenton's line and the normal neck shaft angle of 120 to 130 deg (obtained by measuring the angle of the intersection of lines drawn down the axis of the femoral shaft and the femoral neck) should be checked in all suspicious injuries.

Differential Diagnosis

Pelvic fracture, femoral shaft fracture, stress fracture, and hip dislocation are sometimes mistaken for a hip fracture prior to radiographic examination.

ED Treatment and Disposition

Once the patient is stabilized, the hip fracture is reduced via traction. Femoral head fracture dislocations are an orthopedic emergency and require immediate reduction. A neurovascular exam-

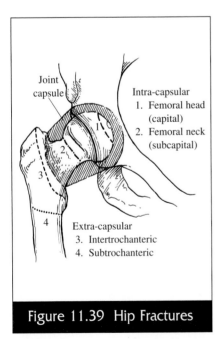

Figure 11.39 Hip Fractures

This illustration depicts the different types of proximal femur fractures.

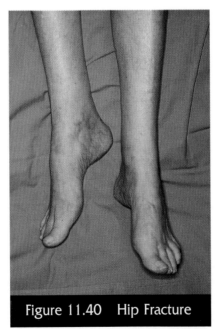

Figure 11.40   Hip Fracture

Patients with hip fractures often present with the affected extremity shortened, externally rotated, and abducted. Note the rotation and shortening in this patient with a right intertrochanteric fracture. (Courtesy of Cathleen M. Vossler, MD.)

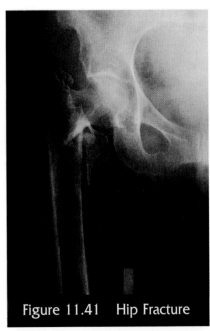

Figure 11.41   Hip Fracture

Radiographic examination reveals an intertrochanteric fracture. (Courtesy of Cathleen M. Vossler, MD.)

ination should be carefully performed before and after any reduction attempts. Orthopedic consultation should be obtained early, since these patients will require admission and in most cases surgical reduction and fixation.

Clinical Pearls

1. Hip pain can be referred to other areas. Therefore, in any patient complaining of knee or thigh pain consider the possibility of a hip fracture.
2. Fracture dislocation of the femoral head requires great forces, and associated injuries such as chest, intraabdominal, and retroperitoneal injuries should be considered.
3. Intracapsular fractures usually have much less blood loss than extracapsular fractures because of hematoma containment within the capsule.
4. Fractures of the hip may be diagnosed by auscultation of differences in bone conduction between the patient's two extremities. This is performed by placing the stethoscope's diaphragm on the anterior superior iliac spine and giving the patella several soft taps.
5. In the elderly, hip fractures are usually secondary to a fall. Be sure to address the cause of the fall to rule out a pathologic etiology (i.e., acute myocardial infarction, syncope, etc.).

PELVIC FRACTURE

DIAGNOSIS

Associated Clinical Features

Pelvic fractures range in severity from stable pubic rami fractures to unstable fractures with hemorrhagic shock. Pain is the most frequently encountered complaint. Blood at the urethral meatus, a high riding prostate, gross hematuria, or a scrotal hematoma (Fig. 11.42) are all signs of associated urinary tract injury. Ecchymosis of the anterior abdominal wall, flank, sacral, or gluteal region should be regarded as a sign of serious hemorrhage. Blood found during rectal examination may indicate puncture of the wall of the rectum from a pelvic fracture. Leg shortening may also be seen. A careful neurologic examination is necessary since there may be compromise of the sciatic, femoral, obturator, or pudendal nerves.

Differential Diagnosis

Femur fracture, hip fracture, or intraabdominal or retroperitoneal pathology (including hemorrhage, perforated viscous) can be confused with pelvic fractures.

ED Treatment and Disposition

Management includes initial stabilization and evaluation for any life-threatening injuries. Patients require multiple large-bore IVs and type and cross-

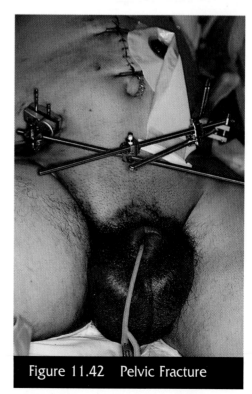

Figure 11.42   Pelvic Fracture

Pelvic fractures may require emergent external fixation to help control hemorrhage. Scrotal hematoma, or Destot's sign, suggests a pelvic fracture. (Courtesy of Cathleen M. Vossler, MD.)

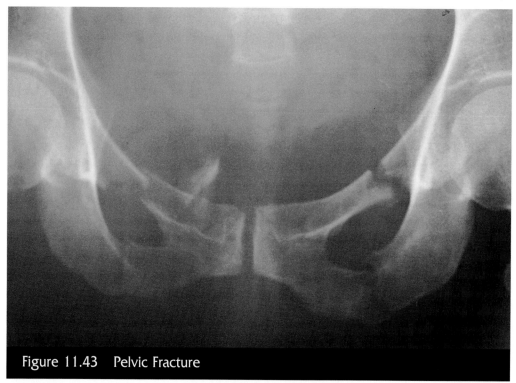

Figure 11.43   Pelvic Fracture

Radiographic examination reveals bilateral sacroiliac joint diastasis, complete transverse fracture of the sacrum, and comminuted fractures of the right superior and inferior pubic rami. (Courtesy of Cathleen M. Vossler, MD.)

match with blood readily available. Hemorrhagic shock occurs secondary to bleeding from a pelvic fracture and is the major cause of death in these patients. Retroperitoneal bleeding is unavoidable and up to 6 L of blood can easily be lost. Early orthopedic consultation is critical for emergent external fixation placement. Angiography should be performed to control small bleeding sites if there is continued exsanguination.

Clinical Pearls

1. Pelvic fractures may cause or be associated with serious abdominal, thoracic, genitourinary, or neurovascular injury.
2. Don't assume that a pelvic fracture is the sole cause of hemorrhagic shock in a patient. Look for other sources.
3. Posterior pelvic fractures are more likely to result in hemorrhage and neurovascular damage. Anterior pelvic fractures are more likely to cause urogenital damage.
4. Urinary tract injury is highly associated with pelvic fracture and must be ruled out. If there are any signs of genitourinary injury, a Foley catheter should not be placed until a retrograde urethrogram has been performed.
5. Displacement of pelvic ring fractures is usually associated with fracture or dislocation of another ring element (Fig. 11.43).

Lower Extremity

FEMUR FRACTURE

Associated Clinical Features

Femur fractures occur secondary to great forces, like those associated with motor vehicle accidents. The diagnosis is usually evident on visualization of the thigh (Fig. 11.44) and confirmed radiographically (Fig. 11.45). The position of the leg can help determine at which point the femur is fractured. Commonly associated injuries include hip fracture and dislocation as well as ligamentous injury to the knee. Hematoma formation is common.

Differential Diagnosis

Pelvic fracture, hematoma, hip fracture, hip dislocation, and contusion can be mistaken for femur fracture prior to radiographic examination.

ED Treatment and Disposition

Initial management includes stabilization and evaluation for any life-threatening injuries. It is important to keep in mind that a large amount of blood loss can occur (average blood loss for a femoral shaft fracture is 1000 cc). These patients should have two large-bore IVs and be cross-matched for blood products should they become necessary. The extremity should be immobilized and splinted with a traction device such as a Hare splint. Once this is accomplished, radiographic evaluation of the extremity should be performed. Orthopedic consultation should be obtained and admission arranged. The majority of intertrochanteric and subtrochanteric fractures require operative fixation and stabilization. An open fracture is an orthopedic emergency; these patients require tetanus prophylaxis, antibiotic coverage, as well as emergent irrigation and debridement in the operating room.

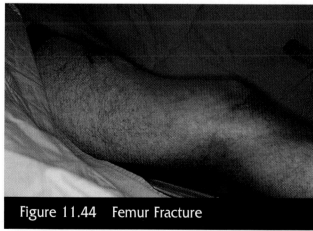

Figure 11.44   Femur Fracture

A closed midshaft femur fracture is seen. Note the deformity in the middle of the thigh consistent with this injury. (Courtesy of Daniel L. Savitt, MD.)

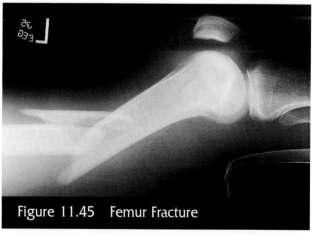

Figure 11.45   Femur Fracture

Radiographic examination reveals a comminuted displaced distal femur fracture. (Courtesy of Cathleen M. Vossler, MD.)

Clinical Pearls

1. Pain can be referred. Any injury between the lumbosacral spine and the knee can be referred to the thigh or knee.
2. Vascular compromise can occur and should be suspected with an expanding hematoma, absent or diminished pulses, or progressive neurologic signs. Neurovascular status needs to be assessed frequently.
3. Femoral shaft fractures can mask the clinical findings of a hip dislocation; thus radiographs of the pelvis and hips should be obtained routinely.

DIAGNOSIS   # PATELLAR DISLOCATION

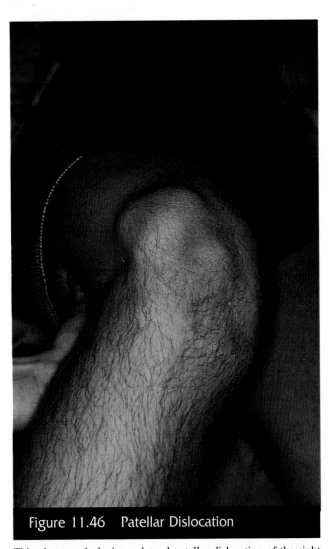

Figure 11.46   Patellar Dislocation

This photograph depicts a lateral patellar dislocation of the right knee. Note the obvious lateral deformity of the right patella. (Courtesy of Cathleen M. Vossler, MD.)

Associated Clinical Features

Patellar dislocations result from direct trauma to the patella. A force is applied to the upper portion of the patella at the same time as a rotational force to the knee. The most common dislocations are lateral, but horizontal, superior, and intercondylar also occur. Dislocations tend to be recurrent due to the resultant increased laxity of the supporting structures. Patients who have had recurrent dislocations often reduce the dislocation prior to arrival to the ED. Common complaints include pain, swelling, and a deformity in the knee. Physical examination reveals fullness or deformity in the lateral aspect of the knee (Fig. 11.46). Fractures of the patella or femoral condyle occur in 5% of patients.

Differential Diagnosis

Distal femur fracture, quadriceps and/or patellar tendon rupture, patellar fracture, or knee dislocation can be mistaken for a patellar dislocation.

ED Treatment and Disposition

Reduction is easily accomplished and results in immediate relief of pain. Lateral dislocations are reduced by flexing the hip, extending the knee, and gently directing pressure medially on the patella. Other dislocations generally require open reduction. Radiographic examination should be obtained to document patellar position as well as evaluate for fracture. These patients require a knee immobilizer or long leg cast in full extension for 4 to 6 weeks. Orthopedic consultation should be obtained, since these patients require further evaluation.

Clinical Pearls

1. A dislocated patella may reduce spontaneously prior to presentation and should be addressed as a possibility in any patient who presents with knee pain. This can be elucidated in the history by inquiring about a deformity of the knee at the time of the injury that is no longer present.
2. Complications of patellar dislocation include degenerative arthritis, recurrent dislocations and subluxations, and fractures.
3. The patellar apprehension test should be performed on these patients; patients have the sensation that the patella will dislocate when there is a lateral pressure placed on the patella, at which point they grab for their knee.

FRACTURE BLISTERS

DIAGNOSIS

Associated Clinical Features

Fracture blisters are vesicles or bullae that arise secondary to swelling from soft-tissue injury and fracture formation (Fig. 11.47). The most commonly affected areas include the tibia, ankle, and elbow. Patients note blister formation within 1 to 2 days after the initial trauma. Patients complain of pain, swelling, ecchymosis, and decreased range of motion. Complications include infection, deep vein thrombosis, and compartment syndrome.

Differential Diagnosis

Sprain, fracture, cellulitis, necrotizing fasciitis, compartment syndrome, or burns could be confused with fracture blisters.

ED Treatment and Disposition

Blisters are generally left intact, and the underlying fracture is treated.

Clinical Pearls

1. Although blisters can be seen with other conditions including barbiturate overdose, in the setting of trauma they frequently indicate an underlying fracture.
2. Blisters are managed in a similar fashion to second-degree burns.

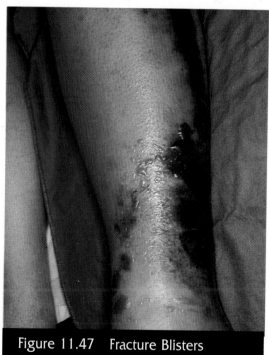

Figure 11.47   Fracture Blisters

Fracture blisters in a patient who fell down four steps on the evening prior to presentation. The patient had initially complained of ankle pain, decreased range of motion, and an inability to bear weight. Upon awakening the next morning, he noted ecchymosis, swelling, and blister formation. Radiographics revealed fracture of the fibula. (Courtesy of Cathleen M. Vossler, MD.)

Associated Clinical Features

Rupture of the Achilles' tendon occurs most frequently in middle-aged males involved in athletic activities. There are three mechanisms that result in this injury: a direct blow to the tendon, forceful dorsiflexion of the ankle, or increased tension on an already taut tendon. Rupture occurs 2 to 3 cm above its attachment to the calcaneus (Fig. 11.48). Patients complain of a feeling of being hit in the posterior aspect of the lower leg. They may hear or feel a pop. There is weakness when pushing off of the foot; pain, edema, and ecchymosis develop. A Thompson's test can be diagnostic of an Achilles' rupture (Fig. 11.49). The patient should be placed in a prone position; the gastrocnemius muscle should be grasped and squeezed. If the Achilles' tendon is even partially intact, then the ankle will plantar flex; if ruptured, there will be no movement of the ankle.

Differential Diagnosis

Partial Achilles' tendon tear, plantaris tendon rupture, ankle sprain, and partial gastrocnemius muscle rupture have been confused with an Achilles' tendon rupture.

ED Treatment and Disposition

Treatment is either operative or conservative. In either case, the extremity is immobilized without weight bearing for 6 weeks, followed by 6 weeks of partial weight bearing. ED treatment consists of elevation, analgesia, ice, and immobilization with a posterior splint. Orthopedic consultation should be obtained so that a plan of treatment can be chosen. These patients can be discharged home with close orthopedic follow-up or can be admitted for acute repair. Partial tears are generally treated conservatively.

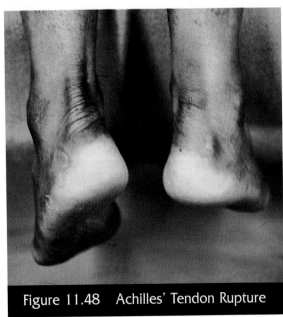

Figure 11.48   Achilles' Tendon Rupture

This photograph depicts a patient with a right Achilles' tendon rupture. Note the loss of the normal resting plantar flexion on the right owing to disruption of the tendon. This is seen with the patient in a non-weight-bearing position. Swelling is also apparent over the site of the tendon injury. (Courtesy of Kevin J. Knoop, MD, MS.)

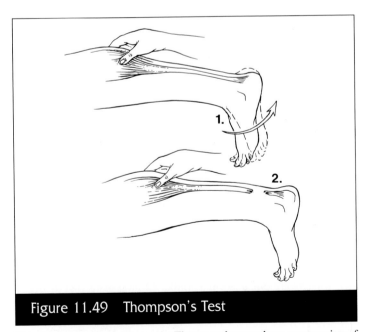

Figure 11.49   Thompson's Test

This illustration demonstrates the Thompson's test where compression of the gastrocnemius-soleus complex normally produces plantar flexion of the foot (1). If the tendon is completely ruptured, then this will not occur (2).

Clinical Pearls

1. Advantages to surgical repair are increased strength and mobility, and a decreased rate of re-rupture.
2. Approximately 25% of these injuries are initially misdiagnosed as ankle sprains.
3. These patients maintain the ability to plantar flex the foot in a non-weight-bearing position owing to the action of the tibialis posterior, toe flexor, and peroneal muscles.
4. Palpation of the tendon alone may not detect rupture as the tendon sheath is often intact.

ANKLE DISLOCATION

DIAGNOSIS

Associated Clinical Features

Ankle dislocations require forces of great magnitude. Posterior dislocation is the most common, but the ankle can also dislocate laterally, medially, superiorly, or anteriorly (Figs. 11.50, 11.52). A posteriorly dislocated ankle is locked in plantar flexion with the anterior tibia easily palpable. The foot has a shortened appearance with the ankle very edematous. Anterior dislocations present with the foot dorsiflexed and elongated. Lateral dislocations present with the entire foot displaced laterally. Ankle dislocations are commonly associated with malleolar fractures.

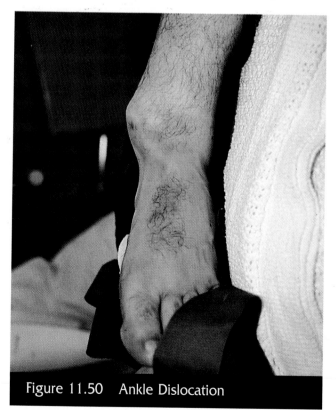

Figure 11.50   Ankle Dislocation

A posterior ankle dislocation is pictured. Radiographs showed an associated fracture. (Courtesy of Mark Madenwald, MD)

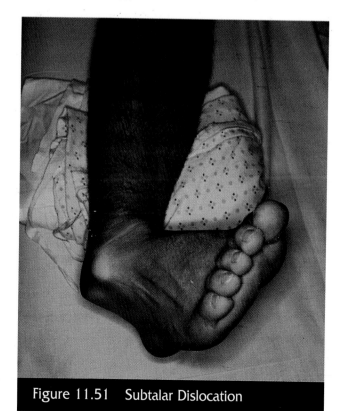

Figure 11.51   Subtalar Dislocation

This patient landed on his foot while playing basketball. Neurovascular status was intact, and the ankle was promptly reduced after x-ray showed no associated fracture. (Courtesy of Kevin J. Knoop, MD, MS.)

Differential Diagnosis

Fractures of the tibia, fibula, or talus, as well as ankle sprains, are all commonly mistaken for ankle dislocation on initial examination. A subtalar foot dislocation (Fig. 11.51) resembles ankle dislocation.

ED Treatment and Disposition

Routine radiographs should be obtained to identify any fractures. Reduction should occur before radiography if circulatory compromise exists. To reduce the ankle, gentle traction is applied to the foot, in an opposite direction of the force that caused the injury. Neurovascular status should be checked before and after any attempts at reduction or immobilization. Reduction usually requires conscious sedation, a Bier block, or general anesthesia. Patients should be placed in a posterior splint with immediate referral to an orthopedic surgeon for hospitalization.

Clinical Pearls

1. These injuries are commonly associated with malleolar fractures and often require open reduction and internal fixation.
2. Fifty percent of ankle dislocations are open and require surgical debridement.
3. There is an increased incidence of avascular necrosis following ankle dislocation.

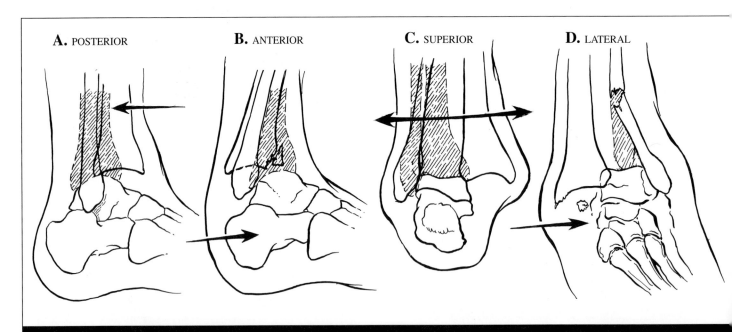

A. POSTERIOR   **B.** ANTERIOR   **C.** SUPERIOR   **D.** LATERAL

Figure 11.52   Ankle Dislocations

This illustration depicts different types of ankle dislocations. Arrows denote direction of the injury force. (Adapted with permission from Simon *Emergency Orthopedics: The Extremities.* New York, Appleton and Lange, 1987, p 402.)

Associated Clinical Features

Patients complain of pain, swelling, decreased range of motion, and tenderness over the lateral aspect of the foot (Fig. 11.53). Fractures of the fifth metatarsal base have been generically referred to as Jones fractures (Fig. 11.53). However, the fractures can be divided into three types, depending on their anatomic location. Treatment is determined by this division.

The classic Jones fracture is a transverse fracture of the fifth metatarsal diaphysis (Figs. 11.54(b), 11.55). It occurs when a force is applied to a plantar flexed and inverted foot. It is also referred to as a proximal shaft stress fracture and is usually due to repetitive stress injury. Patients often have prodromal symptoms.

A fracture at the metaphyseal-diaphyseal junction has been termed a pseudo-Jones fracture. It is always an acute injury.

The last type is an avulsion fracture of the fifth metatarsal base caused by sudden inversion of the foot (Fig. 11.54(A), 11.56). The avulsion injury is caused by traction on the lateral cord of the plantar aponeurosis.

Differential Diagnosis

Care must be taken to avoid confusing the two sesamoid bones in this area with a fracture. The more common of the two, the os peroneum (present in

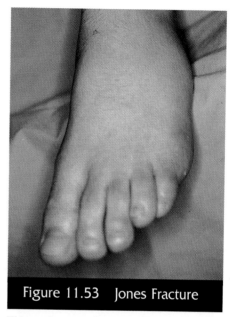

Figure 11.53   Jones Fracture

This patient sustained an injury of the fifth metatarsal and presented with pain and swelling over this site. His radiograph revealed a fracture. (Courtesy of Cathleen M. Vossler, MD.)

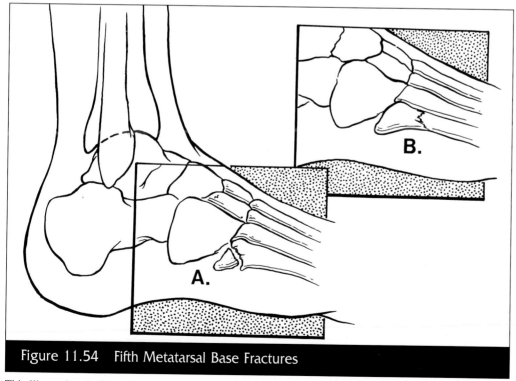

Figure 11.54   Fifth Metatarsal Base Fractures

This illustration depicts an avulsion fracture (A) and a classic Jones fracture (B).

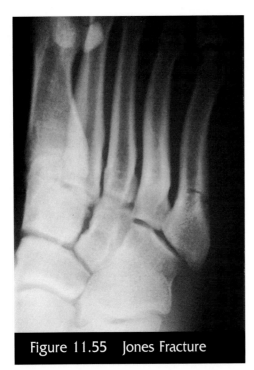

Figure 11.55   Jones Fracture

Radiograph with typical appearance for a diaphyseal fracture of the fifth metatarsal base. (Courtesy of Alan B. Storrow, MD.)

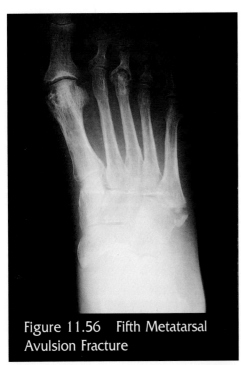

Figure 11.56   Fifth Metatarsal Avulsion Fracture

Radiograph illustrating an avulsion type fracture of the fifth metatarsal base, sometimes referred to as a ballet dancer's fracture (See Fig. 11.54). (Courtesy of Alan B. Storrow, MD.)

approximately 15%), lies within the peroneus longus tendon. More rare is the os vesalianum, which lies in the peroneus brevis tendon. Both have smooth, rounded surfaces and usually occur bilaterally. The fifth metatarsal base apophysis might also be confused as a fracture. It usually fuses by 16 years of age, although some fail to fuse.

Other entities to consider include ankle sprain, other metatarsal fractures, and foot dislocations.

ED Treatment and Disposition

A Jones fracture should be splinted and referred to orthopedics for definitive repair. It may heal slowly and cause permanent pain and disability. Surgical treatment is sometimes recommended, particularly since the stress involved with these fractures usually occurs in the sporting activities of young patients.

A pseudo-Jones fracture usually heals without complication, although more slowly than the avulsion fracture. Referral to orthopedics for a walking, or non-weight-bearing, cast according to local preference, is indicated.

The avulsion fracture usually heals rapidly and seldom leads to permanent disability. Most orthopedic physicians treat these patients symptomatically with a short leg walking cast or hard sole shoe for 2 to 3 weeks. Surgery is rarely indicated.

Clinical Pearls

1. It is important to differentiate between the different types of fifth metatarsal base fractures; treatment and disposition are dictated by these categories.
2. The original description of these fractures was by Sir Robert Jones, who personally sustained an injury while dancing. The avulsion fracture is sometimes referred to as the ballet dancer's fracture.
3. The classic Jones fracture has a high incidence of delayed healing and nonunion.

Associated Clinical Features

Ankle sprains are extremely common problems in the ED. Classification of these injuries based on physical examination and radiography helps guide management and definitive treatment.

The most common mechanism is an inversion stress that injures, in order, the joint capsule, anterior talofibular ligament, calcaneofibular ligament, and posterior talofibular ligament. Since the medial deltoid ligament is quite strong and elastic, serious eversion injuries usually result in avulsion of the medial malleolus or fracture of the lateral malleolus.

A first-degree sprain is defined by a stretch injury, or microscopic damage, to ligaments resulting in pain, tenderness, minimal swelling, and maintenance of the ability to bear weight. A second-degree sprain is defined by a partial tear of the ligamentous structures resulting in pain, swelling (Fig. 11.57), local hemorrhage (Fig. 11.58), and moderate degree of functional loss. A third-degree sprain is a complete tear of the ligament or ligaments and presents with positive stress testing, significant swelling, and an inability to bear weight.

Differential Diagnosis

Malleolar and fifth metatarsal fractures can be confused with ankle sprains prior to radiographs. Any patient with joint pain should have an infectious etiology considered.

ED Treatment and Disposition

First-degree injuries are treated with ice packs, elevation, woven elastic (Ace) wrap, and early mobilization. For patients with mild second-degree sprains, immobilization for 72 h, followed by use of an ankle support has been advocated. More serious second-degree and all third-degree sprains should receive immobilization, ice, and elevation and be referred to orthopedics. In younger patients surgery is an option, although clear recommendations are lacking.

Another option for patients with marked swelling, in whom grading is uncertain, is immobilization, ice, elevation, and a reassessment at 72 h.

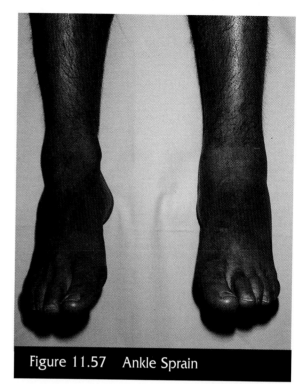

Figure 11.57   Ankle Sprain

Comparison view of a patient with a second-degree left lateral ankle sprain. Note the swelling and asymmetry of the affected area. (Courtesy of Kevin J. Knoop, MD, MS.)

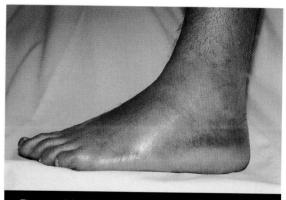

Figure 11.58   Ankle Sprain

Note the dependent ecchymosis and swelling in this patient with a second-degree left lateral ankle sprain. (Courtesy of Lawrence B. Stack, MD.)

Clinical Pearls

1. Ankle injuries are the most common orthopedic problem in emergency medicine.
2. Complications of ankle sprains include instability, persistent pain, recurrent sprains, and peroneal tendon dislocation.

3. The most common eversion injury is a fracture of the lateral malleolus. Since inversion injuries also produce lateral problems, the most common injuries to the ankle involve the lateral side.
4. Both malleoli, the proximal fibula, and the fifth metatarsal should be examined for injury when evaluating a patient with an ankle sprain.

CHAPTER 12

EXTREMITY CONDITIONS

Selim Suner
Daniel L. Savitt

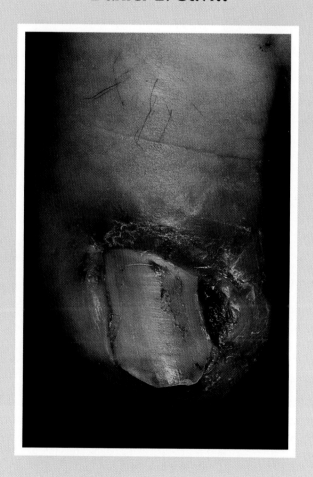

Associated Clinical Features

Inorganic arsenic compounds as well as sodium and potassium arsenite and arsenate are found in insecticides, wood preservatives, and in glass manufacturing. Arsine gas is produced with metal refining, galvanizing, etching, lead plating and in the silicone microchip industry. Acute arsenic poisoning, the most common cause of acute heavy metal poisoning, is encountered in accidental ingestion, industrial accidents, suicide, and homicide attempts. Low-dose exposure in industry or from contaminated water and food products may lead to chronic poisoning. Arsenic poisoning produces a syndrome involving the skin, hair, nails, GI system, bone marrow, liver, peripheral and central nervous systems, and kidneys. Acute symptoms of arsenic poisoning include violent gastroenteritis, hypotension, prolonged QT interval, seizures, and coma. Other symptoms such as hair loss (Fig. 12.1), raindrop hyperpigmentation, characteristic Mees' lines on the nails (Fig. 12.2), anemia and leukopenia, jaundice, subacute sensorimotor polyneuropathy, paralysis, hematuria, and renal failure are characteristic of chronic arsenic poisoning. Arsine gas exposure results in hemolysis and secondary renal failure. Arsenic binds with tissue sulfhydryl groups, causes direct capillary injury, has direct toxicity on large organs, and causes uncoupling of oxidative phosphorylation.

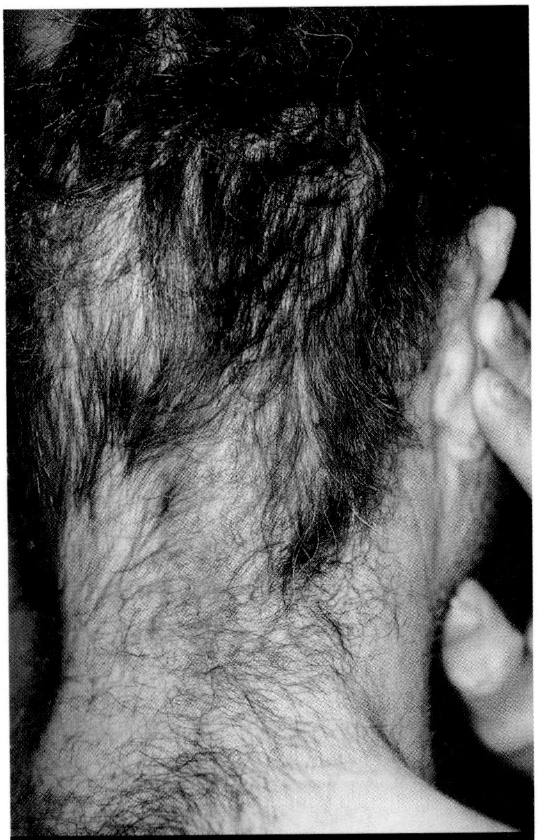

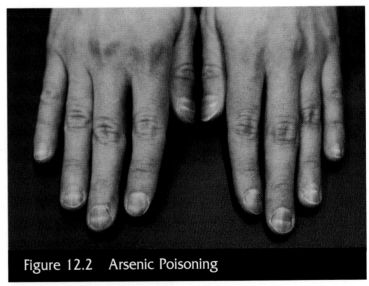

Figure 12.1   Arsenic Poisoning

The patchy hair loss seen in this photograph is from chronic arsenic poisoning. (Courtesy of Selim Suner, MD, MS.)

Figure 12.2   Arsenic Poisoning

Characteristic Mees' lines of chronic arsenic poisoning. Note the transverse white lines on all the nails of both hands. Mees' lines are often seen in conjunction with polyneuropathy of arsenic poisoning. (Courtesy of Robert Hoffman, MD.)

Differential Diagnosis

Similar symptoms may be seen with other heavy metal ingestions including thallium toxicity, food-borne toxins, bacterial diarrhea, renal failure, malaria, psoriasis, and Hodgkin's disease.

ED Treatment and Disposition

In the setting of acute arsenic poisoning, the first priority is to institute advanced life support measures to stabilize vital signs. Acute ingestion commonly requires resuscitation with intravenous fluids. Attention is directed to hydration status, cardiac monitoring, and gathering routine laboratory data. Standard gastric decontamination techniques, including gastric lavage and administration of activated charcoal, have been recommended. Although activated charcoal adsorbs arsenic poorly, it may be effective against coingestions. Toxicologic consultation should be obtained to determine the choice of chelating agents, which include dimercaprol (BAL), dimercaptosuccinic acid (DMSA), and D-penicillamine. Hemodialysis is indicated in the setting of renal failure. Diagnosis is based on clinical findings and 24-h urine arsenic level greater than 100 μg. CBC, liver function tests, electrolytes, BUN, creatinine, and urinalysis may be helpful in the diagnosis. The level of care is determined by the presentation, but most require admission and observation for a minimum of 24 h. A 24-h urine collection should be initiated on all admitted patients.

Clinical Pearls

1. Consider the diagnosis of acute arsenic poisoning in any patient with unexplained hypotension accompanied by or preceded by severe gastroenteritis.
2. Consider the diagnosis of chronic arsenic poisoning in any patient with a peripheral neuropathy, typical skin or hair manifestations, or recurrent gastroenteritis.
3. Remote arsenic exposure can be elucidated by obtaining levels in scalp and pubic hair.
4. There is a garlic odor on the breath or skin with arsenic poisoning. 5-Arsenic is absorbed through the skin, lungs, and GI tract and crosses the placenta.

CELLULITIS

DIAGNOSIS

Associated Clinical Features

Cellulitis is infection of the skin or subcutaneous tissues from local invasion, traumatic wounds, or hematogenous dissemination. The local inflammatory response is characterized by erythema with poorly defined borders, edema, warmth, pain, and limitation of movement (Figs. 12.3 and 12.4). Fever and constitutional symptoms may be present and are commonly associated with bacteremia. Trauma, lymphatic or venous stasis, immunodeficiency, and foreign bodies are predisposing factors. There may be enlarged regional lymph nodes. Organisms commonly causing cellulitis are group A beta hemolytic *Streptococcus* and *Staphylococcus aureus* in nonintertriginous skin not associated with an ulcer, gram-negative organisms in intertriginous skin and ulcerations, and *Haemophilus influenzae* in children younger than 3 years. In immunocompromised hosts *Escherichia coli*, *Klebsiella* species, *Enterobacter* species, and *Pseudomonas aeruginosa* may be the etiologic agents.

Differential Diagnosis

Deep venous thrombosis of the lower extremities, erythema nodosum, septic or inflammatory arthritis, osteomyelitis, herpes zoster, allergic reactions, arthropod envenomation, and burns are included in the differential diagnosis of cellulitis.

ED Treatment and Disposition

Treatment of minor cases commonly consists of immobilization, elevation, analgesia, and oral antibiotics with reevaluation in 48 h. Admission and parenteral administration of antibiotics may be necessary for immunocompromised or toxic appearing patients or those who do not initially respond to outpatient therapy.

Clinical Pearls

1. Aggressive treatment of cellulitis with parenteral antibiotics in immunocompromised patients (e.g., diabetes mellitus) is warranted.
2. Fever is uncommon and associated with bacteremia.
3. Radiography for the presence of foreign body or gas in the tissue should be considered.
4. Leading edge aspirates are of low yield, but may be of help in a toxic-appearing patient.

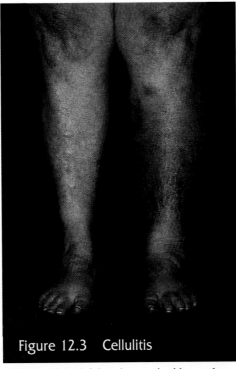

Figure 12.3   Cellulitis

Cellulitis of the left leg characterized by erythema and mild swelling. (Courtesy of Frank Birinyi, MD.)

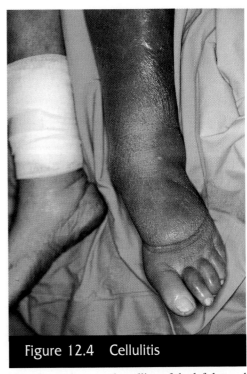

Figure 12.4   Cellulitis

Note the erythema and swelling of the left leg and foot secondary to cellulitis. The leg and foot were hot and exquisitely tender on physical examination. (Courtesy of Selim Suner, MD, MS.)

Associated Clinical Features

A felon is a pyogenic infection of the distal pulp space often caused by staphylococci or streptococci. A felon has no way of decompressing itself because the collection of pus is trapped between the septa that attach the skin to the distal phalanx. This condition is characterized by severe pain, exquisite tenderness, and tense swelling of the distal pulp with erythema (Fig. 12.5). There may be a visible collection of pus or palpable fluctuance. Complications include deep ischemic necrosis, osteomyelitis, septic arthritis, and septic tenosynovitis.

Differential Diagnosis

In the differential diagnosis of a felon, hematoma following traumatic injury, paronychia and herpetic whitlow should be considered.

ED Treatment and Disposition

There are several incision and drainage techniques employed in the treatment of a felon, and there is controversy surrounding which technique is the best to use. Incision and drainage utilizing a midlateral incision along the nondominant side of the finger or over the area of greatest fluctuance is commonly used to drain a felon. An alternative technique is to make a longitudinal volar incision directly through the finger pad into the pulp space and pus collection. To ensure complete drainage of the abscess cavity, all compartments should be entered. The packing of the abscess space is made with a small, loose-fitting wick to facilitate drainage. Oral antibiotics directed against gram-positive organisms should be used for 10 days and the packing removed or replaced after 24 to 48 h.

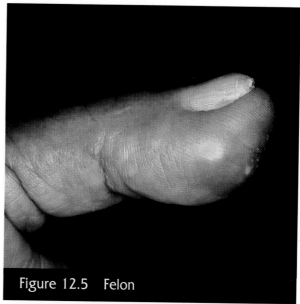

Figure 12.5　Felon

Note the area of purulence at the center of the palmar pad in this thumb with a felon. There is also swelling and erythema. (Courtesy of Daniel L. Savitt, MD.)

Clinical Pearls

1. Do not extend the incision proximal to the distal flexion crease.
2. Incisions should be made dorsal to the neurovascular bundle, and the pincer surfaces (radial aspects of the index and long fingers and ulnar aspect of the thumb and small finger) should be avoided when possible.
3. "Hockey stick" and "fish mouth" incisions are associated with increased occurrence of unnecessary sequelae and are not recommended.
4. If there is radiographic evidence of osteomyelitis, bone debridement along with antibiotic coverage is required.

Associated Clinical Features

Gangrene denotes an area of tissue that has lost its blood supply and is undergoing tissue necrosis. The term *dry gangrene* (Figs. 12.6 and 12.7) is used for tissues undergoing sterile ischemic coagulative necrosis, whereas *wet gangrene* is seen when liquidative necrosis from bacterial and leukocytic action is pronounced. *Streptococcus pyogenes* is often implicated in rapidly developing (6 h to 2 days) gangrene in traumatic and surgical wounds. Clostridia, anaerobic streptococci, and mixed aerobic and anaerobic flora can also be seen in wounds caused by trauma, surgery, or diabetic ulcers.

Differential Diagnosis

Gas gangrene, frostbite, cyanosis, traumatic ecchymosis, and subungual hematoma are some conditions that should be included in the differential diagnosis of gangrene.

ED Treatment and Disposition

The treatment consists of amputation, debridement, and antibiotic therapy as needed. Underlying vascular pathology must be evaluated by arteriography and corrected surgically. Hospitalization is usually required, and patients who present with systemic toxicity may require resuscitation in the ED.

Clinical Pearls

1. Obtain radiographs to rule out clostridial myonecrosis and osteomyelitis.
2. Soft-tissue infection may complicate this condition.

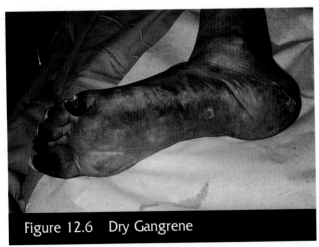

Figure 12.6   Dry Gangrene

Dry gangrene of the toes showing the areas of total tissue death appearing black and lighter shades of discoloration of the skin demarcating areas of impending gangrene. (Courtesy of Lawrence B. Stack, MD.)

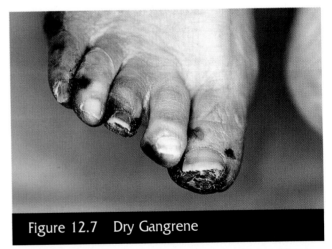

Figure 12.7   Dry Gangrene

Dry gangrene of the toes as a result of vascular disease. (Courtesy of Selim Suner, MD, MS.)

Associated Clinical Features

Also called clostridial myonecrosis, this infection causes rapid necrosis and liquefaction of fascia, muscle, and tendon. The vast majority of cases involve *Clostridium perfringens,* which produces a lethal necrotizing hemolytic alpha exotoxin. Myonecrosis is classically associated with trauma and diabetes. It is also seen in association with colon cancer, atherosclerotic disease, and abdominal surgery. The inoculation of the bacteria occurs either directly into the wound or by hematogenous spread. There is edematous bronze to purple discoloration, flaccid bullae with watery brown nonpurulent fluid (Fig. 12.8), and a foul odor. The most important clinical presentation is pain due to edema and the rapid production of gas in the infected muscle (Fig. 12.9). Pain out of proportion to the appearance of the injury is classic. Low-grade fever, which is an unreliable index of the severity of the infection, and tachycardia out of proportion to the fever are often present.

Crepitance and appearance of gross pockets of air in the tissue may be appreciated, but are not present early in the course of the illness. The incubation period for clostridia ranges between 1 and 4 days, but it can be as early as 6 h. Decreased tissue oxygen tension along with wound contamination are required for the infection to progress. Factors favoring decreased tissue oxygen tension include decreased blood supply, foreign body, tissue necrosis, or wound bacteria, which consume oxygen.

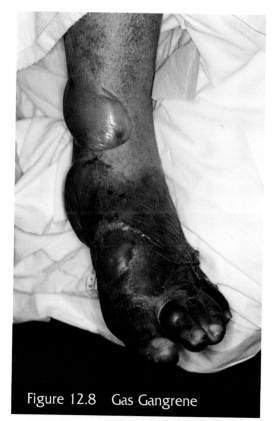

Figure 12.8   Gas Gangrene

A gangrenous foot with large bullae, areas of skin which are sloughing, and necrotic skin. There is also significant swelling. (Courtesy of Daniel L. Savitt, MD.)

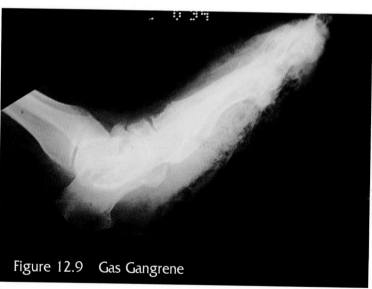

Figure 12.9   Gas Gangrene

Lateral view radiograph of the foot seen in Fig. 12.8. In addition to the swelling, there is air within the soft tissues best seen in the plantar portion of the foot. (Courtesy of Selim Suner, MD, MS.)

Differential Diagnosis

Crepitant cellulitis, synergistic necrotizing cellulitis, acute streptococcal hemolytic gangrene, and streptococcal myositis are some conditions that may be confused with clostridial myositis. Aspiration and Gram's stain showing gram-positive rods and few leukocytes may help, but often surgical exploration of the fascia and muscle is required to make the correct diagnosis.

ED Treatment and Disposition

Aggressive resuscitation with intravenous fluids is initiated, and consideration is given to packed red blood cell transfusion. Broad spectrum antibiotics in conjunction with penicillin G, in the non-penicillin-allergic patient, is given in the ED. Tetanus prophylaxis must not be overlooked. Surgical debridement or amputation, the mainstays of therapy, must be initiated promptly. Hyperbaric oxygen therapy in conjunction with surgical and antibiotic therapy has been shown to have a synergistic effect in preventing progression of the infection and production of toxin.

Clinical Pearls

1. Clostridial infection should be considered in patients presenting with low-grade fever, tachycardia out of proportion to the fever, and pain out of proportion to physical findings.
2. Mortality is 80 to 90% if untreated, 10 to 25% when treated appropriately.
3. Mixed gram-negative rods and enterococci are found in nonclostridial gas gangrene, which is exclusively seen in diabetics and carries a mortality of only 4% when treated.
4. Gram's stain yielding gram-positive bacilli with a relative lack of leukocytes can rapidly confirm clinically suspected clostridial myonecrosis.

DIAGNOSIS

CRYSTAL-INDUCED SYNOVITIS (GOUT AND PSEUDOGOUT)

Associated Clinical Features

Gout is an inflammatory disease characterized by deposition of sodium urate monohydrate crystals in cartilage, subchondral bone, and periarticular structures. Gout is most frequently associated with inborn errors of metabolism, myeloproliferative disorders, leukemia, hemolytic anemia, glycogen storage disease, hypertension, diabetes mellitus, obesity, heavy alcohol intoxication, and worsening renal function (gouty nephropathy). An acute attack is characterized by sudden onset of monarticular arthritis most commonly in the metatarsophalangeal (MTP) joint of the great toe (Named after the bad-tempered virgin foot goddess Podagra) (Fig. 12.10). There is swelling, erythema, and tenderness of the affected joint. There may be deposits of monosodium urate monohydrate (tophi) on the external ear and elbows and along tendons (Fig. 12.11).

In pseudogout, calcium pyrophosphate dihydrate (rod- or rhombus-shaped, weakly birefringent) crystals are deposited. Pseudogout is most frequently seen in association with hyperparathyroidism, hemochromatosis, hypophosphatasia, hypomagnesemia, myxedematous hypothyroidism, and ochronosis. Although any joint may be involved, knees and wrists are the most common. After joint deposition, the crystals are phagocytized by leukocytes that release proteolytic enzymes. The acute presenting signs and symptoms are identical with those of gout, but tophi formation is not seen with pseudogout. Fever, pain, and erythema are common to both entities.

Differential Diagnosis

Cellulitis and septic arthritis must be excluded. 2,000–50,000 WBCs with polymophonuclear neutrophil leukocyte (PMN) predominance is expected in the cell count of the synovial fluid obtained from an inflamed joint. Rheumatoid arthritis, sarcoidosis, hyperparathyroidism, cellulitis, septic arthritis, and traumatic injury may present similar to crystalline-induced synovitis. The diagnosis is made by seeing negatively birefringent urate crystals or rod (or rhombus)-shaped, weakly birefringent calcium pyrophosphate dihydrate crystals on polarized microscopy (See Figs. 17.1 and 17.2) with negative Gram's stain and cultures. Punched out lesions on subchondral bone may be seen on radiography in chronic tophaceous gout. Chondrocalcinosis may be seen in pseudogout.

ED Treatment and Disposition

Nonsteroidal anti-inflammatory medications are used with excellent results in the acute setting (e.g., indomethacin, 50 mg PO tid if renal function is normal) with immobilization of the joint and rest. Colchicine is a reasonable alternative but often has intolerable side effects such as nausea, vomiting, and diarrhea, and is associated with serious toxicity including bone marrow suppression, neuropathy, myopathy, and death (particularly when given intravenously). Intramuscular injection of adrenocorticotropic hormone (ACTH, 40–80 units IM or SC) or steroids may be used in patients with contraindications to colchicine and nonsteroidal anti-inflammatory medications. Intraarticular injection of steroids will alleviate symptoms rapidly without systemic side effects. Allopurinol or probenecid are used in chronic management of gout and play no role in acute treatment.

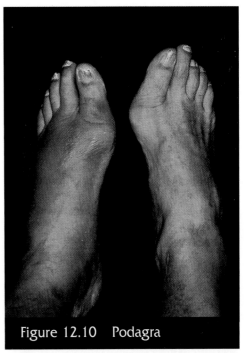

Figure 12.10   Podagra

Podagra denotes gouty inflammation of the first MTP joint. Note the swelling and erythema of the right first MTP. (Courtesy of Kevin J. Knoop, MD, MS.)

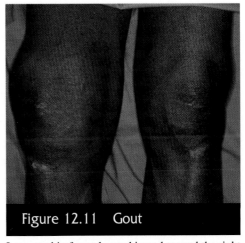

Figure 12.11   Gout

Large tophi of gout located in and around the right knee. (Courtesy of Daniel L. Savitt, MD.)

Clinical Pearls

1. Most (90%) of patients with crystalline-induced synovitis are male and older than 40 years.
2. Serum urate may be elevated or normal during acute episode.
3. Polyarticular presentation becomes increasingly more common with long-standing disease.
4. Acute gouty arthritis attacks may be triggered by minor trauma, diuretic or salicylate use, alcohol abuse, or dietary indiscretion.

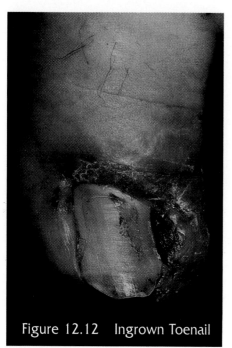

Figure 12.12   Ingrown Toenail

An ingrown toenail on the medial aspect of the left great toe. (Courtesy of Frank Birinyi, MD.)

Associated Clinical Features

This painful condition is the result of impingement and puncture of the medial or lateral nail fold epithelium by the nail plate. Tenderness and swelling of the nail fold is followed by granulation tissue growth causing sharp pain, erythema, and further swelling (Fig. 12.12). If not promptly treated, the granulation tissue becomes epithelialized, preventing elevation of the nail above the medial or lateral nail groove. Often there is secondary bacterial or fungal infection.

Differential Diagnosis

Paronychia, felon, and benign or malignant mass should be considered in the differential diagnosis of an ingrown toenail.

ED Treatment and Disposition

Early: Elevation of the nail out of nail fold and placement of gauze under nail to prevent contact in conjunction with warm soaks is the initial mode of therapy. *Late:* Surgical management involves removal of part of the nail and the inflamed tissue and destruction of the involved nail matrix. In the ED, the lateral portion of the affected nail is removed after digital block followed by packing of the paronychial fold with petroleum gauze or other nonadherent dressing. Dressing changes should be done daily with follow-up by a podiatrist until nail plate growth is complete. The destruction of the nail matrix is required only in patients with recurrent infected ingrown toenails and is not part of the emergency department management, which is designed to prevent injury to the nail matrix.

Clinical Pearls

1. Ingrown toenail is most common in the great toe, is associated with tight-fitting footwear, and may result from improper nail trimming (i.e., cutting the nail too short).
2. Antibiotics are indicated only if cellulitis is suspected or if the patient is a diabetic or has peripheral vascular disease.
3. Use of antibiotics is not a substitute for surgical excision and will result in only transient improvement of symptoms.

Associated Clinical Features

Inflammation of lymphatic channels in the subcutaneous tissues is commonly caused by the spread of local bacterial infection. Group A streptococcus is the most frequently implicated agent. Lymphangitis is characterized by red linear streaks (Figs. 12.13 and 12.14) extending from the site of infection (e.g., finger, toe) to regional lymph nodes (e.g., axilla, groin). The lymph nodes are often enlarged and tender. There may be associated peripheral edema of the involved extremity. Lymphangitis may develop within 24 to 48 h of the initial infection.

Differential Diagnosis

Cellulitis, trauma, and superficial thrombophlebitis are in the differential diagnosis of lymphangitis.

ED Treatment and Disposition

Rest, elevation, and immobilization in addition to antibiotics are the mainstays of treatment. Lymphangitis may be treated with oral antibiotics in afebrile patients who are not immunocompromised. Coverage for *Streptococcus* and *Staphylococcus* is appropriate. Toxic-appearing patients require admission for parenteral antibiotics. Any patient sent home with oral antibiotics should be followed up in 24 to 48 h. Patients who subsequently do not show improvement require admission for parenteral antibiotic therapy.

Clinical Pearls

1. Consider *Pasteurella multocida* with cat bites, *Spirillum minus* with rat bites, and *Mycobacterium marinum* in association with swimming pools and aquaria.
2. Chronic lymphangitis may be associated with mycotic, mycobacterial, and filarial infection.
3. In Africa and Southeast Asia, filariasis (*Wuchereria bancrofti*) is the most common etiologic agent.

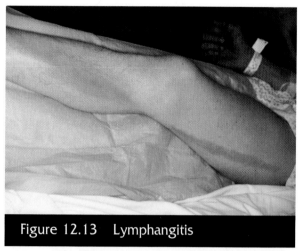

Figure 12.13 Lymphangitis

Severe lymphangitis is seen in the lower extremity. The red streak extends from the ankle to the groin and follows lymphatic channels. The site of infection, in this case, was located on the great toe. (Courtesy of Liudvikas Jagminas, MD.)

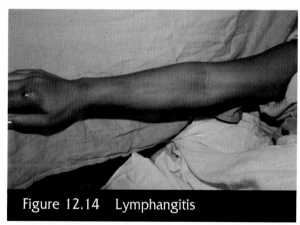

Figure 12.14 Lymphangitis

The lymphangitis extends from the wrist to the upper arm. Lymphangitis in the upper extremity commonly arises from nail biting. (Courtesy of Daniel L. Savitt, MD.)

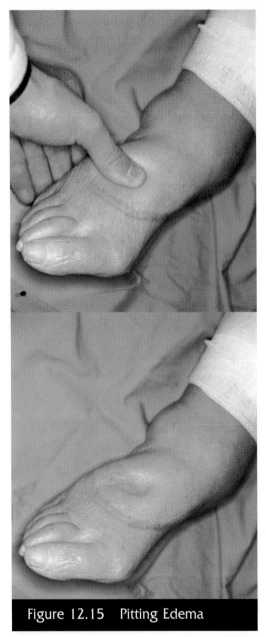

Figure 12.15   Pitting Edema

Pitting edema is seen in a woman with lymphedema of her lower extremities. Note how the impression of the thumb remains on the foot. (Courtesy of Daniel L. Savitt, MD.)

Associated Clinical Features

Lymphedema is a congenital or acquired childhood (praecox) and adult (tarda) obstruction of lymphatic channels associated with malignancy, radiation, trauma, surgery inflammation, infection, parasitic invasion, paralysis, renal insufficiency, congestive heart failure, cirrhosis, and malnutrition. Lymphedema is characterized by painless nonpitting edema (Fig. 12.15), fatigue, increase in limb size particularly during the day, and presence of lymph vesicles. The skin becomes thickened and brown in the late stages.

Differential Diagnosis

Cellulitis, DVT, lymphangitis, traumatic hematoma, right heart failure, tuberculosis, and lymphogranuloma venereum should be considered when the diagnosis of lymphedema is made. Subcutaneous dye injection, radiographic lymphography, and radionuclide lymph clearance may be used to aid in the diagnosis.

ED Treatment and Disposition

Control of edema with elevation, pneumatic compression boots and firm elastic stockings, maintenance of healthy skin, and avoidance of cellulitis and lymphangitis are the mainstays of treatment. Treatment of the underlying disease may be curative.

Clinical Pearls

1. Swelling usually starts distally and progresses proximally.
2. The dorsum of the toes and feet is always involved in lymphedema, unlike other causes of edema.
3. Careful examination for right heart failure and screening for renal insufficiency should be completed for all patients with lymphedema.

Associated Clinical Features

Olecranon or patellar bursitis is an inflammatory reaction of the bursa over the olecranon process (Fig. 12.16) or the patella (Fig. 12.17). It is associated with chronic irritation, trauma, or infection. The fluid collection may be infectious (septic bursitis, Fig. 12.18), gouty, or inflammatory. It is most commonly caused by repetitive minor trauma to the joint and is characterized by progressive pain, tenderness, and swelling. There may be erythema, warmth, and limited flexion of the joint secondary to pain. It is critical to differentiate septic from benign inflammation since the signs and symptoms can be similar. Prepatellar bursitis, also termed *housemaid's knee,* involves the prepatellar bursa, which is anterior to the infrapatellar tendon. Characterized by a warm, swollen tender knee, it may result from kneeling. It is important to distinguish this condition from a knee effusion.

Differential Diagnosis

Septic arthritis, crystal synovitis, fracture, and traumatic effusion may all mimic this condition. Aspiration and fluid analysis with Gram's stain, culture, and polarized microscopy are diagnostic in both instances. Synovial fluid with greater than 50,000 WBC, polymorphonuclear neutrophil leukocyte (PMN) predominance, and a positive Gram's stain and culture is associated with septic arthritis. High WBC count and PMN predominance with negative Gram's stain and sterile cultures may be seen in rheumatoid and seronegative arthritides. There are commonly fewer than 50,000 WBCs without PMN predominance and a negative Gram's stain with inflammatory bursitis. Crystals seen under polarized microscopy differentiate this condition from crystalline-induced synovitis.

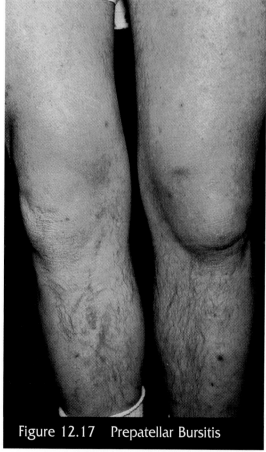

Figure 12.17   Prepatellar Bursitis

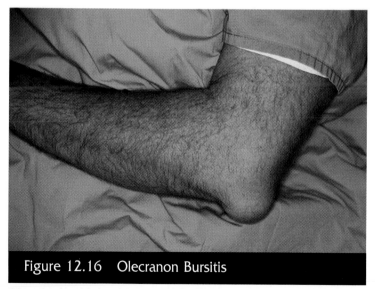

Figure 12.16   Olecranon Bursitis

Olecranon bursitis is evident in this flexed elbow. (Courtesy of Selim Suner, MD, MS.)

Local bursal swelling is evident over the left knee. (Courtesy of Kevin J. Knoop, MD, MS.)

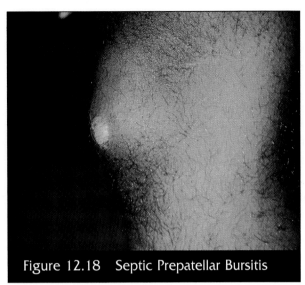

Figure 12.18   Septic Prepatellar Bursitis

This patient with diabetes presented with systemic signs of infection and required operative drainage of this pus-filled bursa. (Courtesy of Alan B. Storrow, MD.)

ED Treatment and Disposition

Rest, bulky dressings, and nonsteroidal anti-inflammatory medications are used to treat both conditions. If bursa is infected, repeated aspirations along with gram-positive antibiotic coverage is the treatment. The rare cases resistant to treatment may require incision and drainage or excision. Most patients can be treated as outpatients with close follow-up.

Clinical Pearls

1. The most important diagnostic dilemma is to differentiate between bursitis and a septic joint.
2. Patients with arthritis, unlike bursitis, will allow passive range of motion of the joint, and joint effusion is usually absent.
3. The olecranon and patellar bursa have a propensity to become infected. Infected bursae may have lower total cell counts than are commonly associated with septic joints.
4. Local steroid injection into the bursa may be used in aseptic bursitis. Complications of steroid injections include infection, local atrophy, bleeding, and tendon rupture.
5. Incision and drainage are not recommended for routine bursitis.

DIAGNOSIS	PALMAR SPACE INFECTION

Associated Clinical Features

Palmar space infections are infections within the deep soft-tissue planes of the hand involving the midpalmar space, the web spaces (collar button abscess), and the thenar (Fig. 12.19) or hypothenar spaces. These infections commonly arise from callus, fissures, puncture wounds to the palm, and rupture of flexor tenosynovitis of the digits. The palm loses its concavity, and there is dorsal swelling. In addition, tenderness, erythema, swelling, warmth, and fluctuance are evident in the palm. A *thenar space* infection is characterized by swelling over the thenar eminence and pain with abduction of the thumb. With a *midpalmar space* infection, motion is limited and painful for the middle and ring fingers. *Hypothenar space* infections are extremely rare. There is an extremely high morbidity associated with these infections.

Differential Diagnosis

Cellulitis, local traumatic injury, fractures, and soft-tissue mass are included in the differential diagnosis of palmar space infections.

ED Treatment and Disposition

All deep space infections of the hand should be managed by a hand surgeon. Prompt incision and drainage in the operating room is necessary for the best outcome. Frequently both palmar and dorsal incisions are necessary. Loose packing and antibiotic treatment follow surgery. Parenteral antibiotics against *Staphylococcus aureus* as well as anaerobes should be started in the ED.

Clinical Pearls

1. Palmar space infections may cause swelling on the dorsal hand.
2. In general, erythema, fluctuance, or tenderness are seen on the palmar aspect with very little seen dorsally.

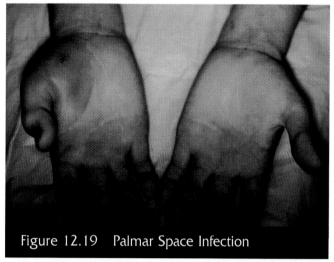

Figure 12.19   Palmar Space Infection

Thenar space infection following injury to the thumb. In this palmar view erythema and swelling in the thenar area and abduction of the thumb are evident. (Courtesy of Richard Zienowicz, MD.)

TENOSYNOVITIS   DIAGNOSIS

Associated Clinical Features

Tenosynovitis is inflammation of the tendon and the surrounding synovial sheath characterized by pain and tenderness. Pyogenic flexor tenosynovitis is infection of the tendon sheath from hematogenous origin, puncture wounds, or local extension. Tenosynovitis is characterized by the four signs of Kanavel (described for a finger flexor tendon): mild flexion contracture (Fig. 12.20), fusiform swelling along the volar finger surface, tenderness along the entire tendon sheath especially at the palmar surface of the metacarpophalangeal (MCP) joint, and severe pain with passive extension. Tenosynovitis may be complicated by fibrosis and adhesions leading to stiffness, loss of function, and tendon necrosis from destruction of the blood supply.

Differential Diagnosis

Cellulitis, traumatic injury, lymphangitis, osteomyelitis, septic arthritis, carpometacarpal arthritis, and allergic reactions may mimic some of the signs and symptoms of tenosynovitis.

ED Treatment and Disposition

It is difficult to distinguish infectious and noninfectious etiologies early in the course of the illness. Early (24 to 48 h) management of tenosynovitis, thought to be noninfectious, is accomplished with immobilization and nonsteroidal anti-inflammatory medications. Parenteral antibiotics, rest, immobilization, elevation, compressive dressing, and early consultation with a hand surgeon for incision and drainage within 24 to 48 h are mandated with pyogenic flexor tenosynovitis.

Clinical Pearls

1. *Staphylococcus aureus* is the most common organism but *Streptococcus,* gram-negative, and anaerobic organisms may also be responsible.
2. The most specific sign of tenosynovitis is pain with passive extension of the digit.
3. The abductor pollicis longus (APL) and the extensor pollicis brevis (EPB) (de Quervain's tenosynovitis) and the wrist are the most common sites for tenosynovitis.
4. Finkelstein's test is used to support the diagnosis of de Quervain's tenosynovitis (Fig. 12.21). The patient is instructed to make a fist with the thumb tucked inside the other fingers and the wrist is passively deviated to the ulnar side. Sharp pain along the APL and EPB tendons denotes a positive Finkelstein's test and is strong evidence of de Quervain's tenosynovitis.

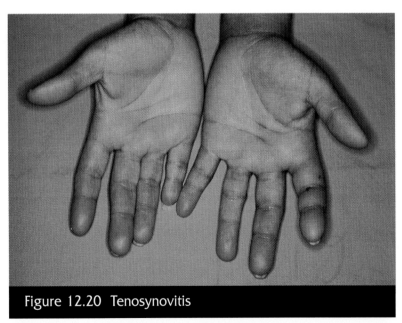

Figure 12.20 Tenosynovitis

Flexor tenosynovitis of the left index finger (after patient sustained a paper cut). Note the flexion and mild swelling of the index finger with the hand in the resting position. (Courtesy of Selim Suner, MD, MS.)

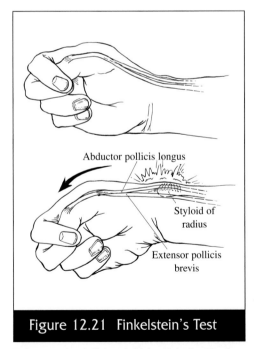

Abductor pollicis longus

Styloid of radius

Extensor pollicis brevis

Figure 12.21 Finkelstein's Test

Pain over the radial styloid is elicited with ulnar deviation of the wrist as shown.

Associated Clinical Features

Thrombophlebitis is superficial thrombosis and inflammation of veins or varicosities characterized by redness, tenderness, and palpable, indurated cordlike venous segments (Fig. 12.22). Common causes of thrombophlebitis are intravenous catheter insertion, irritant solutions through the intravenous line, and trauma. There is little risk of embolism when associated with varicose veins or superficial veins distal to the popliteal fossa; however, pulmonary embolism can occur secondary to propagation of the thrombus of more proximal veins into the deep venous system.

Differential Diagnosis

Septic superficial thrombophlebitis, lymphangitis, deep vein thrombosis, and cellulitis should be included in the differential diagnosis of thrombophlebitis. The patient must be evaluated for the possibility of deep venous thrombosis if no underlying cause of superficial thrombosis is elucidated.

ED Treatment and Disposition

Elevation with warm compresses, rest, and analgesia are sufficient treatment for uncomplicated superficial thrombophlebitis. Superficial thrombophlebitis and involvement of the saphenofemoral or iliofemoral system requires admission to the hospital with anticoagulation and treatment as a DVT. Also, admission to the hospital is warranted if there is extensive involvement, septic signs, progression of symptoms despite treatment, or severe inflammatory reactions.

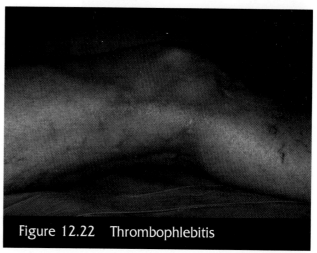

Figure 12.22   Thrombophlebitis

This photograph shows thrombophlebitis of the superficial veins in the leg. The thrombosed veins are erythematous, close to the surface, and palpable. (Courtesy of Lawrence B. Stack, MD.)

Clinical Pearls

1. Sixteen percent involve deep veins. There is a 40% risk of pulmonary embolism from superficial thrombophlebitis without underlying cause.
2. This condition is frequently associated with malignancy; this association is known as Trousseau's syndrome.
3. Since lymphatic drainage follows the greater saphenous vein, Doppler studies or venography may be needed to distinguish superficial thrombophlebitis from lymphangitis in this area.

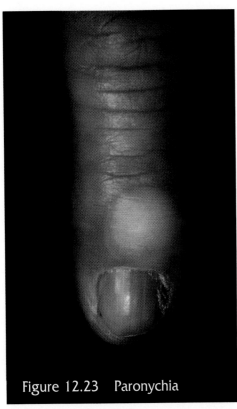

Figure 12.23   Paronychia

A paronychia involving one lateral fold and the eponychium. There is swelling, erythema and tenderness on the dorsum of the distal phalanx. (Courtesy of Frank Birinyi, MD.)

Associated Clinical Features

Paronychia is the most common infection seen in the hand and is characterized by infection and pus accumulation along the lateral nail fold. Paronychia may spread to involve the eponychium (Fig. 12.23) at the base of the nail and the opposite lateral nail fold if untreated. *Staphylococcus aureus* is the most frequently implicated organism.

Differential Diagnosis

Felon, dactylitis, herpetic whitlow, and traumatic injury should be considered when making the diagnosis of paronychia.

ED Treatment and Disposition

If recognized early, warm soaks with or without oral antibiotics may be sufficient. After 2 to 3 days, there may be sufficient pus accumulation along the eponychial fold to warrant incision and drainage. After digital block, a longitudinal incision is made along the eponychial fold. If the affected portion begins under the nail, removal of the proximal nail may be necessary. Another technique is elevation of the infected eponychium and lateral nail fold with a number 11 scalpel blade. The incisions should be packed open with gauze (removed in 24 to 48 h). Oral antibiotics should be prescribed, and the finger should be reevaluated in 2 to 3 days.

Clinical Pearls

1. Paronychia is typically associated with nail biting, manicure trauma, and small foreign bodies.
2. Superinfection with fungal agents may occur with immunocompromised patients or neglected paronychia.
3. Damage to the germinal matrix during excision of the nail plate results in nail deformity.
4. It is important to distinguish a paronychia from herpetic whitlow where incision and drainage is contraindicated.

Associated Clinical Features

This patient presented with discrete palpable purpuric lesions with central necrosis (Fig. 12.24) surrounded by a rim of erythema. Biopsies of the lesions demonstrated leukocytoclastic vasculitis consistent with hypersensitivity vasculitis.

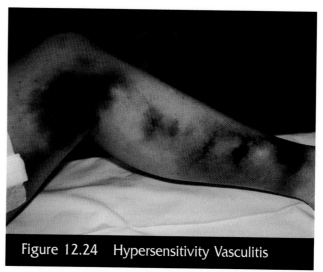

Figure 12.24   Hypersensitivity Vasculitis

The palpable purpura of a patient with hypersensitivity vasculitis secondary to new use of a nonsteroidal anti-inflammatory medication. (Courtesy of Lawrence B. Stack, MD.)

The eruption typically begins or is limited to the lower extremities. The palpable, nonblanching purpura or petechiae are usually secondary to a primary vasculitis or an embolic event which activates complement proteins. These proteins cause small blood vessel wall segmental inflammation, necrosis, and fibrin deposition, much like Henoch-Schönlein purpura (HSP). Features typical of this problem include self-limited palpable purpura, adult age, equal sexual incidence, and lack of other examination or laboratory abnormalities. There may be systemic involvement of the muscles, joints, gastrointestinal tract, or kidney, as well as pruritus and pain. The duration can be acute (especially drug-induced), subacute, or chronic.

Hypersensitivity vasculitis is more likely if the patient has recently received a new drug, or one known to cause purpura (Fig. 12.24). It can also be caused by sensitivity to infectious antigens. The cause is idiopathic in approximately 40 to 60% of patients.

Differential Diagnosis

The differential of purpura must include infections (bacterial and viral), hematologic abnormalities [e.g., thrombotic thrombocytopenic purpura, idiopathic thrombocytopenic purpura, disseminated intravascular coagulation], collagen-vascular diseases [e.g., systemic lupus erythematosus, rheumatoid arthritis, Sjogren's syndrome], and neoplasm. The primary vasculitides, such as HSP, polyarteritis nodosa, Wegener's granulomatosis, and temporal arteritis must also be considered.

The diagnostic criteria for hypersensitivity vasculitis includes at least three of the following: age >16 years, related medication, palpable purpura, maculopapular rash, and appropriate biopsy.

ED Treatment and Disposition

Since the differentiation of hypersensitivity vasculitis with a vasculitis of bacterial origin is often difficult, initial antibiotic therapy, blood cultures, and admission are usually indicated. Multiple episodes, especially if idiopathic, can occur. The suspected medication should be discontinued immediately, and the use of steroids can be considered. Other treatment modalities include the use of immunosuppressive medications and plasmapheresis.

Clinical Pearls

1. Diagnosis of the primary vasculitides is almost always made histopathologically.
2. There may be overlap between the causes of purpura.
3. Self-limited or irreversible damage may occur to the kidneys.
4. Synonyms for this entity include necrotizing vasculitis and allergic vasculitis.

DIAGNOSIS   SUBCLAVIAN VEIN THROMBOSIS

Associated Clinical Features

Thrombosis of the subclavian vein (Paget-Von-Schroetter syndrome) is an uncommon condition usually of iatrogenic origin. It may also be seen in young patients following exercise and results from compression injury to the subclavian or axillary vein from a narrow thoracic outlet (effort thrombosis). Symptoms of pain, discomfort, and tightness or swelling in the arm are manifested within a day of the thrombosis (Fig. 12.25). Pitting edema develops in the fingers, hand, and forearm. There is no arterial insufficiency, and the pulses are palpable. There is a 15% risk of developing pulmonary embolism from thrombosis of veins in the upper extremity; however, large or fatal emboli from this source are very rare. Ascending venography is the gold standard for diagnosis. Duplex scan, impedance plethysmography, and Doppler studies are also used, but the accuracy of these studies have not been studied in the upper extremity.

Differential Diagnosis

Superior vena cava syndrome, trauma to the upper extremity, congestive heart failure, angioedema, and lymphatic obstruction must be considered in the differential diagnosis.

ED Treatment and Disposition

Treatment consists of elevation, local heat, analgesia, and anticoagulation with intravenous heparin for patients presenting with long-term thrombosis. Patients should be admitted to the hospital. In cases of acute thrombosis (within 5 days of symptom onset), the treatment is thrombolysis with direct catheter infusion of urokinase or streptokinase. Surgical thrombectomy has also been employed. Operative correction of anatomic abnormalities should be accomplished to prevent long-term morbidity.

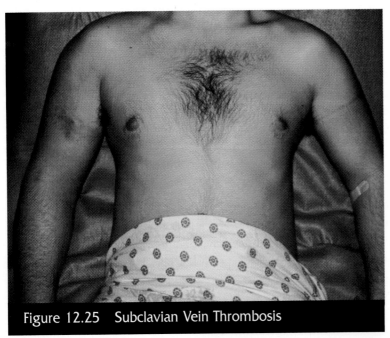

Figure 12.25   Subclavian Vein Thrombosis

Right subclavian vein thrombosis is manifested in this patient by swelling of the upper right extremity. (Courtesy of Douglas R. Landry, MD.)

Clinical Pearls

1. Swelling of the neck and face signifies thrombosis of the superior vena cava.
2. The superficial veins in the upper extremity are often distended and do not collapse when the arm is elevated.
3. There is greater incidence of subclavian vein thrombosis in men and in the right arm.
4. There may be late sequelae related to the thrombus such as pain, recurrent swelling, and early fatigue of the upper extremity.
5. Balloon angioplasty has been used to correct stenosis of the subclavian vein.

NECROTIZING FASCIITIS   DIAGNOSIS

Associated Clinical Features

This uncommon severe infection involves the subcutaneous soft tissues including the superficial and deep fascial layers. It is most commonly seen in the lower extremities, abdominal wall, perianal and groin area, and postoperative wounds, but can manifest in any body part. The infection is spread most commonly from a site of trauma or surgical wound, abscess, decubitus ulcer, or intestinal perforation. Alcohol and parenteral drug abuse and diabetes mellitus are predisposing factors. Omphalitis may progress to necrotizing fasciitis in the newborn. Pain and tenderness, erythema, swelling, warmth, shiny skin, lymphangitis, and lymphadenitis are early clinical findings. There is rapid progression with changes in skin color, bullae formation with pink and purple fluid (Fig. 12.26), and cutaneous necrosis (Fig. 12.27) within 48 h. The skin becomes anesthetic and subcutaneous gas may be present in the affected area.

There is systemic toxicity manifested by high fever, dehydration, leukocytosis, and frequently positive blood cultures. Fournier's gangrene is a form of necrotizing fasciitis occurring in the groin and genitalia of male patients. It is rapidly progressive and is associated with a high mortality rate, particularly in diabetics. The infection can pass through Buck's fascia of the penis, dartos fascia of the scrotum and penis, Colles' fascia of the perineum, and Scarpa's fascia of the abdominal wall. Necrotizing fasciitis of the face, eyelids, neck, and lips are rare but acutely life-threatening infections which compromise the airway. There are two groups of organisms implicated in necrotizing fasciitis. Type I includes anaerobic species (*Bacteroides* and *Peptostreptococcus* species) and type II group A streptococci alone or with *Staphylococcus aureus.*

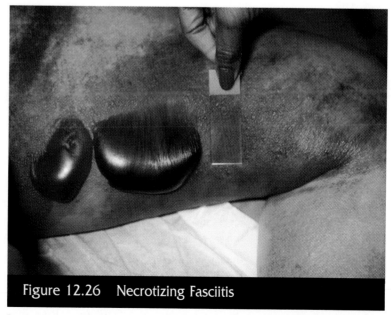

Figure 12.26   Necrotizing Fasciitis

Large cutaneous bullae are seen on the leg of this patient with necrotizing fasciitis. Note the dark purple fluid in the bullae. (Courtesy of Lawrence B. Stack, MD.)

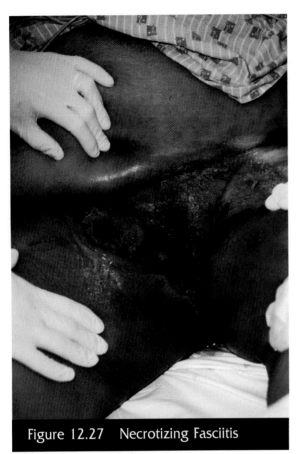

Figure 12.27   Necrotizing Fasciitis

Necrotizing fasciitis with cutaneous necrosis can be seen in the inner thigh of this patient. (Courtesy of Lawrence B. Stack, MD.)

Differential Diagnosis

Cellulitis, osteomyelitis, gas gangrene, streptococcal myonecrosis, infected vascular gangrene, and trauma should all be considered.

ED Treatment and Disposition

Prompt diagnosis is critical in the treatment of this condition. If the diagnosis is made within 4 days from the onset of symptoms, the mortality rate is reduced from 50 to 12%. The initial treatment involves resuscitation with volume expansion. One recommended initial antibiotic regimen includes a combination of ampicillin, gentamicin, and clindamycin. Prompt surgical excision is essential.

Clinical Pearls

1. Intravenous calcium replacement may be necessary to reverse hypocalcemia from subcutaneous fat necrosis.
2. Radiographs may be used to detect subcutaneous gas that is not palpable.
3. Hemolysis and disseminated intravascular coagulation (DIC) may be seen in association with necrotizing fasciitis.
4. Necrotizing fasciitis does not involve muscle, whereas gas gangrene has extensive muscle involvement.

DIAGNOSIS   CERVICAL RADICULOPATHY

Associated Clinical Features

Cervical radiculopathy is often caused by compression of a nerve root by a laterally bulging or herniated intervertebral disk. Osteoarthritis and spondylosis may also cause radiculopathy in the cervical spine. Pain results from injury of the sinuvertebral nerves innervating the nerve roots, dura and ligaments, facet joints, and bone. Common clinical features associated with cervical radiculopathy include pain, paresthesia, and root signs (sensory loss, lower motor neuron muscle weakness, impaired reflexes, and trophic changes). The pain is sharp and stabbing and worse with cough, and it radiates over the shoulder down the arm. There is often numbness and tingling following a dermatomal distribution. Root signs may be found corresponding to anatomic distribution of nerves (e.g., triceps muscle weakness, pinprick deficit along the middle finger, and atrophy with loss of triceps jerk associated with C-7 radiculopathy). MRI and CT myelogram are the commonly used modalities to evaluate cervical radiculopathy from disk and bone disease. Electromyelogram studies may also be helpful in ruling out other disease processes.

Differential Diagnosis

Trauma, myelopathy, plexopathy, neurofibromatosis, metastatic tumor infiltration of nerve roots, neoplasm, shingles, and central cord syndrome should be considered in the differential diagnosis of cervical radiculopathy.

ED Treatment and Disposition

The mainstay of ED treatment is pain control and referral to an orthopedic surgeon or neurosurgeon. Since prolonged nerve root compression can lead to permanent neurologic deficits, immediate referral is necessary for progressive neurologic signs. Patients with intractable pain, progressive weakness in the upper extremities, and myelopathy should be admitted to the hospital.

Clinical Pearls

1. Most radiculopathies resulting from cervical disk disease is seen in the 30 to 60 year age group and in the C-5 to C-7 region.
2. Risk factors for cervical radiculopathy include heavy lifting, cigarette smoking, frequent diving from a board, and prior trauma to the neck.
3. Patients with acute cervical radiculopathy may present with their upper extremity supported by their head to counteract the cervical root distraction caused by the weight of their dependent extremity (Fig. 12.28).

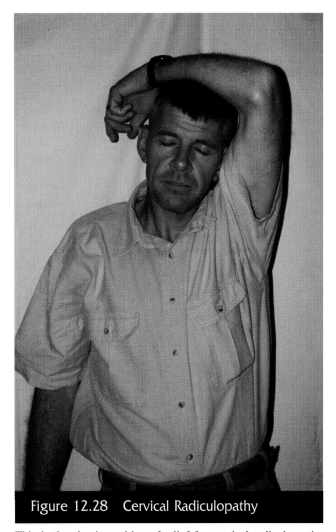

Figure 12.28   Cervical Radiculopathy

This is the classic position of relief for cervical radicular pain. This patient presented with severe pain in the neck with radiation to the extremity. The only relief the patient was able to feel was by holding his arm over his head in the position shown. This patient has a C-5 to C-6 herniated nucleus pulposus. (Courtesy of Kevin J. Knoop, MD, MS.)

Associated Clinical Features

Digital clubbing results from increase in soft-tissue density at the tips of the fingers, particularly on the dorsum. Associated with the increased tissue mass is enhanced blood flow, excessive curvature of the fingernails, and hyperemic and swollen skin folds around the fingernail (Fig. 12.29). Clubbing may also be seen in the toes. The mechanism underlying clubbing is not known, but it is postulated that the end result is dilatation of the distal digital blood vessels with soft-tissue hypertrophy. Clubbing may be hereditary, idiopathic, or acquired and is associated with multiple medical conditions including carcinoma, intrathoracic sepsis, bacterial endocarditis, cyanotic congenital heart disease, esophageal disorders, cirrhosis, inflammatory bowel disease, pulmonary disorders, atrial myxoma, repeated pregnancies, and pachydermoperiostosis. The incidence of clubbing with each of these conditions is variable. Digital clubbing may be reversible in certain disease processes.

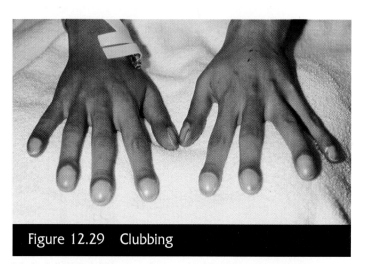

Figure 12.29   Clubbing

Marked digital clubbing can be seen in this patient. Note the hyperemia in the skin folds around the nail. (Courtesy of Alan B. Storrow, MD.)

Differential Diagnosis

Hypertrophic osteoarthropathy, infection, and trauma should be considered in the differential diagnosis of clubbing.

ED Treatment and Disposition

Treatment of the underlying condition is indicated. The disposition depends on the underlying diagnosis and condition of the patient.

Clinical Pearls

1. Bone radiographs can be used to diagnose hypertrophic osteoarthropathy. Subperiosteal formation of bone is seen in the distal diaphyses of long bones.
2. Patients rarely observe clubbing in their own fingers even if the fingers are markedly clubbed.

Associated Clinical Features

Phlegmasia alba dolens (painful white leg, or milk leg) is caused by extensive thrombosis of the iliofemoral veins and characterized by pitting edema of the entire lower extremity, tenderness in the inguinal area, and a pale extremity due to reflex spasm of the femoral artery. Phlegmasia cerulea dolens (painful blue leg, Fig. 12.30) arises from thrombosis of the veins in the lower extremity including the perforating and collateral veins resulting in a cool, painful, swollen, tense, and cyanotic lower extremity occasionally with bullae formation. Compartment syndrome and gangrene may follow.

Differential Diagnosis

Arterial insufficiency or thrombosis, aortic dissection, abdominal aortic aneurysm, deep venous thrombosis, cellulitis, and lymphedema may mimic these conditions. Doppler ultrasound, impedance plethysmography, and venography (most accurate for determining extent) are used in the diagnosis.

ED Treatment and Disposition

Systemic anticoagulation with intravenous heparin is indicated for this condition. If there is no improvement in 12 to 24 h, then iliofemoral venous thrombosis should be suspected. The role of intravenous thrombolytic therapy is controversial.

Clinical Pearls

1. Pregnancy is one risk factor for phlegmasia alba dolens.
2. Forty-four percent of patients with phlegmasia cerulea dolens have an underlying malignancy.
3. Phlegmasia dolens is seen in fewer than 10% of patients with venous thrombosis.
4. Hypotension may result from venous pooling of blood in the lower extremity and diminished venous return to the heart.
5. Petechiae on the skin of the lower extremity may be present.

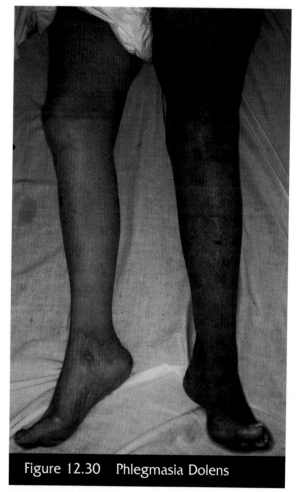

Figure 12.30   Phlegmasia Dolens

Phlegmasia cerulea dolens of the left lower extremity. Note the bluish discoloration and swelling in the left lower extremity. (Courtesy of Daniel L. Savitt, MD.)

Associated Clinical Features

Porphyrias are problems associated with enzymatic defects in heme biosynthesis. Porphyria cutanea tarda (PCT) presents as a condition of fragile skin and vesicles found on the dorsum of the hands, especially after trauma. The classic symptoms are easily traumatized skin leading to blisters in sun-exposed areas, erosions, milia, and hypertrichosis (Fig. 12.31). It may be induced by ethanol, estrogens, oral contraceptives, iron overload, and certain environmental exposures. The typical bullae and erosions may also occur in other areas, especially the feet and nose. In contrast to other porphyrias, PCT is not associated with life-threatening respiratory failure or abdominal pain or peripheral autonomic neuropathies. Confirmation of the diagnosis requires special 24-h urine testing for various porphyrins.

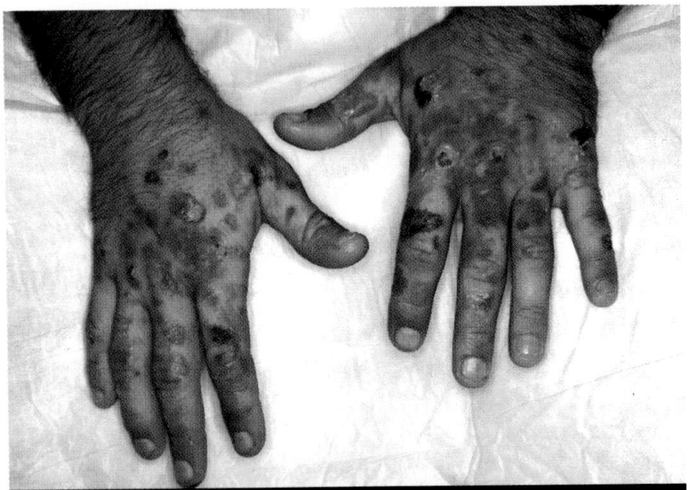

Figure 12.31   Porphyria Cutanea Tarda

Blisters and erosions of porphyria cutanea tarda. (Courtesy of Selim Suner, MD, MS.)

Differential Diagnosis

Other forms of porphyria, other bullous diseases, systemic lupus erythematosus (SLE), sarcoidosis, and Sjogren's syndrome must be considered.

ED Treatment and Disposition

Laboratory examination may begin in the ED with blood chemistries, porphyrin studies, and consideration of appropriate biopsies. Treatment includes discontinuation of any drugs which might initiate PCT. Phlebotomy and the use of chloroquine can be considered.

Clinical Pearls

1. PCT is the most common type of porphyria.
2. Examination of the urine may reveal orange-red fluorescence with a Wood's lamp.
3. This condition is sometimes termed *fragile skin.*

CHAPTER 13

CUTANEOUS CONDITIONS

Christopher R. Sartori
Michael B. Brooks

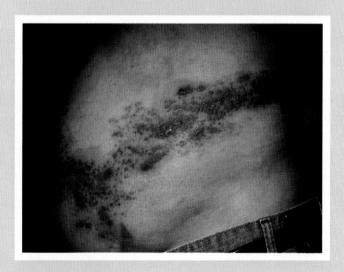

Associated Clinical Features

Considered a hypersensitivity syndrome, erythema multiforme (EM) presents with characteristic target or iris-shaped papules and vesicobullous plaques (Figs. 13.1 and 13.2). These lesions are frequently cutaneous manifestations of a drug reaction or herpes simplex infection. These plaques are usually symmetric, pruritic, and painful, often involving the mucous membranes and extremities including the palms and soles. The milder form of the disease has minimal mucosal involvement, no bullae, and no systemic symptoms. Fever, malaise, and other constitutional symptoms are noted in the severe form of EM, known as Stevens-Johnson syndrome (see next diagnosis).

Differential Diagnosis

The maculopapular presentation may be confused with urticaria or fixed drug eruption, whereas the oral vesicobullous plaques resemble herpetic gingivostomatitis. However, the cutaneous target lesions and their symmetry are typical of EM.

ED Treatment and Disposition

Elimination of any possible etiology (idiopathic cause noted approximately 50%) and supportive measures to allay the burning and itching is basic to treating this disorder. Milder forms of the disease usually resolve spontaneously within 2 to 3 weeks. Corticosteroids are reserved for the severest presentations. Erythema multiforme minor can be treated on an outpatient basis. However, patients with significant systemic illness

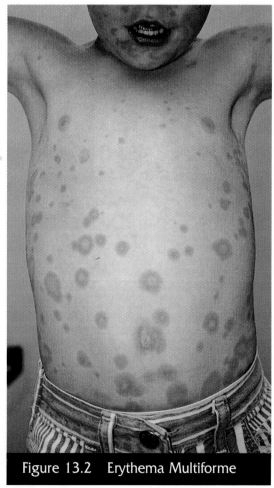

Figure 13.2   Erythema Multiforme

Note the symmetric distribution of the targetoid macules. (Courtesy of Michael Redman, PA-C.)

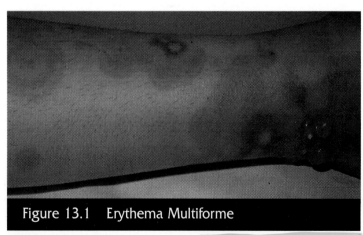

Figure 13.1   Erythema Multiforme

Note the characteristic target eruption, an erythematous macule with central clearing. Distally located on the extremity is a vesicobullous plaque, a common variation in presentation. (Courtesy of Dept. of Dermatology, Wilford Hall USAF Medical Center and Brooke Army Medical Center, San Antonio, TX.)

and additional eruptions involving the mucosal surfaces (Stevens-Johnson syndrome) may require admission and supportive care.

Clinical Pearls

1. Symmetrically distributed target lesions on the extensor surfaces of the extremities and a lack of significant systemic manifestations are classified as erythema multiforme minor.
2. Drug-associated erythema multiforme usually begins within 2 to 3 weeks of initiating therapy. Sulfonamides and penicillins are most often the culprits.
3. Many clinicians empirically treat idiopathic cases with a trial of acyclovir therapy owing to the high incidence of subclinical herpes simplex infections as the cause of the EM.

STEVENS-JOHNSON SYNDROME (EM MAJOR)   DIAGNOSIS

Associated Clinical Features

Stevens-Johnson syndrome is a severe, rarely fatal variety of erythema multiforme. An abrupt onset of constitutional symptoms precedes the hemorrhagic bullae found on multiple mucosal surfaces and the edematous, erythematous cutaneous plaques (Fig. 13.3). The bullae erode producing stomatitis, conjunctivitis, vulvovaginitis, or balanitis. Patients appear extremely ill and may develop pneumonia, arthritis, seizures, coma, and hepatic dysfunction. Death, when it occurs, is usually due to overwhelming sepsis.

Differential Diagnosis

Meningococcemia must be considered in the differential diagnosis. The severe involvement of mucous membranes is characteristic of Stevens-Johnson syndrome.

ED Treatment and Disposition

Patients presenting with significant evidence of toxicity should be admitted to the hospital. Supportive measures and selective use of systemic corticosteroids are the cornerstone of therapy.

Clinical Pearls

1. Thick, hemorrhagic crusts of the mucosal surfaces are diagnostic of Stevens-Johnson syndrome.
2. Sulfonamides, penicillins, and anticonvulsants are common causes of Stevens-Johnson syndrome.

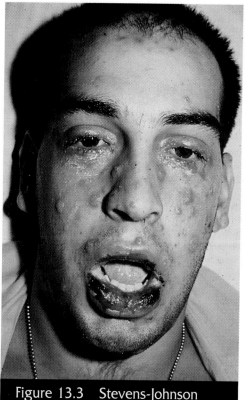

Figure 13.3 Stevens-Johnson Syndrome

Note the multiple mucosal surface involvement of the face resulting in thick, hemorrhagic crusts on the lips. (Courtesy of Dept. of Dermatology, Wilford Hall USAF Medical Center and Brooke Army Medical Center, San Antonio, TX.)

Associated Clinical Features

Toxic epidermal necrolysis (TEN) is characterized by the formation of widespread bullae (Fig. 13.4), usually a cutaneous manifestation of a drug reaction. The epidermis eventually becomes necrotic, leading to extensive exfoliation and exposure of the raw dermis (Fig. 13.5). A prodrome of fever, fatigue, myalgias, and skin tenderness occur in the majority of patients. The mortality rate approaches 25%, with death usually due to sepsis. TEN is generally considered to be the most severe form of erythema multiforme.

Differential Diagnosis

Early in its course TEN may resemble scarlet fever, toxic shock syndrome, or erythema multiforme. In children staphylococcal scalded-skin syndrome closely mimics TEN; however, it involves only the superficial epidermis without extension to the dermis.

ED Treatment and Disposition

Supportive care includes debridement of necrotic tissue, pain control, aggressive hydration, and appropriate antibiotic therapy. These patients are best managed in burn treatment centers.

Clinical Pearls

1. Patients generally present with widespread skin and mucous membrane involvement, significant constitutional symptoms, and painful skin.
2. The initial bullae coalesce, leading to exfoliation of the entire epidermis.

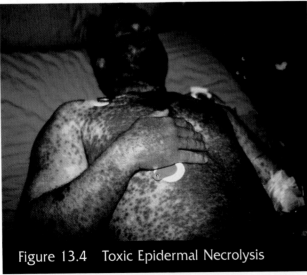

Figure 13.4   Toxic Epidermal Necrolysis

Note the widespread erythematous bullae and blisters on this ill-appearing patient. (Courtesy of Dept. of Dermatology, Wilford Hall USAF Medical Center and Brooke Army Medical Center, San Antonio, TX.)

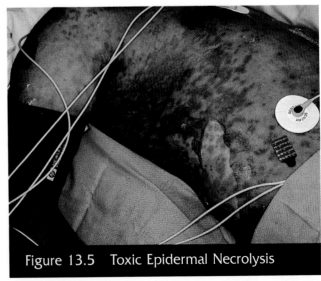

Figure 13.5   Toxic Epidermal Necrolysis

The initial bullae have coalesced, leading to extensive exfoliation of the epidermis. (Courtesy of Keith Batts, MD.)

Associated Clinical Features

Necrotizing vasculitis is a hypersensitivity vasculitis in adults associated with infectious agents, connective tissue diseases, and drugs. Symptoms may be confined to the skin in the form of symmetric petechiae and palpable purpura over the distal third of the extremities (Fig. 13.6). Systemic vascular involvement occurs in the kidneys (glomerulonephritis), muscles, joints, gastrointestinal tract (abdominal pain and bleeding), and peripheral nerves (neuritis). Henoch-Schönlein purpura (HSP) (Fig. 13.7) is the classic example of vasculitis in children, consisting of a clinical triad of palpable purpura, arthritis, and abdominal pain. It is usually a benign, self-limited disease that most commonly occurs in children after a bacterial or viral infection.

Differential Diagnosis

Idiopathic thrombocytopenic purpura (ITP), disseminated intravascular coagulation (DIC), meningococcemia, gonococcemia, Rocky Mountain spotted fever, staphylococcal septicemia, and embolic endocarditis must all be considered in the differential diagnosis; however, patients with septic vasculitis are generally more severely ill with rapidly progressive symptoms. Also, the purpura of septic vasculitis tend to be fewer in number, asymmetric, and distal in location. Biopsy of the purpura is helpful in distinguishing necrotizing vasculitis from septic vasculitis, DIC, and embolic endocarditis.

ED Treatment and Disposition

A majority of cases are self-limited and require only rest, elevation, and analgesics. Severe cases with systemic manifestations may require admission for supportive care, corticosteroids, and cytotoxic immunosuppressive therapy. Antibiotics should be utilized if the vasculitis follows an infection (i.e., after streptococcal infection).

Clinical Pearls

1. The petechiae and purpura of necrotizing vasculitis are usually localized to the lower third of the extremities.
2. A patient presenting with purpura and the signs and symptoms of serum sickness should lead to the suspicion of necrotizing vasculitis.

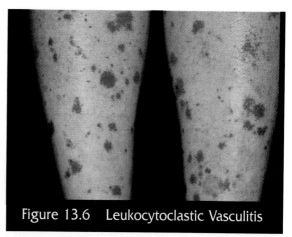

Figure 13.6 Leukocytoclastic Vasculitis

Multiple symmetric petechiae and palpable purpura are noted over the lower third of the extremities. (Courtesy of Dept. of Dermatology, Wilford Hall USAF Medical Center and Brooke Army Medical Center, San Antonio, TX.)

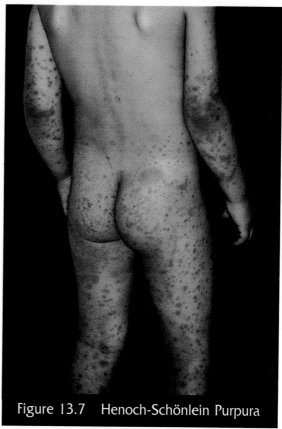

Figure 13.7 Henoch-Schönlein Purpura

Note the classic acral distribution of HSP. It is immunoglobulin A (IgA)-mediated and most commonly occurs in children after a streptococcal or viral infection. (Courtesy of Kevin J. Knoop, MD, MS.)

Associated Clinical Features

Rickettsia rickettsii is transmitted via the bite of an infected tick. Prodromal symptoms of fever, rigors, headache, myalgias, and weakness occur 7 to 10 days after inoculation. The initially blanching macular eruption begins on the distal extremities and somewhat later on the palms and soles (Fig. 13.8). It soon becomes purpuric as it spreads centrally to involve the trunk and abdomen. However, it can also present without obvious cutaneous manifestations.

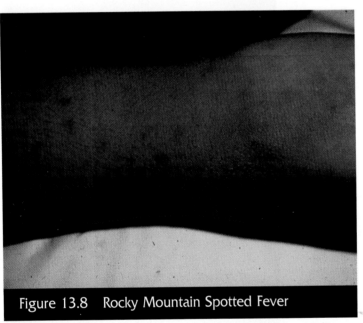

Figure 13.8   Rocky Mountain Spotted Fever

This acral exanthem is characterized by erythematous macules which soon progress to petechiae. (Courtesy of Dept. of Dermatology, Wilford Hall USAF Medical Center and Brooke Army Medical Center, San Antonio, TX.)

Differential Diagnosis

Viral exanthems, drug eruptions, necrotizing vasculitis, purpuric bacteremia, and atypical measles syndrome may all resemble this potentially fatal illness.

ED Treatment and Disposition

Tetracycline or chloramphenicol is required for this potentially fatal illness. Tetracycline is the drug of choice, yet it should be avoided in pregnant or lactating females and children younger than 8 years of age. Mildly ill patients may be treated with oral antibiotics on an outpatient basis as long as close follow-up can be arranged. More severely ill patients should be admitted because their care can be complicated by circulatory collapse and coma. Approximately 20% of untreated patients will die.

Clinical Pearls

1. Systemic manifestations of the illness may present without obvious cutaneous manifestations.
2. Palmar and plantar petechiae in a severely ill patient should be treated as Rocky Mountain spotted fever until proved otherwise.
3. Most cases occur between April and October, with the highest incidence occurring in the Southeast and South-Central states.
4. Atypical measles syndrome occurs in individuals vaccinated with a measles virus vaccine between 1963 and 1968 and subsequently exposed to the virus.

Associated Clinical Features

Disseminated gonococcus (GC) is a systemic infection with septic vasculitis following the hematogenous dissemination of the organism *Neisseria gonorrhoeae*. The spectrum of disease varies from skin lesions alone to skin lesions with tenosynovitis or septic arthritis. The initial lesion is an erythematous macule that evolves into a necrotic, purpuric vesicopustule (Fig. 13.9). These purpura are few in number, asymmetric, and predominantly distal in location.

Differential Diagnosis

The purpura may resemble meningococcemia, staphylococcal septicemia, necrotizing vasculitis, or endocarditis with emboli. Infectious arthritis or tenosynovitis must be considered when the patient presents with joint complaints. It is important to obtain Gram's stain of the contents of the vesicopustule, as well as all other body sites and fluids. Biopsy of the vesicopustule is helpful in distinguishing this entity from necrotizing vasculitis and embolic phenomenon.

ED Treatment and Disposition

Ceftriaxone is the agent of choice for initial management. Therapy consists of intravenous or intramuscular ceftriaxone or cefotaxime until symptoms either improve or resolve, followed by an additional 7 days of orally administered ciprofloxacin or cefuroxime. Hospitalization is recommended for noncompliant patients or cases noted to have an associated septic arthritis.

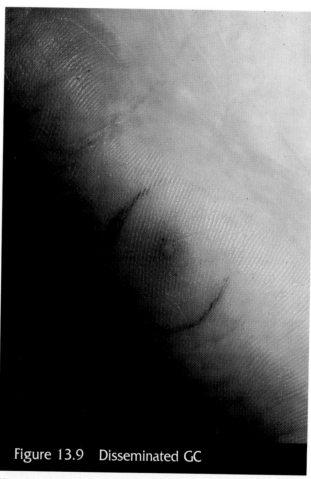

Figure 13.9   Disseminated GC

Here involving the hypothenar eminence of the hand is the characteristic, asymmetric, purpuric vesicopustule of disseminated GC. (Courtesy of Dept. of Dermatology, Wilford Hall USAF Medical Center and Brooke Army Medical Center, San Antonio, TX.)

Clinical Pearls

1. The most common symptom of disseminated GC is arthralgia of one or more joints, primarily involving the hands or knees.
2. Skin lesions develop in up to 70% of cases and will resolve within 4 days regardless of antibiotics.
3. The initial erythematous macule of disseminated GC evolves into a necrotic, purpuric vesicopustule.
4. The purpura of septic vasculitis (of whatever bacterial etiology) tend to be fewer in number, asymmetric, and distal in location.

Associated Clinical Features

Infective endocarditis is an illness characterized by fever, valve destruction, and peripheral embolization manifested by rare, usually distal purpura. *Streptococcus viridans* is the most common causative organism. Janeway lesions (Fig. 13.10) occur in 5% of cases and consist of nontender, small, erythematous macules on the palms or soles. Osler's nodes (Fig. 13.11) occur in 10% of cases and consist of transient, tender, purplish nodules on the pulp of the fingers and toes. Splinter hemorrhages are black, linear discolorations beneath the nail plate (Fig. 13.12). They are present in 20% of cases and are more suggestive of subacute bacterial endocarditis (SBE) if present at the proximal or middle nail plate. Murmurs, retinal hemorrhages, septic arthritis, and significant embolic episodes such as pulmonary embolism or stroke may also be present.

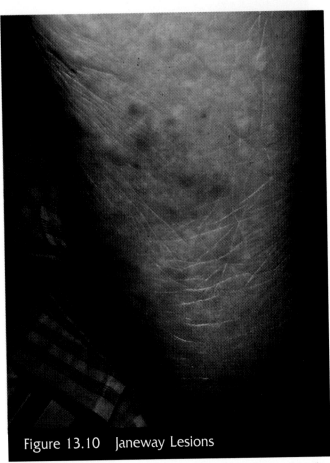

Figure 13.10   Janeway Lesions

Peripheral embolization to the sole resulting in a cluster of erythematous macules known as Janeway lesions. (Courtesy of Dept. of Dermatology, Wilford Hall USAF Medical Center and Brooke Army Medical Center, San Antonio, TX.)

Differential Diagnosis

Meningococcemia, gonococcemia, staphylococcal septicemia, and necrotizing vasculitis must all be considered in the differential diagnosis. Biopsy of the purpura is helpful in distinguishing this condition from septic vasculitis and necrotizing vasculitis. Echocardiogram can aid in the diagnosis.

ED Treatment and Disposition

Antibiotics must be appropriate for the infectious agent; however, therapy is often required before the diagnosis is confirmed or the infecting organism is known. All toxic patients require admission, as do all febrile patients who have prosthetic valves or who are intravenous drug abusers. These patients should receive gentamicin with nafcillin or vancomycin empirically pending the blood culture results. Patients with rheumatic or congenital valve abnormalities may receive streptomycin with penicillin or vancomycin.

Clinical Pearls

1. Janeway lesions, Osler's nodes, and splinter hemorrhages in a febrile patient with a murmur are virtually diagnostic of infective endocarditis.
2. Rheumatic heart disease is the most common predisposing factor, with the mitral valve being the most common site of damage.
3. Congenital heart disease, intravenous drug abuse, and prosthetic heart valves are additional predisposing factors to the development of infective endocarditis.

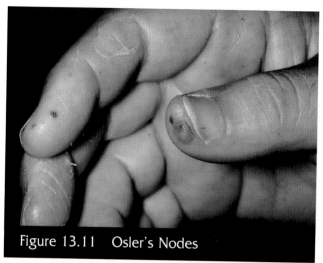

Figure 13.11 Osler's Nodes

Subcutaneous, purplish, and tender nodules in the pulp of the fingers known as Osler's nodes. (Courtesy of the Armed Forces Institute of Pathology, Bethesda, MD.)

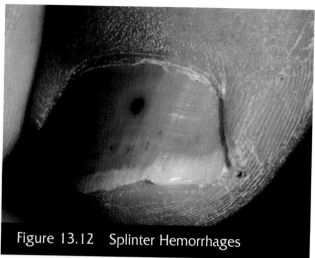

Figure 13.12 Splinter Hemorrhages

Note the splinter hemorrhages along the distal aspect of the nail plate due to emboli from subacute bacterial endocarditis. (Courtesy of the Armed Forces Institute of Pathology, Bethesda, MD.)

IDIOPATHIC THROMBOCYTOPENIC PURPURA   DIAGNOSIS

Associated Clinical Features

Idiopathic thrombocytopenic purpura (ITP) occurs as the result of platelet injury and destruction. Pinpoint, red, nonblanching petechiae or nonpalpable purpura and ecchymoses are found on the skin (Fig. 13.13) and mucous membranes, either spontaneously (platelets <10,000/mm^3) or at the site of minimal trauma (platelets <40,000/mm^3). Melena, hematochezia, menorrhagia, and severe intracranial hemorrhages may also occur in conjunction with the purpura. The acute form affects children 1 to 2 weeks after a viral illness; the chronic form occurs most often in adults and may present with an associated splenomegaly.

Differential Diagnosis

Nonhemorrhagic vascular dilatations like telangiectasia or true petechiae and purpura as found in scurvy or posttraumatic purpura must be differentiated from this potentially debilitating illness. Assessment of the platelet count aids in making the diagnosis.

ED Treatment and Disposition

Hospitalization at the time of diagnosis is recommended because the differential diagnosis is extensive and the bleeding risks are significant. Platelets are transfused only if there is life-threatening bleeding or the total count is <10,000/mm^3. Immunosuppressive drugs and cortico-steroids are of benefit in the acute cases; splenectomy is utilized in chronic cases.

Clinical Pearls

1. Petechiae and purpura in a thrombocytopenic patient with splenomegaly make the diagnosis.

2. The acute form of ITP has an excellent prognosis (90% spontaneous remission), whereas the course of chronic ITP is one of varying severity with little hope of remission.

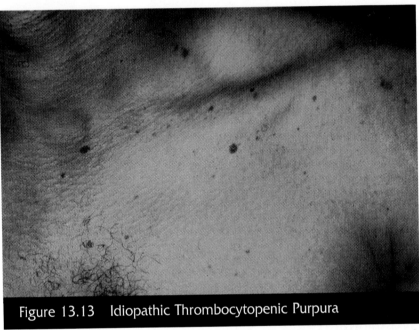

Figure 13.13   Idiopathic Thrombocytopenic Purpura

This thrombocytopenic patient with splenomegaly has pinpoint, nonblanching, nonpalpable petechiae. (Courtesy of Dept. of Dermatology, Wilford Hall USAF Medical Center and Brooke Army Medical Center, San Antonio, TX.)

DIAGNOSIS   LIVEDO RETICULARIS

Associated Clinical Features

Livedo reticularis presents as a macular, reticulated (lacelike) patch of nonpalpable cutaneous vasodilatation (Fig. 13.14) in response to a variety of vascular occlusive processes. This pattern predominates in the peripheral or acral areas and may or may not be associated with purpura. In time, the overlying epidermis and dermis may infarct and form ulcerations or develop palpable dermal papules or nodules. Livedo reticularis is usually representative of a severe underlying systemic disease. Inflammatory vascular diseases (livedo vasculitis, polyarteritis nodosa, lupus erythematosus), septic emboli (meningococcemia), tumors (pheochromocytoma), and systemic illnesses associated with mechanical vessel blockage (anticardiolipin antibody syndrome, polycythemia vera, sickle cell anemia, cholesterol embolus) are a few diseases associated with or responsible for livedo reticularis. It can also occur independent of any disease association.

Differential Diagnosis

The most important consideration in making this diagnosis is to rule out an associated vascular occlusion of whatever etiology.

ED Treatment and Disposition

The treatment of livedo reticularis is treatment of the underlying disorder.

Clinical Pearls

1. Livedo vasculitis is an inflammatory vascular disease usually found on the ankles and dorsum of the feet. It consists of painful stellate-shaped ulcerations surrounded by an erythematous livedo pattern.
2. A toxic child with stellate-shaped purpura covering much of the body is diagnostic of meningococcemia.
3. Cholesterol emboli usually occur after an intraarterial procedure. Pain often precedes the livedo pattern of purpura on the distal extremities.
4. Patients with anticardiolipin antibody syndrome have extensive livedo reticularis and recurrent arterial and venous thromboses involving multiple organ systems.

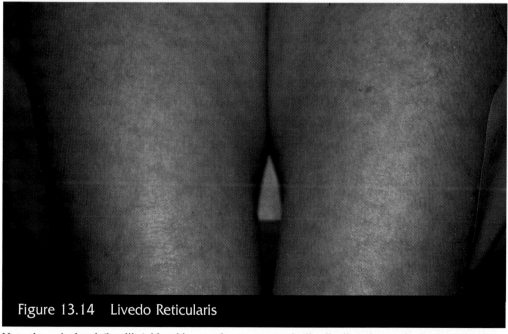

Figure 13.14   Livedo Reticularis

Note the reticulated (lacelike) blanching erythema symmetrically distributed over the lower extremities. (Courtesy of Dept. of Dermatology, Wilford Hall USAF Medical Center and Brooke Army Medical Center, San Antonio, TX.)

Associated Clinical Features

Herpes zoster is a dermatomal, unilateral reactivation of the varicella-zoster virus. Pain, tenderness, and dysesthesias usually precede the eruption composed of umbilicated, grouped vesicles on an erythematous, edematous base (Fig. 13.15). The vesicles may become purulent or hemorrhagic. Nerve involvement may actually occur without cutaneous involvement. Ophthalmic zoster involves the nasociliary branch of the fifth cranial nerve and presents with vesicles on the nose and cornea. Ramsay-Hunt syndrome is a herpes zoster infection of the geniculate ganglion that presents with decreased hearing and facial palsy.

Differential Diagnosis

The most likely differential diagnosis is herpes simplex infection, which is usually recurrent. Herpes zoster recurs in fewer than 5% of immunocompetent patients. The eruption may resemble contact dermatitis, localized cellulitis, or grouped insect bites. The prodromal pain must be differentiated from potential pleural, cardiac, or abdominal origin. Tzank smear of the floor of a vesicle demonstrating multinucleated giant cells makes the diagnosis of a herpes family infection (Fig. 13.16). Cultures may be necessary to distinguish herpes zoster forms.

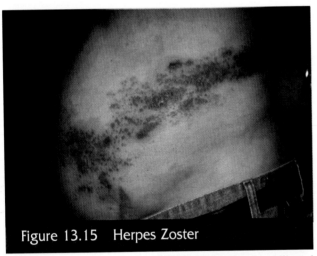

Figure 13.15   Herpes Zoster

This eruption consists of a dermatomal distribution of umbilicated vesicles on an erythematous base. Note the occasional cluster of hemorrhagic vesicles. Tzank smear is positive. (Courtesy of Dept. of Dermatology, Wilford Hall USAF Medical Center and Brooke Army Medical Center, San Antonio, TX.)

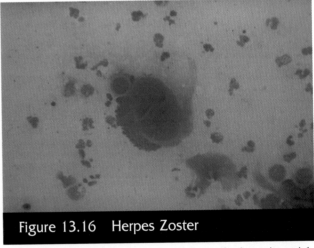

Figure 13.16   Herpes Zoster

A Tzank smear of both the roof and floor of a herpetic vesicle demonstrating a multinucleated giant cell. (Courtesy of Dept. of Dermatology, Wilford Hall USAF Medical Center and Brooke Army Medical Center, San Antonio, TX.)

ED Treatment and Disposition

Uncomplicated cases of herpes zoster can be managed with supportive care, especially pain control. Admission to the hospital for intravenous acyclovir is usually reserved for complicated cases involving multiple dermatomal distribution or the ophthalmic branch of the trigeminal nerve, disseminated disease, or immunocompromised patients. Acyclovir or famciclovir hasten the healing and decreases the pain if started within 72 h of appearance of the vesicles. These agents have also been shown to reduce the duration of post–herpetic neuralgia. Herpes zoster keratitis requires immediate opthalmologic consultation to avoid any potential vision loss.

Clinical Pearls

1. Dermatomally grouped, umbilicated vesicles on an erythematous base are diagnostic of herpes zoster.
2. The thorax is the most common area involved, followed by the face (trigeminal nerve).
3. The nonimmune or immunocompromised should avoid lesional contact from prodrome until reepithelialization, since the crusts can contain the varicella-zoster virus.
4. An infected patient is able to transmit chicken pox, but not herpes zoster, to a nonimmune individual.

HERPETIC WHITLOW

DIAGNOSIS

Associated Clinical Features

Herpetic whitlow is a painful herpes simplex infection of the distal finger characterized by edema, erythema, vesicles, and/or pustules grouped on an erythematous base (Fig. 13.17). Fever, lymphangitis, and regional adenopathy often accompany the lesion.

Differential Diagnosis

Paronychia, felon, and contact dermatitis must be differentiated from this contagious illness. A Tzank smear of the floor of the vesicle demonstrating multinucleated giant cells makes the diagnosis.

ED Treatment and Disposition

Acyclovir in addition to analgesics and antipyretics are useful. To be most effective, acyclovir must be started within 72 h of the appearance of the eruption. Topical antibiotic ointments help prevent secondary infection and may speed healing.

Clinical Pearls

1. Grouped, umbilicated vesicles on an erythematous base are diagnostic of a herpes family infection.
2. Wear protective gloves; herpetic whitlow is an occupational hazard in the medical and dental professions.

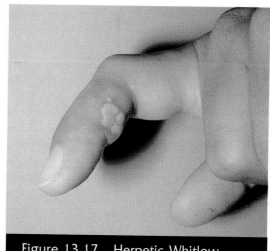

Figure 13.17   Herpetic Whitlow

Note the cluster of vesicles on an erythematous base located at the distal finger. Tzank smear is positive. (Courtesy of Lawrence B. Stack, MD.)

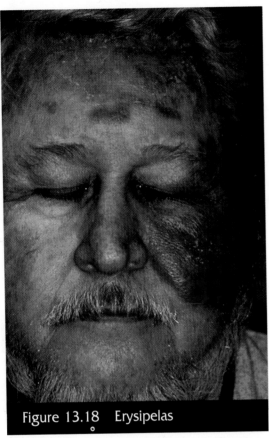

Figure 13.18 Erysipelas

Note the well demarcated, edematous, erythematous, shiny plaque. (Courtesy of Dept. of Dermatology, Wilford Hall USAF Medical Center and Brooke Army Medical Center, San Antonio, TX.)

Associated Clinical Features

Erysipelas is a group A streptococcal cellulitis involving the skin to the level of the dermis. The plaque is typically erythematous, edematous, and painful with an elevated, well demarcated border (Fig. 13.18). The associated edema tends to make the plaque appear shiny. Erysipelas frequently occurs on the face and lower extremities.

Differential Diagnosis

Other significant illnesses, such as deep venous thrombosis, thrombophlebitis, and necrotizing fasciitis, must be ruled out.

ED Treatment and Disposition

All infections require rest, elevation, heat, and antibiotics. Mild presentations may be treated on an outpatient basis with oral dicloxacillin or erythromycin in penicillin-allergic patients. More severe illness or toxicity requires hospitalization and intravenous antibiotics.

Clinical Pearls

1. The well demarcated, tender, shiny, erythematous plaque is diagnostic of erysipelas.
2. This same shiny, erythematous plaque on the face of a febrile child may be caused by *Haemophilus influenzae,* necessitating intravenous chloramphenicol or a cephalosporin.

Associated Clinical Features

Hot tub folliculitis is a pruritic, follicular, pustular eruption confined to the hair follicle and is secondary to a cutaneous infection with *Pseudomonas aeruginosa* (Fig. 13.19). Headache, sore throat, earache, and fever may accompany the pustules, which usually localize to the trunk and proximal extremities.

Differential Diagnosis

Other forms of folliculitis (including those caused by *Staphylococcus aureus*), acne, and miliaria rubra are usually considered in the differential diagnosis.

ED Treatment and Disposition

The folliculitis usually involutes in 7 to 10 days without treatment. Acetic acid compresses and local wound cleansing may speed recovery. In addition, the hot tub or source of exposure must be decontaminated to avoid recurrent exposure.

Clinical Pearls

1. Pruritic pustules confined to the hair follicles of the trunk and proximal extremities is diagnostic of folliculitis.
2. This most commonly occurs in individuals who use hot tubs, whirlpools, or saunas.
3. This may also result from contact with chemicals (exfoliative beauty aids) or repetitive physical trauma (friction from tight clothing).

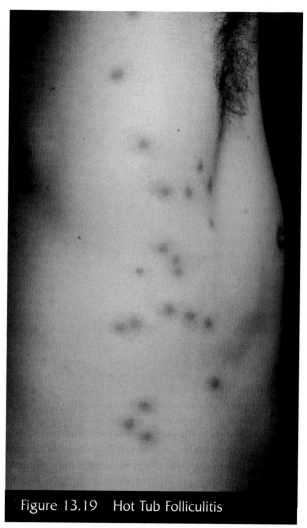

Figure 13.19   Hot Tub Folliculitis

Note the pustules localized to the hair follicles of the trunk and proximal extremity. (Courtesy of Jeffrey S. Gibson, MD.)

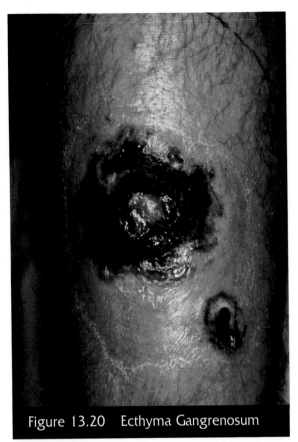

Figure 13.20 Ecthyma Gangrenosum

The initial pustule surrounded by an erythematous halo becomes hemorrhagic and necrotic, forming this painless ulcer. (Courtesy of Dept. of Dermatology, Wilford Hall USAF Medical Center and Brooke Army Medical Center, San Antonio, TX.)

Associated Clinical Features

Ecthyma gangrenosum is a *Pseudomonas aeruginosa* infection which usually occurs in the septic, immunocompromised, or neutropenic patient. The initially erythematous macules develop bullae or pustules surrounded by violaceous halos. The pustules become hemorrhagic and rupture, forming painless ulcers with necrotic, black centers (Fig. 13.20).

Differential Diagnosis

Necrotizing vasculitis, fixed drug eruptions, pyoderma gangrenosum, and brown recluse spider bites must all be considered in the differential diagnosis.

ED Treatment and Disposition

These patients are usually septic and immunocompromised. Admission is usually required for the patient to receive antipseudomonal antibiotics and general supportive care.

Clinical Pearls

1. Consider ecthyma gangrenosum when examining a septic patient who presents with bullae or pustules that rupture and form painless, necrotic ulcers.
2. It is important to consider underlying immunodeficiency when making this diagnosis.

Associated Clinical Features

Pityriasis rosea is a mild inflammatory, exanthematous, papulosquamous eruption. The pathognomonic finding is an oval salmon-colored papule with a central collarette of scale. It primarily occurs on the trunk with the long axis of the oval papule following the lines of cleavage in a Christmas tree–like distribution (Fig. 13.21). A herald patch, consisting of a much larger plaque with central clearing and scales, frequently precedes the exanthematous phase by 1 to 2 weeks (Fig. 13.22). The eruption usually lasts 4 to 6 weeks and is frequently pruritic.

Differential Diagnosis

This must be differentiated from the secondary lesions of syphilis, tinea versicolor, and some drug eruptions.

ED Treatment and Disposition

Symptomatic treatment is usually all that can be offered to the patient. Antihistamines may alleviate the associated pruritus. Ultraviolet light has also been used with some success.

Clinical Pearls

1. A salmon-colored papule with central scale, negative KOH examination for hyphae, and negative serologic testing for syphilis makes the diagnosis of pityriasis rosea.
2. It frequently appears very atypical in dark-skinned individuals (acral, face, and genital location).

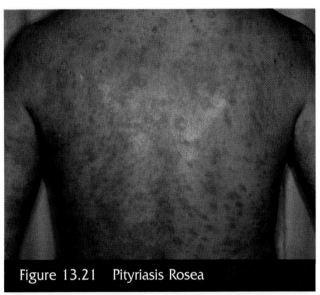

Figure 13.21   Pityriasis Rosea

An exanthematous, papulosquamous eruption with the long axis of the oval papules following the lines of cleavage in a Christmas tree–like distribution. (Courtesy of Dept. of Dermatology, Wilford Hall USAF Medical Center and Brooke Army Medical Center, San Antonio, TX.)

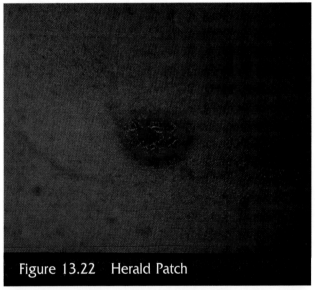

Figure 13.22   Herald Patch

A herald patch precedes the exanthematous phase: a larger, oval, salmon-colored patch with a central collarette of scale. (Courtesy of Dept. of Dermatology, Wilford Hall USAF Medical Center and Brooke Army Medical Center, San Antonio, TX.)

Associated Clinical Features

The initial papules of secondary syphilis are usually asymptomatic and appear 2 to 10 weeks after the primary chancre. Headache, sore throat, fever, arthralgias, myalgias, and a generalized lymphadenopathy may also be present. These exanthematic papules are symmetric and nondestructive, usually forming a pityriasis rosea–like pattern on the trunk, palms, and soles (Fig. 13.23). Later lesions are firm, pigmented papules with a coppery tint and adherent scales (Fig. 13.24). Macerated papules may form on the mucous membranes (mucous patch, Fig. 13.25), "motheaten" alopecia may occur on the scalp, and condylomata lata may occur in the intertriginous areas.

Differential Diagnosis

Syphilis is "the great imitator." It may resemble psoriasis, drug eruptions, pityriasis rosea, viral exanthems, tinea corporis, tinea versicolor, and condyloma acuminata. A positive serologic test for syphilis makes the diagnosis.

ED Treatment and Disposition

Penicillin is the agent of choice for treatment, with tetracycline or erythromycin used in cases of penicillin allergy. A Jarisch-Herxheimer reaction may occur several hours after treatment with antibiotics, correlating with the clearance of spirochetes from the bloodstream. This reaction lasts approximately 24 h, yet it may be more threatening than the disease itself. Increasing fever, rigors, myalgias, headache, tachycardia, hypotension, and a drop in the leukocyte and platelet count may be encountered. Fluid resuscitation to maintain the blood pressure and supportive care may be needed.

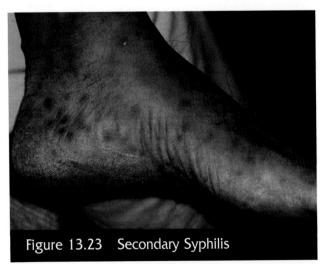

Figure 13.23   Secondary Syphilis

These eruptive, scaly, copper-colored papules on the foot may be the initial presentation of secondary syphilis. They are usually symmetric, asymptomatic, and nondestructive. (Courtesy of Dept. of Dermatology, Wilford Hall USAF Medical Center and Brooke Army Medical Center, San Antonio, TX.)

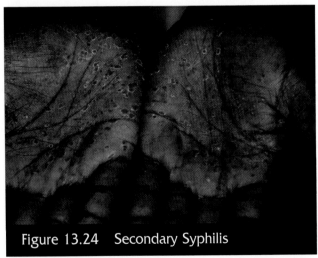

Figure 13.24   Secondary Syphilis

These firm, pigmented papules with a coppery tint and adherent scale are characteristic. (Courtesy of Dept. of Dermatology, Wilford Hall USAF Medical Center and Brooke Army Medical Center, San Antonio, TX.)

Clinical Pearls

1. Scaly palmar and plantar papules are strongly suggestive of secondary syphilis, the incidence of which is rising.

2. These scaling red-brown papules appear 2 to 10 weeks after the spontaneous resolution of the initial painless chancre.

3. The latent stage follows the resolution of the papules, characterized by a positive serology and an absence of signs and symptoms.

4. Tertiary syphilis occurs in untreated or poorly treated patients and may manifest itself as general paresis, tabes dorsalis, optic atrophy, and aortitis with aneurysms.

5. It is important to consider the prozone phenomenon (falsely negative agglutination in undiluted serum) in an AIDS patient with presumed syphilis in whom the serologic test is negative.

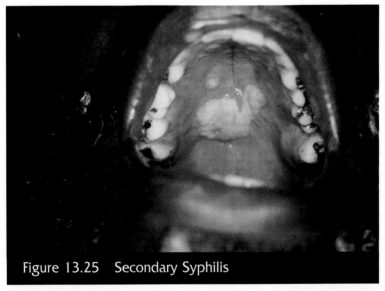

Figure 13.25   Secondary Syphilis

Two other lesions found late in the course of secondary syphilis. The mucous patch is the sharply defined, macerated plaque on the floor of the mouth. Condylomata lata are the broad-based, erosive nodules found around the oral commissures. Both eruptions are commonly found in the HIV-infected population with secondary syphilis. (Courtesy of Dept. of Dermatology, Wilford Hall USAF Medical Center and Brooke Army Medical Center, San Antonio, TX.)

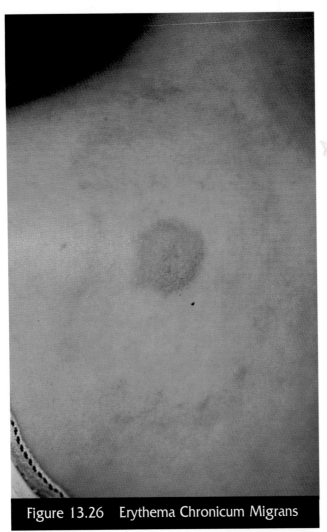

Figure 13.26 Erythema Chronicum Migrans

This pathognomonic eruption of Lyme disease forms at the site of the tick bite. The initial plaque expands its well defined border and clears centrally, forming an annular appearance. (Courtesy of David W. Munter, MD.)

Associated Clinical Features

Borrelia burgdorferi is the tick-borne spirochete responsible for Lyme borreliosis, and erythema chronicum migrans (ECM) is the pathognomonic rash of Lyme disease occuring early in the infection. The initial prodromal symptoms of fever, myalgias, arthralgias, and headache are followed by a macule or papule progressing to a plaque at the site of the bite. This plaque expands its red, raised border as it clears centrally, leading to an annular appearance (Fig. 3.26). The plaque may burn and is rarely pruritic.

Differential Diagnosis

This annular plaque may resemble a fixed drug eruption, tinea corporis, urticaria, or the herald patch of pityriasis rosea. The multiple, secondary annular papules and plaques that may rarely form can resemble secondary syphilis. However, the Lyme-related eruption spares the palms and soles.

ED Treatment and Disposition

The duration of antibiotic treatment (10 to 30 days) depends on the severity of the symptoms. Tetracycline or doxycycline are the drugs of choice. Pregnant or lactating females and children younger than 8 years of age should be treated with penicillin or amoxicillin. Erythromycin is a suitable alternative. Patients with minimal symptoms may be treated on an outpatient basis. Those patients with significant toxicity and complications require admission, supportive care, and parenteral antibiotics.

Clinical Pearls

1. An annular plaque arising at the site of a tick bite in a patient with systemic symptoms should be treated as Lyme disease until proved otherwise.
2. Stage I of Lyme disease consists of constitutional symptoms and the characteristic rash of ECM.
3. Stage II of Lyme disease consists of neurologic (aseptic meningitis, encephalitis, bilateral Bell's palsy) and cardiac (myocarditis, conduction blocks) manifestations.
4. Stage III of Lyme disease consists of an asymmetric, episodic, oligoarticular arthritis.

Associated Clinical Features

Tinea corporis includes all dermatophyte infections excluding the scalp, face, hands, feet, and groin. The dermatophytosis is pruritic and consists of well circumscribed scaly plaque with a slightly elevated border and central clearing (Fig. 13.27). This annular configuration is most commonly found on the trunk and neck. Skin scrapings viewed with a KOH preparation exhibit septate hyphae.

Tinea faciale is a dermatophyte infection of the facial skin. It commonly appears as a well circumscribed erythematous patch (Fig. 13.28). Tinea manus is a dermatophyte infection of the hands (Fig. 13.29).

Differential Diagnosis

Pityriasis rosea, secondary syphilis, psoriasis, seborrheic dermatitis, and tinea versicolor are all usually considered in the differential diagnosis. A KOH examination of the scale demonstrating hyphae confirms the diagnosis.

ED Treatment and Disposition

Small, localized plaques may be treated with a topical antifungal cream. Extensive or resistant infection requires systemic griseofulvin or ketoconazole. It is important to treat for 2 weeks beyond the point of clinical cure to ensure successful eradication of the fungus.

Clinical Pearls

1. The scale is usually located at the leading edge of erythema and provides the best yield for scraping as part of the KOH examination.
2. If it scales, scrape it and look for hyphae.

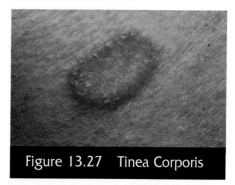

Figure 13.27   Tinea Corporis

This dermatophytosis is known as ringworm, a well defined, pruritic, scaly plaque with a raised border and central clearing (annular). KOH preparation is positive. (Courtesy of Dept. of Dermatology, Wilford Hall USAF Medical Center and Brooke Army Medical Center, San Antonio, TX.)

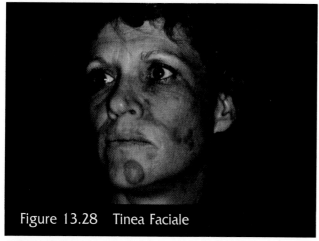

Figure 13.28   Tinea Faciale

Note the sharply marginated, polycyclic, scaly plaque with central clearing localized to the face. KOH preparation is positive. (Courtesy of Dept. of Dermatology, Wilford Hall USAF Medical Center and Brooke Army Medical Center, San Antonio, TX.)

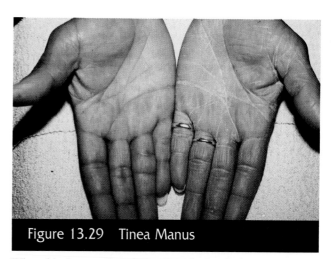

Figure 13.29   Tinea Manus

When this dermatophytosis involves the hands, it is usually unilateral. Note the diffuse hyperkeratosis of the palm of the left hand. KOH preparation is positive. (Courtesy of Dept. of Dermatology, Wilford Hall USAF Medical Center and Brooke Army Medical Center, San Antonio, TX.)

Associated Clinical Features

Tinea cruris, or "jock itch," is a pruritic dermatophytosis of the intertriginous areas, usually excluding the penis and scrotum. The scaly, erythematous plaque spreads peripherally with central clearing (Fig. 13.30). The borders of the plaque are well defined.

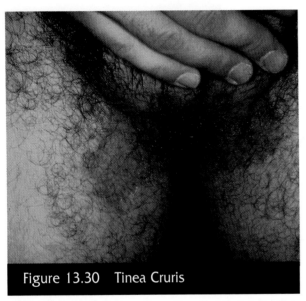

Figure 13.30 Tinea Cruris

This dermatophytosis is commonly called jock itch. Note that the erythematous, scaly plaque with its well defined border does not involve the skin of the scrotum or penis. KOH preparation is positive. (Courtesy of Dept. of Dermatology, Wilford Hall USAF Medical Center and Brooke Army Medical Center, San Antonio, TX.)

Differential Diagnosis

Erythrasma, *Candida albicans,* seborrheic dermatitis, and psoriasis are usually considered in the differential diagnosis. A KOH examination of the scale demonstrating hyphae confirms the diagnosis.

ED Treatment and Disposition

Initial treatment consists of topical antifungal medications. Griseofulvin or ketoconazole are reserved for resistant cases. It is important to treat for 1 week beyond the point of clinical cure to ensure successful eradication of the fungus. Decreasing the amount of perspiration by using topical powders may help prevent recurrences.

Clinical Pearls

1. A less well defined, pruritic, intertriginous plaque which typically involves the scrotum is usually erythrasma. It is caused by *Nocarelia minutissimus* and is treated with topical erythromycin.
2. If it scales, scrape it and look for hyphae.

Associated Clinical Features

Tinea pedis, or "athlete's foot," is a pruritic dermatophytosis. It consists of erythema and scaling of the sole, maceration, occasional vesiculation, and fissure formation between and under the toes (Fig. 13.31). These pruritic, painful fissures may become secondarily infected with gram-negative organisms. Frequently the toenails are also affected.

Differential Diagnosis

Foot eczema, psoriasis, and Reiter's syndrome are considered in the differential diagnosis. A KOH examination of the scale demonstrating hyphae confirms the diagnosis.

ED Treatment and Disposition

Topical antifungal creams are the initial treatment of choice. Antibiotics may be used to treat secondary infection. Griseofulvin, then ketoconazole, are used for chronic or resistant cases. It is important to treat for 1 week beyond the point of clinical cure to ensure successful eradication of the fungus.

Clinical Pearls

1. If it scales, scrape it and look for hyphae.
2. Macerated areas may become secondarily infected by bacteria.

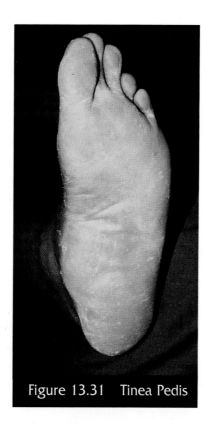

Figure 13.31   Tinea Pedis

This diffuse, pruritic, scaling hyperkeratosis of the sole of the foot extending to the interdigital spaces is known as athlete's foot. KOH preparation is positive. (Courtesy of Dept. of Dermatology, Wilford Hall USAF Medical Center and Brooke Army Medical Center, San Antonio, TX.)

TINEA CAPITIS   DIAGNOSIS

Associated Clinical Features

Tinea capitis is scalp ringworm, or a dermatophytosis of the scalp. It presents as a pruritic, erythematous, scaly plaque with broken or missing hairs frequently referred to as "gray patch" or "black dot" ringworm (Fig. 13.32). This may develop into a kerion. A kerion is a delayed-type hypersensitivity reaction to the fungus where the initial erythematous, scaly plaque becomes boggy with inflamed, purulent nodules and plaques (Fig. 13.33). The hair follicle is frequently destroyed by the inflammatory process in a kerion leading to a scarring alopecia.

Differential Diagnosis

Various inflammatory follicular conditions, such as folliculitis, impetigo, psoriasis, alopecia areata, and seborrheic dermatitis, may resemble tinea capitis. The diagnosis is made by a KOH examination of a scraping of the area revealing hyphae and spores.

ED Treatment Disposition

Systemic griseofulvin is usually required for several weeks to successfully treat tinea capitis. Systemic antibiotics and corticosteroids are usually added when treating a kerion. Selenium sulfide lotion used as a shampoo may actually decrease the duration of the infection. It is important to treat for 2 weeks beyond the point of clinical cure to ensure successful eradication of the fungus. Ketoconazole is reserved for resistant cases.

Clinical Pearls

1. Tinea capitis is a disease of childhood; it is rare in immunocompetent adults.
2. It is epidemic in many African American communities.
3. The KOH scrape is aided by using a disposable urethral brush or similar device.

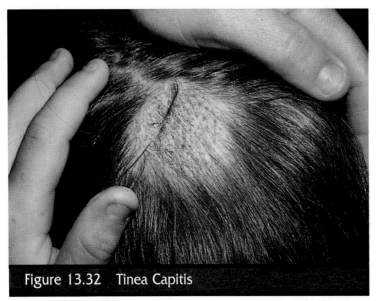

Figure 13.32   Tinea Capitis

This dermatophytosis is characterized by a pruritic, circular area of hair loss covered by adherent scales. KOH preparation is positive. (Courtesy of Dept. of Dermatology, Wilford Hall USAF Medical Center and Brooke Army Medical Center, San Antonio, TX.)

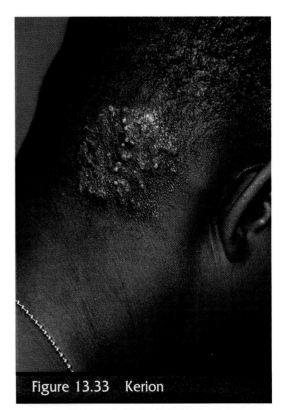

Figure 13.33   Kerion

This collection of boggy, inflamed, purulent nodules and papules is the result of a delayed-type hypersensitivity reaction to the fungus. Scarring alopecia will follow as a result of the actual destruction of the hair follicle. (Courtesy of Dept. of Dermatology, Wilford Hall USAF Medical Center and Brooke Army Medical Center, San Antonio, TX.)

Associated Clinical Features

Onychomycosis is an invasion of the nails by any fungus. Four clinical subtypes are noted. *Distal subungual* presents as discolorations of the free edge of the nail with hyperkeratosis leading to a subungual accumulation of friable keratinaceous debris (Fig. 13.34). *White superficial* consists of sharply outlined white areas on the nail plate which leave the surface friable. *Proximal subungual* presents as discolorations which start proximally at the nail fold. *Candidal onychomycosis* encompasses the entire nail plate, leaving the surface rough and friable.

Differential Diagnosis

Psoriasis and various other nail dystrophies such as distal onycholysis caused by excessive water exposure or drugs must be differentiated from this fungal infection. Pseudomonal nail infection is characterized by the subungual accumulation of green debris. A KOH examination of the keratinaceous debris demonstrating hyphae confirms onychomycosis.

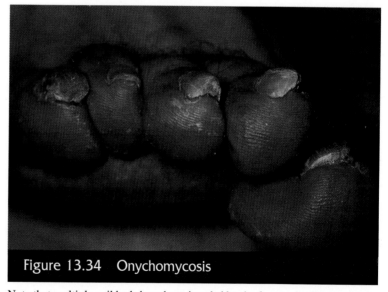

Figure 13.34   Onychomycosis

Note that multiple nail beds have been invaded by the fungus, leading to chronic hyperkeratosis and subungual accumulation of friable keratinaceous debris. (Courtesy of Dept. of Dermatology, Wilford Hall USAF Medical Center and Brooke Army Medical Center, San Antonio, TX.)

ED Treatment and Disposition

The most common treatment consists of oral griseofulvin. Candidal infections require oral ketoconazole. Toenail onychomycosis is very difficult to eradicate. Recently, itraconazole has shown promise as a drug for curing toenail onychomycosis.

Clinical Pearls

1. All that causes the nail plate to separate from the nail bed is not necessarily fungus.
2. If it scales, scrape it and look for hyphae.

Associated Clinical Features

Tinea versicolor is a chronic, superficial fungal infection that involves the trunk and extremities, with little or no involvement of the face. Finely scaling brown macules are present in fair-skinned patients, whereas scaly hypopigmented macules are often noted in dark-skinned patients (Fig. 13.35). These sharply demarcated macules are intermittently pruritic.

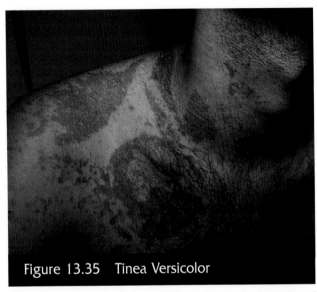

Figure 13.35   Tinea Versicolor

This chronic superficial fungal infection leads to the formation of multiple well defined, scaly, hypopigmented macules on the trunk and extremities. (Courtesy of Dept. of Dermatology, Wilford Hall USAF Medical Center and Brooke Army Medical Center, San Antonio, TX.)

Differential Diagnosis

Pityriasis rosea, secondary syphilis, and some drug eruptions must all be considered in the differential diagnosis. A KOH examination of a scraping of the area revealing hyphae and spores makes the diagnosis (Fig. 17.15).

ED Treatment and Disposition

Treatment consists of short applications of selenium sulfide lotion, topical antifungal creams, or topical ketoconazole. Resistant cases require oral ketoconazole. Ultraviolet exposure is required to regain any lost pigment.

Clinical Pearls

1. If it scales, scrape it and look for hyphae.
2. Clinically active areas or areas colonized with the fungus may be identified by the orange fluorescence noted on Wood's light examination.

Associated Clinical Features

Basal cell carcinoma is a malignancy of the basal cell layer of the epidermis, presenting as a translucent, pearly papule with central ulceration and rolled borders with fine superficial telangiectasias (Fig. 13.36). It is most frequently located on the head, neck, and upper trunk. The patient frequently notes easy bleeding of the papule with poor to nonhealing. There are several variants of basal cell carcinomas. Pigmented basal cell carcinoma consists of a brownish-black, firm nodule with irregular surface and central ulceration (Fig. 13.37). Superficial multicentric basal cell carcinoma is psoriasiform in nature, consisting of a flat, erythematous, scaly translucent plaque without central ulceration or raised border (Fig. 13.38).

Differential Diagnosis

Pigmented basal cell carcinoma resembles nodular melanoma. Superficial multicentric basal cell carcinoma resembles psoriasis, tinea corporis, and squamous cell carcinoma in situ.

ED Treatment and Disposition

Excisional surgery, cryosurgery, or electrosurgery are recommended forms of treatment. If there is a potential for disfigurement, radiation therapy is usually instituted instead of surgery. Prompt dermatologic consultation must be arranged when evaluating any suspicious lesion.

Clinical Pearls

1. Basal cell carcinoma is the most common form of skin cancer.
2. This malignancy forms in the epidermis that has developing hair follicles; therefore, it is not found on the vermilion border of the lips or the genital mucosal membranes.
3. The pearly, rolled, telangiectatic border with central ulceration is diagnostic of basal cell carcinoma.
4. Despite being locally invasive, basal cell carcinoma does not metastasize.

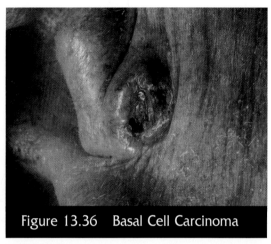

Figure 13.36   Basal Cell Carcinoma

Nodular basal cell carcinoma consists of a firm, centrally ulcerated (rodent ulcer) nodule with a raised, rolled, pearly, telangiectatic border. (Courtesy of Dept. of Dermatology, Wilford Hall USAF Medical Center and Brooke Army Medical Center, San Antonio, TX.)

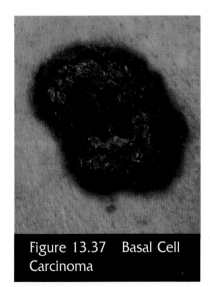

Figure 13.37   Basal Cell Carcinoma

This pigmented basal cell carcinoma consists of a firm, translucent, brownish-black, ulcerated nodule with an irregular surface and asymmetry of its border. (Courtesy of Dept. of Dermatology, Wilford Hall USAF Medical Center and Brooke Army Medical Center, San Antonio, TX.)

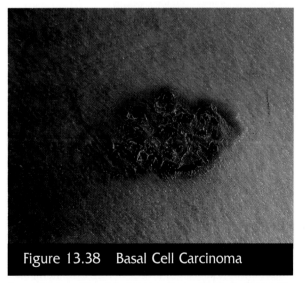

Figure 13.38   Basal Cell Carcinoma

Superficial multicentric basal cell carcinoma is frequently psoriasiform in nature. Note the flat, erythematous, scaly plaque with its elevated, irregular border. (Courtesy of Dept. of Dermatology, Wilford Hall USAF Medical Center and Brooke Army Medical Center, San Antonio, TX.)

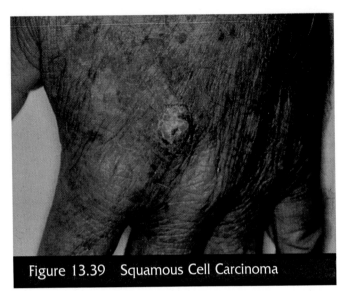

Figure 13.39   Squamous Cell Carcinoma

Note the single erythematous, scaly plaque on the dorsal aspect of this sun-exposed hand. (Courtesy of Dept. of Dermatology, Wilford Hall USAF Medical Center and Brooke Army Medical Center, San Antonio, TX.)

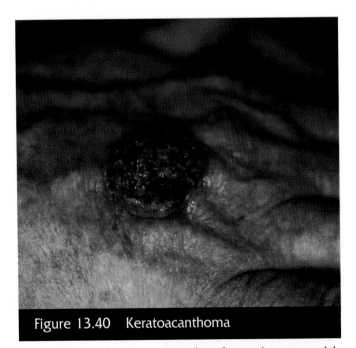

Figure 13.40   Keratoacanthoma

This rapidly evolving neoplasm consists of an erythematous nodule with a hyperkeratotic core. It most closely resembles a squamous cell carcinoma, although it is a benign epithelial neoplasm. Biopsy serves to differentiate these two conditions. (Courtesy of Dept. of Dermatology, Wilford Hall USAF Medical Center and Brooke Army Medical Center, San Antonio, TX.)

Associated Clinical Features

Squamous cell carcinoma varies from erythematous, hyperkeratotic, sharply demarcated plaques to elevated, ulcerative nodules (Fig. 13.39). It may be sun-induced or related to ionizing radiation or industrial carcinogens. Bowen's disease is actually an in situ squamous cell carcinoma consisting of a firm, solitary, erythematous macule or plaque with fine scale and a well defined border. It resembles the superficial multicentric variety of basal cell carcinoma. Erythroplasia of Queyrat consists of the same in situ plaque localized to the penis. Invasive squamous cell carcinoma is characterized by a discrete elevated plaque or nodule with thick keratotic scale and ulceration.

Differential Diagnosis

Squamous cell carcinoma must be differentiated from a benign lesion such as tinea corporis, psoriasis, impetigo, wart, seborrheic keratosis, or keratoacanthoma (Fig. 13.40).

ED Treatment and Disposition

Excisional surgery is required, with radiation therapy utilized in potentially disfiguring cases. All suspicious lesions require prompt dermatologic consultation.

Clinical Pearls

1. Squamous cell carcinoma is the second most common type of cutaneous malignancy.
2. This malignancy develops more commonly in fair-skinned people with a significant history of sun exposure.
3. Most lesions are found on the lips or other sun-exposed areas.
4. A rapidly evolving (2 to 4 weeks) nodule or plaque with a dense hyperkeratotic core is a keratoacanthoma. It is closely related to squamous cell carcinoma and frequently occurs at a site of trauma. Treatment is the same.

Associated Clinical Features

Melanoma is a malignancy involving the melanocytes of the epidermis. Asymmetry, an irregular border, a mottled display of color, a diameter greater than 5 to 6 mm, and an elevation or distortion of the surface are five signs that a lesion may be a melanoma (Fig. 13.41). Melanoma may or may not occur in sun-exposed areas.

Differential Diagnosis

Lentigo maligna is characterized by a single, flat, frecklelike macule with an irregular border, usually on the face (Fig. 13.42). This melanoma in situ is often confused with a solar lentigo or a seborrheic keratosis. Superficially spreading melanoma is the most common form of melanoma. It usually presents as a brown macule with irregular borders and variegation in color. Nodular melanoma usually starts as a papule which becomes an elevated nodule with irregular borders and variegation in color (Fig. 13.43). It must be differentiated from a hemangioma, angiokeratoma, or pigmented basal cell carcinoma. Acral lentiginous melanomas are often mistaken for plantar warts or subungual hematomas; they are flat, pigmented, irregularly bordered macules of the palms, soles, and subungual areas (Fig. 13.44).

ED Treatment and Disposition

Melanoma must be surgically excised with adequate margins. Prompt dermatologic consultation is required of all suspicious lesions because the prognosis of melanoma correlates directly with early detection and treatment.

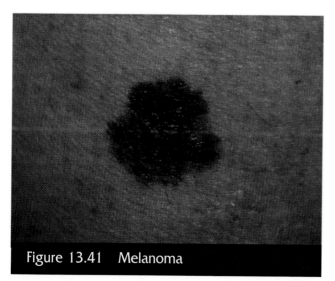

Figure 13.41   Melanoma

Note the asymmetry, irregular border, and focal hyperpigmentation in this melanoma. (Courtesy of Dept. of Dermatology, Wilford Hall USAF Medical Center and Brooke Army Medical Center, San Antonio, TX.)

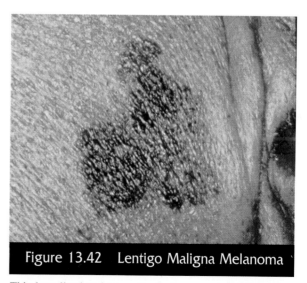

Figure 13.42   Lentigo Maligna Melanoma

This long-lived melanoma in situ has now invaded the dermis, forming a black nodule classified as lentigo maligna melanoma. (Courtesy of Dept. of Dermatology, Wilford Hall USAF Medical Center and Brooke Army Medical Center, San Antonio, TX.)

369

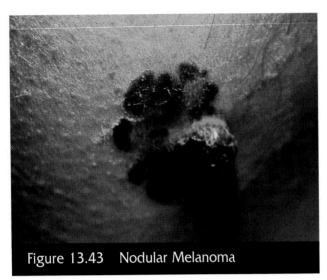

Figure 13.43   Nodular Melanoma

This melanoma has progressed to an exophytic tumor which was deeply invasive histopathologically. (Courtesy of Dept. of Dermatology, Wilford Hall USAF Medical Center and Brooke Army Medical Center, San Antonio, TX.)

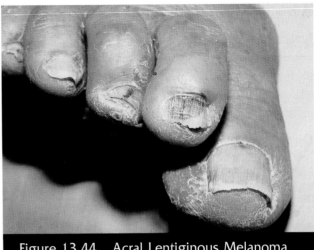

Figure 13.44   Acral Lentiginous Melanoma

The finding of a pigmented, irregularly bordered macule involving the proximal nail fold is called Hutchinson's sign. It represents melanoma of the nail matrix and is therefore classified as an acral lentiginous melanoma. (Courtesy of Dept. of Dermatology, Wilford Hall USAF Medical Center and Brooke Army Medical Center, San Antonio, TX.)

Clinical Pearls

1. Prognosis of melanoma is most dependent on the depth of invasion, therefore, early detection and treatment are essential.
2. Only 20% of melanomas arise from preexisting moles, so the appearance of a new mole, especially after the age of 30, is particularly significant.

DIAGNOSIS   KAPOSI'S SARCOMA

Associated Clinical Features

Kaposi's sarcoma is a vascular neoplasm that is characterized by single or multiple violaceous macules which usually begin on the digits and extend proximally to the trunk (Fig. 13.45). The macules are usually asymptomatic unless they ulcerate and bleed. They may enlarge to form violaceous oval nodules that obstruct lymphatic drainage and cause secondary lymphedema. Mucous membrane involvement is common (Fig. 13.46), as is pulmonary and gastrointestinal involvement. Kaposi's sarcoma is the second most common manifestation of AIDS.

Differential Diagnosis

Multiple lesions resemble pityriasis rosea. Single lesions may resemble malignant melanoma, hemangioma, or ecchymosis.

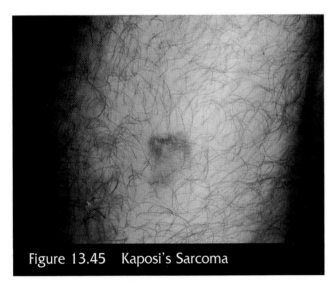

Figure 13.45   Kaposi's Sarcoma

This single, violaceous patch may enlarge to form an obstructive nodule causing secondary lymphedema. It may also ulcerate and bleed. (Courtesy of Dept. of Dermatology, Wilford Hall USAF Medical Center and Brooke Army Medical Center, San Antonio, TX.)

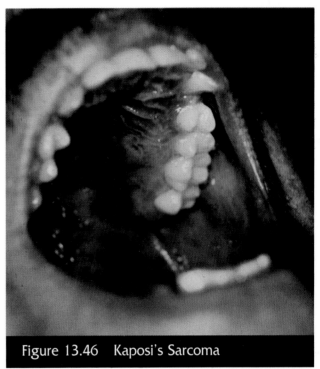

Figure 13.46   Kaposi's Sarcoma

Note the violaceous patch of the oral mucosa, specifically the hard palate. Mucous membrane involvement is very common in AIDS-associated Kaposi's sarcoma. (Courtesy of Dept. of Dermatology, Wilford Hall USAF Medical Center and Brooke Army Medical Center, San Antonio, TX.)

ED Treatment and Disposition

These lesions are exquisitely radiosensitive. Cryotherapy is utilized for single lesions. Multiple lesions may require aggressive chemotherapy.

Clinical Pearls

1. Endemic Kaposi's sarcoma is still primarily a disease of older men of Eastern European and Mediterranean origin.
2. AIDS-associated Kaposi's sarcoma demonstrates a much higher incidence of mucous membrane involvement.

Associated Clinical Features

Pyogenic granuloma is characterized by a solitary, violaceous, pedunculated or sessile, vascular nodule which usually forms at the site of cutaneous injury (Fig. 13.47). The well demarcated nodule consists of exuberant granulation tissue (proud flesh) which may be erosive and encrusted. Pyogenic granuloma commonly occurs on the digits and is particularly common in pregnancy.

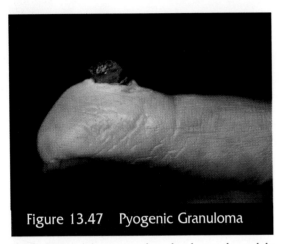

Figure 13.47   Pyogenic Granuloma

This solitary, violaceous, pedunculated, vascular nodule formed at the site of an injury. Note that the nodule is well demarcated by a thin rim of epidermis. (Courtesy of Dept. of Dermatology, Wilford Hall USAF Medical Center and Brooke Army Medical Center, San Antonio, TX.)

Differential Diagnosis

This benign vascular neoplasm resembles a hemangioma; however, it must be differentiated from amelanotic melanoma, squamous cell carcinoma, and metastatic renal cell carcinoma.

ED Treatment and Disposition

Since this neoplasm does not spontaneously resolve, it is usually shaved off with electrodessication of the base.

Clinical Pearls

1. A fine collarette of scale surrounding an exophytic vascular neoplasm is diagnostic.
2. The lesion may exhibit recurrent bleeding episodes.
3. Nearly 25 to 33% of these benign lesions follow some form of minor trauma.

Associated Clinical Features

Fixed drug eruption is a cutaneous reaction to an ingested drug, usually an over-the-counter laxative, barbiturate, tetracycline, or sulfa drug. The reaction occurs at the identical site with repeated exposure to the same drug, usually on the genital skin or proximal extremity. It presents as a round, pruritic, erythematous, sharply demarcated plaque which may evolve into a painful bulla with secondary erosion (Figs. 13.48 and 13.49). Residual hyperpigmentation frequently follows healing.

Differential Diagnosis

Early cellulitis, erythema multiforme, arthropod assault, and genital herpes are usually considered in the differential diagnosis.

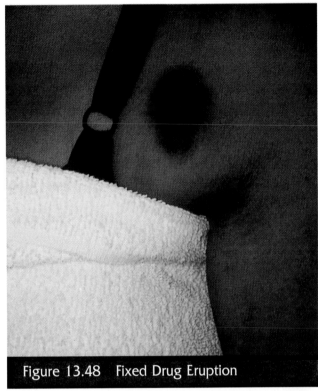

Figure 13.48   Fixed Drug Eruption

This red to violaceous, pruritic, sharply demarcated patch is a cutaneous reaction to a drug. Repeated exposure will cause a similar
reaction in the same location. (Courtesy of Dept. of Dermatology,
Wilford Hall USAF Medical Center and Brooke Army Medical
Center, San Antonio, TX.)

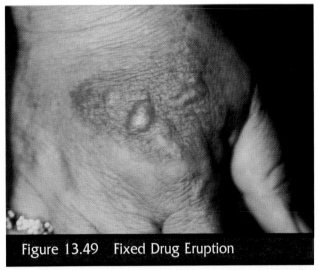

Figure 13.49   Fixed Drug Eruption

The eruption has evolved into a painful bulla which will erode.
This frequently results in residual hyperpigmentation. (Courtesy of
Dept. of Dermatology, Wilford Hall USAF Medical Center and
Brooke Army Medical Center, San Antonio, TX.)

ED Treatment and Disposition

The etiology must be identified and removed before the plaque will resolve. Symptomatic treatment includes antihistamines and analgesics.

Clinical Pearls

1. The identical recurrence of a painful, pruritic, well demarcated violaceous plaque makes the
    diagnosis.
2. This reaction occurs with repeated exposure to the same drug.

Associated Clinical Features

Exanthematous drug eruptions are an adverse hypersensitivity reaction to a drug. This symmetric, pruritic, morbilliform, blanching, erythematous eruption is the most frequent of cutaneous drug eruptions (Fig. 13.50). The initially pruritic macules or papules usually become confluent and may progress to an exfoliative dermatitis.

Differential Diagnosis

Viral exanthem, secondary syphilis, atypical pityriasis rosea, and scarlet fever must all be considered in the differential diagnosis. A serologic test for syphilis, antistreptolysin O titer, and a good history are usually sufficient to make the diagnosis. Severe drug eruptions may be accompanied by eosinophilia, lymphadenopathy, and liver function abnormalities.

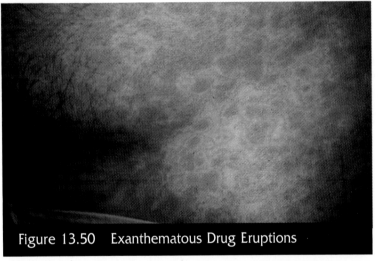

Figure 13.50 Exanthematous Drug Eruptions

This symmetric, morbilliform, blanching eruption was the result of allopurinol. With time, the eruption may become confluent, leading to an exfoliative dermatitis. (Courtesy of Dept. of Dermatology, Wilford Hall USAF Medical Center and Brooke Army Medical Center, San Antonio, TX.)

ED Treatment and Disposition

The eruption may resolve despite the drug's continued use. The drug should be discontinued if considered to be the cause of the rash. It may take as long as 2 weeks for the eruption to fade after discontinuation of the causative drug. Symptomatic management includes antihistamines and topical corticosteroids.

Clinical Pearls

1. Drug eruptions are usually symmetric and pruritic as opposed to viral eruptions, which are usually asymmetric and asymptomatic.
2. Mononucleosis patients taking amoxicillin or AIDS patients taking sulfa drugs frequently experience this reaction.

Associated Clinical Features

Erythema nodosum is a delayed hypersensitivity reaction, usually to certain drugs, infections, or systemic illnesses. This panniculitis (inflammation of the fat) consists of painful, nonulcerated, poorly marginated nodules with overlying erythematous, warm, shiny skin (Fig. 13.51). The lower legs are the most common site; the face is rarely involved. Fever, malaise, and arthralgias often accompany the cutaneous manifestations.

Differential Diagnosis

Erythema induratum, syphilitic gummas, and nodular vasculitis are considered in the differential diagnosis.

ED Treatment and Disposition

Identify and treat the underlying etiology. Oral contraceptives, sulfa drugs, tuberculosis, sarcoidosis, fungal infections, and inflammatory bowel disease are common predisposing factors. Symptomatic treatment includes nonsteroidal antiinflamatory drugs (NSAIDs), bedrest, and compressive dressings.

Clinical Pearls

1. Erythema nodosum most commonly presents in young women secondary to oral contraceptives or sulfa drugs.
2. Its appearance in association with systemic fungal infections (coccidiodomycosis) indicates a likely recovery from the disease.

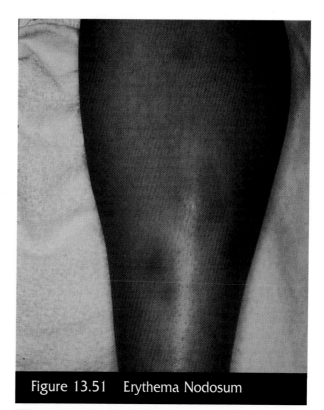

Figure 13.51   Erythema Nodosum

This panniculitis consists of multiple painful, poorly marginated nodules with overlying erythematous, warm, shiny skin. (Courtesy of Dept. of Dermatology, Wilford Hall USAF Medical Center and Brooke Army Medical Center, San Antonio, TX.)

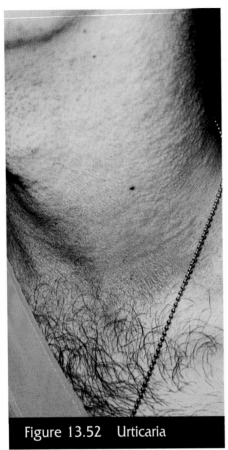

Figure 13.52   Urticaria

Note the edematous papules and wheals covering the skin of the neck. (Courtesy of Alan B. Storrow, MD.)

Associated Clinical Features

Urticaria is a vascular reaction localized to the skin composed of transient, erythematous, edematous, pruritic papules or plaquelike wheals (Figs. 13.52 and 13.53). It tends to favor the covered areas (back, chest, buttocks). Angioedema is a circumscribed edema of the dermis and subcutaneous tissues that usually affects the distensible tissues (lips, eyelids, earlobes, Fig. 13.54). It is usually nonpruritic. There are countless causes of urticaria; the most common being food, medications, and underlying infection. Cholinergic urticaria involves micropapular lesions induced by exercise or heat. Dermatographism presents as linear hives at the site of skin stroking. Cold urticaria can be diagnosed with the ice cube test, and solar urticaria occurs in areas exposed to sunlight. Urticaria may also occur as a result of exposure to pressure, heat, and water. Hereditary angioedema is an autosomal dominant disorder with systemic manifestations secondary to edema of the subcutaneous and mucosal tissues of the respiratory and gastrointestinal tract, in addition to the face and extremities. Mortality rates approach 30%, usually from airway obstruction. There is also an acquired form of angioedema secondary to an underlying malignancy, usually lymphoreticular. Angiotensin converting enzyme inhibitor use is a frequent cause of angioedema.

Differential Diagnosis

Bacterial or viral exanthems, erythema multiforme, and drug eruptions must be considered in the differential diagnosis of urticaria. Edema of any etiology (congestive heart failure, glomerulonephritis, chronic liver disease) must be differentiated from the soft-tissue swelling associated with angioedema.

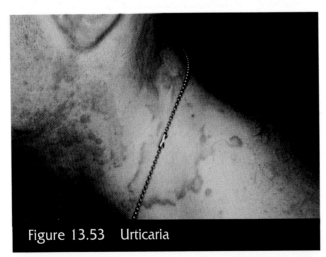

Figure 13.53   Urticaria

This picture demonstrates that the urticarial eruptions may be quite large, forming edematous plaques with central clearing. (Courtesy of Dept. of Dermatology, Wilford Hall USAF Medical Center and Brooke Army Medical Center, San Antonio, TX.)

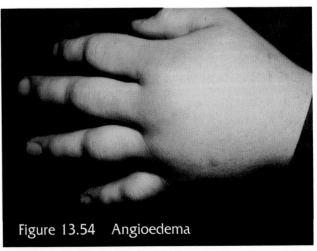

Figure 13.54   Angioedema

This is an example of hereditary angioedema. Note the circumscribed edema of the subcutaneous tissues of the hand, without the presence of urticaria. (Courtesy of Dept. of Dermatology, Wilford Hall USAF Medical Center and Brooke Army Medical Center, San Antonio, TX.)

ED Treatment and Disposition

This involves the identification and elimination of any potential etiology. Antihistamines can be effective for urticaria, often requiring both H_1 and H_2 blockers and steroids for stubborn cases. Life-threatening attacks of hereditary angioedema do not respond well to antihistamines, epinephrine, or steroids. Admission for supportive care and active airway management is the mainstay of treatment. Danazol may be utilized for prophylactic management.

Clinical Pearls

1. Both urticaria and angioedema are acute and evanescent.
2. Urticaria is pruritic and responsive to antihistamines, epinephrine, and steroids.
3. Angioedema is only rarely pruritic and minimally responsive to epinephrine, and may require danazol for long-term treatment.

DYSHIDROTIC ECZEMA (POMPHOLYX)   DIAGNOSIS

Associated Clinical Features

Dyshidrotic eczema is a papulovesicular plaque involving the epidermis of the fingers, palms, and soles. The dermatosis initially consists of pruritic, deep-seated vesicles grouped in clusters (Fig. 13.55). Scaling and painful fissure formation are late complications, as is secondary bacterial infection. Spontaneous remissions and recurrent attacks are usually the rule.

Differential Diagnosis

Acute contact dermatitis must be considered in the differential diagnosis of the acute eruption. Psoriasis and dermatophytosis are considered in the differential diagnosis of the chronic eruption.

ED Treatment and Disposition

Burow's wet dressings should be utilized during the early vesicular stage. High-potency topical steroids are used in all stages of the eruption. Systemic corticosteroids should be

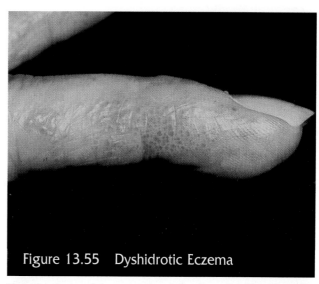

Figure 13.55   Dyshidrotic Eczema

Note the cluster of deep-seated vesicles along the sides of the fingers. Scaling and painful fissure formation may also occur. No overlying erythema is present. (Courtesy of Dept. of Dermatology, Wilford Hall USAF Medical Center and Brooke Army Medical Center, San Antonio, TX.)

avoided except for the most severe cases. Antihistamines treat the pruritus. Dicloxacillin or erythromycin are used to treat secondary bacterial infections. Minimal exposure to water and generous emolliation also hasten healing.

Clinical Pearls

1. Deep-seated, tapioca-like vesicles on the sides of the digits followed by scaling and fissure formation is typical of this disease.
2. Dyshidrotic eczema is frequently associated with psychosocial stressors.
3. The "id reaction," due to fungal infections and drug eruptions, may have similar clinical presentations.

DIAGNOSIS   **ATOPIC DERMATITIS**

Associated Clinical Features

Atopic dermatitis is a broadly defined pruritic inflammation of the epidermis and dermis with approximately 60% of the cases occuring during the first year of life. The characteristic pattern is erythema, papules, and lichenified plaques with excoriation and exudation of wet crusts (Fig. 13.56). Its distribution is the face (sparing of the mouth), the antecubital and popliteal fossae, and the dorsal surfaces of the forearms, hands, and feet. This is generally considered a lifelong condition with gradual improvement toward adulthood.

Differential Diagnosis

Nummular eczema, allergic contact dermatitis, impetigo, dermatophytosis, and psoriasis are usually considered in the differential diagnosis. A KOH examination of the scale rules out dermatophytosis. A biopsy may help differentiate this condition from nummular eczema and contact dermatitis.

ED Treatment and Disposition

Antihistamines treat the pruritus. Unscented emollients prevent xerosis (dry skin). Topical corticosteroids treat the underlying inflammation. Systemic corticosteroids should be avoided except for the most severe cases. Since these patients are frequently colonized with *Staphylococcus aureus*, antistaphylococcal antibiotics are also used during flares of the condition.

Clinical Pearls

1. Flexural surface scaly plaques with excoriation and exudation of crusts is diagnostic of atopic dermatitis.
2. Asthma and allergic rhinitis may develop as the atopic dermatitis improves.

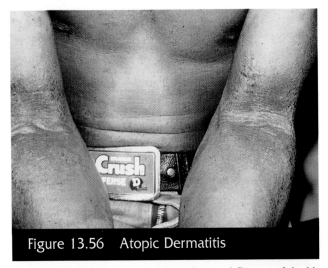

Figure 13.56 Atopic Dermatitis

Note the lichenified plaques with erosions and fissures of the bilateral antecubital fossa. This results from chronic rubbing and scratching. (Courtesy of Dept. of Dermatology, Wilford Hall USAF Medical Center and Brooke Army Medical Center, San Antonio, TX.)

Associated Clinical Features

Nummular eczema is a pruritic eczematous dermatitis consisting of closely grouped vesicles which coalesce into coin-shaped, erythematous plaques with poorly defined borders (Figs. 13.57 and 13.58). These plaques may become encrusted or dry and scaly. They are usually found on the trunk and extremities.

Differential Diagnosis

Allergic contact dermatitis, impetigo, dermatophytosis, and psoriasis must all be considered in the differential diagnosis. If it scales, scrape it and look for hyphae to differentiate a dermatophytosis. A biopsy may help differentiate contact dermatitis from nummular eczema.

ED Treatment and Disposition

Antihistamines treat the pruritus. Unscented emolliants prevent xerosis. Topical corticosteroids treat the underlying inflammation. Systemic corticosteroids should be avoided except for the most severe cases.

Clinical Pearls

1. Coin-shaped, pruritic, eczematous plaques not responsive to antibiotics are diagnostic of nummular eczema.
2. Recurrences tend to occur in previously involved sites.

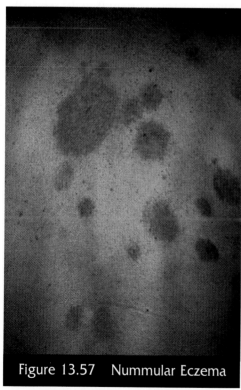

Figure 13.57 Nummular Eczema

An example of multiple erythematous, coin-shaped plaques with fine scales, representative of this pruritic, eczematous dermatitis. (Courtesy of Dept. of Dermatology, Wilford Hall USAF Medical Center and Brooke Army Medical Center, San Antonio, TX.)

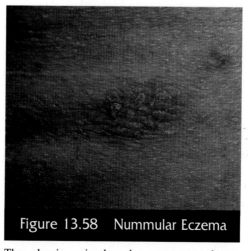

Figure 13.58 Nummular Eczema

The classic coin-shaped eczematous plaque. (Courtesy of Dept. of Dermatology, Wilford Hall USAF Medical Center and Brooke Army Medical Center, San Antonio, TX.)

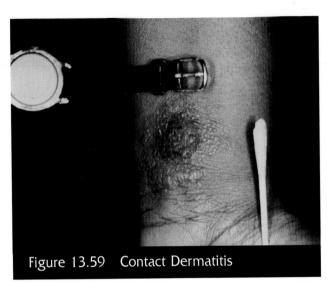

Figure 13.59 Contact Dermatitis

Note that the erythematous, edematous base of the eruption corresponds to the posterior surface of the watch. Superimposed on the erythematous base are multiple vesicles with exudate and crust. (Courtesy of Dept. of Dermatology, Wilford Hall USAF Medical Center and Brooke Army Medical Center, San Antonio, TX.)

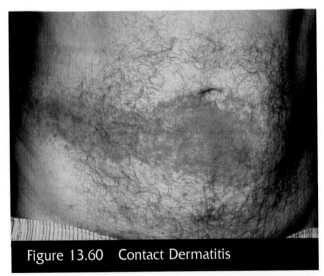

Figure 13.60 Contact Dermatitis

Another example of how the eruption involves only the surface of the skin exposed to the irritant. In this case the irritant is the elastic band of the underwear. Note the linear, well demarcated nature of the eruption, which is classic for contact dermatitis. (Courtesy of Dept. of Dermatology, Wilford Hall USAF Medical Center and Brooke Army Medical Center, San Antonio, TX.)

Associated Clinical Features

Allergic contact dermatitis is an acute or chronic delayed-type hypersensitivity reaction caused by contact exposure to a variety of agents. The acute form is characterized by multiple, closely grouped vesicles with exudative erosions and crust formation on a well defined erythematous, edematous base (Figs. 13.59 and 13.60). Subacute contact dermatitis consists of dry, scaly patches with areas of desquamation, whereas the chronic form consists of hyperkeratosis and pigmentation. All forms of allergic contact dermatitis are pruritic.

Differential Diagnosis

Atopic dermatitis, nummular eczema, impetigo, and dermatophytosis are included in the differential diagnosis. If it scales, scrape it and look for hyphae to differentiate a dermatophytosis. A positive patch test is diagnostic of an allergic contact dermatitis. Contact exposure of the skin to the allergen leading to erythema and vesicle formation is considered a positive test.

ED Treatment and Disposition

Identify and remove any potential allergen. Antihistamines relieve the pruritus. Topical corticosteroids treat the underlying inflammation. Systemic corticosteroids should be avoided except for the most severe cases.

Clinical Pearls

1. Well defined, pruritic areas of erythema superimposed with exudative vesicles and a recent history of exposure to a specific allergen are diagnostic of allergic contact dermatitis.
2. Poison ivy and oak are the most common causes of allergic contact dermatitis.
3. When treating with topical ointments, a worsening of the dermatitis may signify an allergic reaction to the medication.

Associated Clinical Features

Phytophotodermatitis is a pruritic, linear dermatitis that occurs when skin exposed to certain plants becomes exposed to sunlight. Bizarre patterns of pruritic erythema convert into vesicles and bullae that undergo involution, leaving behind a residual intense hyperpigmentation (Fig. 13.61).

Drug-induced photosensitivity is an adverse skin reaction due to simultaneous exposure to certain drugs and ultraviolet radiation. The rash is erythematous and edematous, much like sunburn (Fig. 13.62).

Differential Diagnosis

Rhus dermatitis is most often mistaken for this eruption. Photosensitivity can be caused by other diseases.

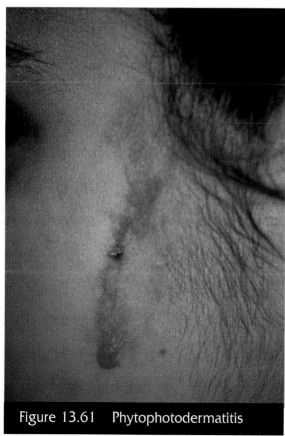

Figure 13.61 Phytophotodermatitis

The linear, photodistributed, eczematous plaque resulted from contact with a plant-derived photosensitizer (lime juice). This frequently resolves with hyperpigmentation. (Courtesy of Dept. of Dermatology, Wilford Hall USAF Medical Center and Brooke Army Medical Center, San Antonio, TX.)

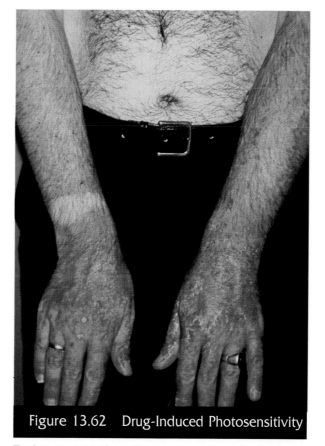

Figure 13.62 Drug-Induced Photosensitivity

Erythematous reaction to ultraviolet radiation associated with carbamazepine use. (Courtesy of Dept. of Dermatology, Naval Medical Center, Portsmouth, VA)

ED Treatment and Disposition

Symptomatic treatment includes wet dressings, antihistamines, calamine lotion, and cortico-steroid creams. For drug-induced photosensitivity, the offending drug should be discontinued. Counsel patients about the use of sunscreens and sun avoidance to prevent recurrences.

Clinical Pearls

1. Linearly distributed, pruritic vesicles in a photodistribution with a history of plant exposure make the diagnosis.
2. The distribution of the rash is limited to sun-exposed areas.
3. Common drugs causing drug-induced photosensitivity are carbamazepine, amiodarone, doxycycline, furosemide, phenothiazines, and sulfonamides.

PART II

SELECTED AREAS

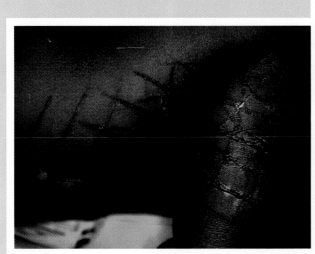

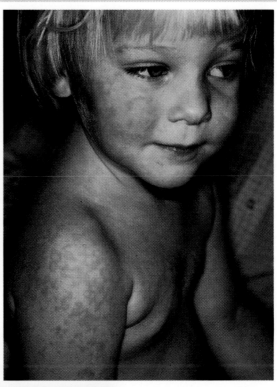

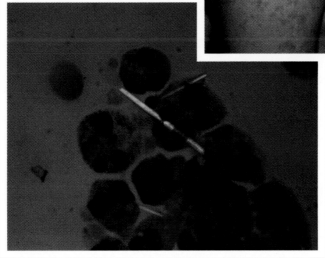

CHAPTER 14

PEDIATRIC CONDITIONS

Javier A. Gonzalez del Rey
Richard M. Ruddy

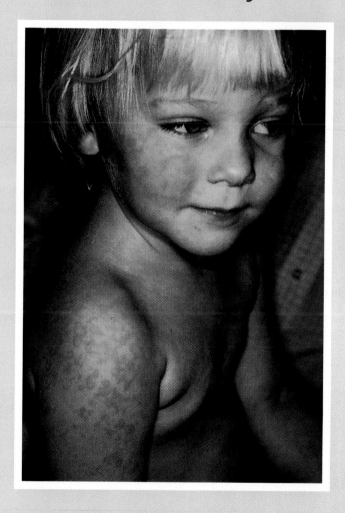

Newborn Conditions

ERYTHEMA TOXICUM

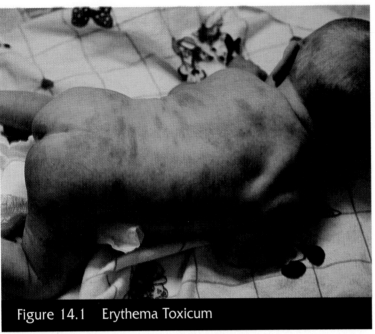

Figure 14.1   Erythema Toxicum

Newborn infant with diffuse macular rash of erythema toxicum. (Courtesy of Kevin J. Knoop, MD, MS.)

Associated Clinical Features

This benign, self-limiting eruption of unknown etiology in newborns is characterized by small, erythematous macules 2 to 3 cm in diameter (Fig. 14.1) with 1- to 3-mm, firm, pale yellow or white papules or pustules in the center. This rash usually presents within the first 2 to 3 days of life. Each individual lesion usually disappears within 4 or 5 days. New lesions may occur during the first 2 weeks of life. Wright-stained slide preparations of the scraping from the center of the lesion demonstrate numerous eosinophils.

Differential Diagnosis

Transient neonatal pustular melanosis, newborn milia, miliaria, herpes simplex, and impetigo of the newborn should be considered.

ED Treatment and Disposition

As this condition is self-limiting, no therapy is indicated in the setting of a well-appearing newborn with normal activity and appetite. In cases in which impetigo, *Candida,* or herpes infections are suspected, a smear from the center of the lesion and culture may be necessary to make a final diagnosis.

Clinical Pearl

1.   Erythema toxicum is the most common rash of the newborn (up to 50% of full terms). The lesions may be present anywhere on the body but tend to spare the palms and soles.

SALMON PATCHES (NEVUS SIMPLEX)

Associated Clinical Features

Nevus simplex (salmon patches) is the most common vascular lesion in infancy, present in about 40% of newborns. It is described as a slightly red, flat, macular lesion on the nape of the neck, the glabella, forehead, or upper eyelids (Figs. 14.2 and 14.3). In general, the eyelid lesions fade within a year and the glabellar within 5 to 6 years. The lesions on the neck often persist.

Differential Diagnosis

Nevus flammeus (port-wine stain) can have a similar appearance.

ED Treatment and Disposition

Parental education and reassurance can be helpful, but no treatment is indicated.

Clinical Pearls

1. In general, flat vascular birthmarks tend to persist through life. Raised vascular birthmarks usually disappear with time.
2. When this lesion is seen on the nape of the neck, it is frequently referred to as a *stork bite*.

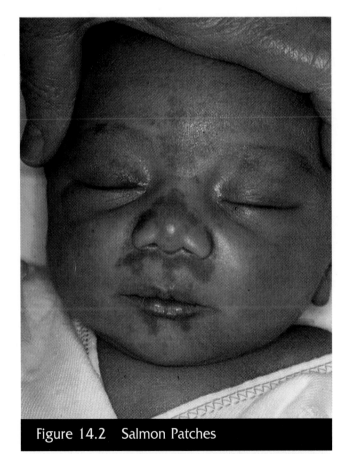

Figure 14.2   Salmon Patches

Newborn with characteristic salmon patches over his face. (Courtesy of Anne W. Lucky, MD.)

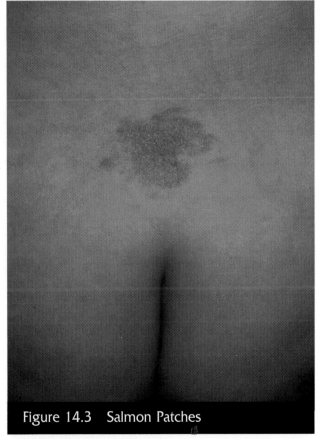

Figure 14.3   Salmon Patches

Child with patch over lower back consistent with salmon patches. (Courtesy of Anne W. Lucky, MD.)

Associated Clinical Features

Physiologic jaundice (Fig. 14.4) is observed in 25 to 50% of term newborns. Most cases are self-limited and generally without sequelae. The physiologic (<12 mg/dL) jaundice of the newborn usually peaks between the second and fourth day. In preterm infants this peak occurs later. Physiologic jaundice is believed to be a combination of factors including an increase of bilirubin production following breakdown of fetal red blood cells associated with a temporary decrease in conjugation of these by-products by the immature newborn liver. Risk factors for unconjugated hyperbilirubinemia include maternal diabetes, prematurity, drugs, polycythemia, traumatic delivery with cutaneous bruising or hematoma, and breast-feeding. Most infants with jaundice have no disease, but a careful history and organized approach is necessary to identify pathologic causes when these patients present to the ED. Kernicterus is a condition resulting from a severe form of unconjugated hyperbilirubinemia and is associated with mental retardation, deafness, seizures, choreoathetosis, and a multitude of other irreversible neurologic abnormalities.

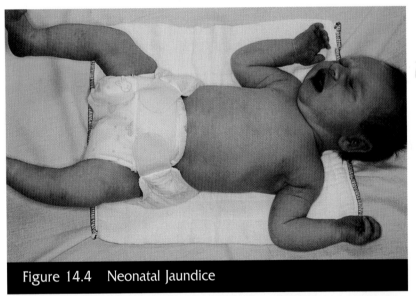

Figure 14.4   Neonatal Jaundice

Newborn with yellowish hue to skin consistent with jaundice. (Courtesy of Kevin J. Knoop, MD, MS.)

Differential Diagnosis

Jaundice within the first 24 h of life is usually associated with sepsis, erythroblastosis fetalis, and bleeding disorders or hemorrhage (traumatic delivery with cutaneous bleeding or hematomas). Physiologic jaundice first appears on the second or third day. Any patient presenting with jaundice after the third day of life should be carefully evaluated for the possibility of sepsis. Late-onset jaundice could be suggestive of septicemia, breast milk jaundice, galactosemia, hemolytic anemias, drug-induced hyperbilirubinemia, pyloric stenosis or duodenal atresia, Crigler-Najjar, or Gilbert's disease.

ED Treatment and Disposition

Initial laboratory work-up should include blood type and Coombs' test, complete blood count with smear for red cell morphology and reticulocyte count, and indirect and direct bilirubin. Other studies may be ordered according to the clinical presentation and history. Initial management should ensure adequate hydration and treatment of the underlying condition. Correct acidosis, since bilirubin precipitates in acid media. In cases of physiologic jaundice the level of serum bilirubin at which to start phototherapy is not clearly defined. The traditional approach is to initiate phototherapy to maintain bilirubin level below 20 mg/dL. Exchange transfusion is considered if the serum level remains elevated (22 to 28 mg/dL) despite appropriate phototherapy.

Clinical Pearls

1. Physiologic jaundice in the presence of a good hemoglobin level is orange in color. It is often visible when the bilirubin level exceeds 8 mg/dL. Jaundice associated with anemia is usually lemon in color.
2. Bilirubin levels should be modified for prematurity, sepsis, low birth weight, and other risk factors when phototherapy or exchange transfusion is considered.

NEONATAL MILK PRODUCTION (WITCH'S MILK)

DIAGNOSIS

Associated Clinical Features

Because of transplacental hormonal effects (maternal estrogens and possibly endogenous prolactin), both sexes are equally liable to breast enlargement. This phenomenon occurs with or without galactorrhea in 60% of normal newborns. After the first 48 h, the hypertrophied breasts may become engorged, and a form of lactation occurs (Fig. 14.5). This engorgement and edema begins to subside after the second week of life. The hypertrophy and galactorrhea may persist up to 6 months in girls. These infants are occasionally predisposed to infections (mastitis or abscess).

Differential Diagnosis

Early mastitis with purulent discharge may resemble normal neonatal milk production.

ED Treatment and Disposition

Treatment is not necessary; reassuring parents is very important.

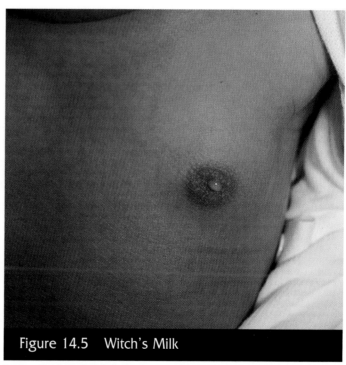

Figure 14.5 Witch's Milk

Milky fluid draining from the nipple in this newborn. (Courtesy of Michael J. Nowicki, MD.)

Clinical Pearl

1. Newborns with hypertrophied mammary tissue and evidence of clear colostrumlike secretion in the absence of erythema, tenderness, and/or fluctuation usually do not present with neonatal mastitis.

Associated Clinical Features

Neonatal mastitis is most common in full-term females, particularly in their second or third week of life. Clinically it manifests as swelling, induration, and tenderness of the affected breast with or without erythema or warmth (Fig. 14.6). In some cases purulent discharge may be obtained from the nipple. Bacteremia and fever are rare. This infection is usually caused by *Staphylococcus aureus,* coliform bacteria, or group B streptococcus. If treatment is delayed, it may progress rapidly with involvement of subcutaneous tissues and subsequent toxicity and systemic findings.

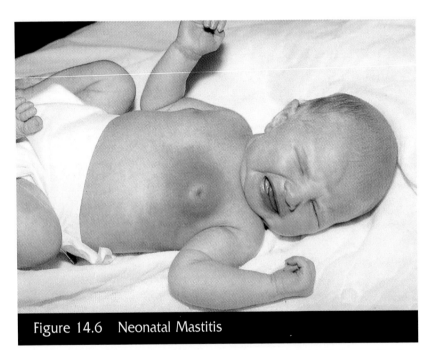

Figure 14.6   Neonatal Mastitis

Neonate with left-sided breast swelling, erythema, and purulent discharge. (Courtesy of Raymond C. Baker, MD.)

Differential Diagnosis

In the initial stages, neonatal mastitis may mimic mammary tissue hypertrophy owing to maternal passive hormonal stimulation. Minor trauma, cutaneous infections, and duct blockage may precede this infection.

ED Treatment and Disposition

Institution of treatment is important to avoid cellulitic spread and breast tissue damage. In cases of mild cellulitis and no fluctuation, nipple discharge culture and antibiotic coverage (semisynthetic penicillin or first-generation cephalosporins) completes the treatment. Adjustment of coverage may be done once results of cultures or Gram's stain are available, especially in the presence of gram-negative bacilli. If no organism is seen initially, semisynthetic penicillin and an aminoglycoside or cefotaxime should be used. In cases of toxicity or subcutaneous spreading, a complete sepsis workup should be performed, and hospitalization is usually indicated. In cases of palpable fluctuation, prompt surgical incision and drainage should be performed by a surgeon to avoid further damage of the mammary tissue. Recovery is usually in 5 to 7 days.

Clinical Pearl

1. Consider mastitis in the neonate with edema, induration, and tenderness of the breast tissue. Erythema and fluctuation to palpation ensue if treatment is delayed.

Associated Clinical Features

Umbilical cord granuloma develops in response to a mild infection at the base of the umbilical cord caused by saprophytic organisms. Usually parents describe a persistent discharge from the base of the cord. The granuloma is soft, pink, and vascular (Fig. 14.7) and is the result of persistence of exuberant granulation tissue.

Differential Diagnosis

An umbilical polyp is a rare anomaly resulting from the persistence of the omphalomesenteric duct (Figs. 14.8 and 14.9) or the urachus and may have a similar appearance. This polyp is usually firm and resistant with a mucoid secretion. Omphalitis, an infection secondary to gram-negative organisms, should be considered.

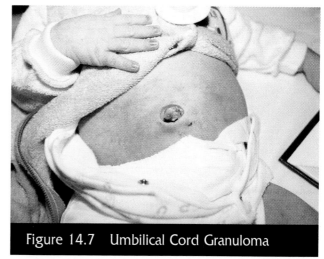

Figure 14.7   Umbilical Cord Granuloma

Newborn infant with umbilical cord demonstrating granuloma on base of umbilical cord. (Courtesy of Michael J. Nowicki, MD.)

ED Treatment and Disposition

Cleaning and drying of the umbilical cord base with alcohol several times a day may prevent granuloma formation. Cauterization of the granuloma with silver nitrate is the treatment of choice. It is important to protect the surrounding skin to avoid chemical burns produced by the excess of silver nitrate.

Clinical Pearls

1. Commonly the only sign of granuloma formation is the presence of nonpurulent discharge noted in the diaper area in contact with the umbilicus.
2. Omphalitis presents with redness on the abdominal wall and often with a purulent discharge from the umbilicus.

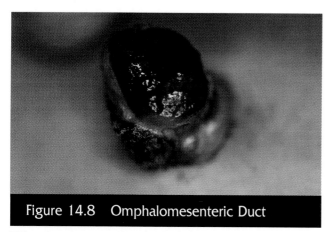

Figure 14.8   Omphalomesenteric Duct

This red mass resembling a granuloma was found to be an omphalomesenteric duct. (Courtesy of Kevin J. Knoop, MD, MS.)

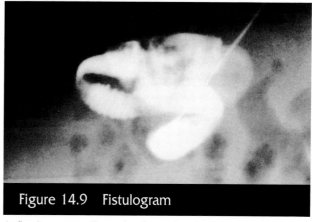

Figure 14.9   Fistulogram

A fistulogram confirms the diagnosis of persistent omphalomesenteric duct. (Courtesy of Kevin J. Knoop, MD, MS.)

Associated Clinical Features

HPS is characterized by postprandial, nonbilious vomiting due to hypertrophy and hyperplasia of the pyloric musculature producing gastric outlet obstruction. It is usually diagnosed in infants from birth to 5 months, most commonly occurring at 2 to 8 weeks of life. The vomiting progresses to forceful and described as projectile (although this pattern is not always present). There is a familial incidence, and white males are more frequently affected. During the physical examination, peristaltic waves may be observed traveling from the left upper to right upper quadrants (Fig. 14.10). The hypertrophy and hyperplasia of the antral and pyloric musculature produces the "olive" to palpation (best palpated after emptying the stomach with a nasogastric tube). Because of persistent vomiting, hypochloremic alkalosis with various degrees of dehydration and failure to thrive may occur when not diagnosed early. The finding of the pyloric olive is pathognomonic. Ultrasound and fluoroscopy are useful diagnostic tools to confirm the diagnosis when the olive is not evident.

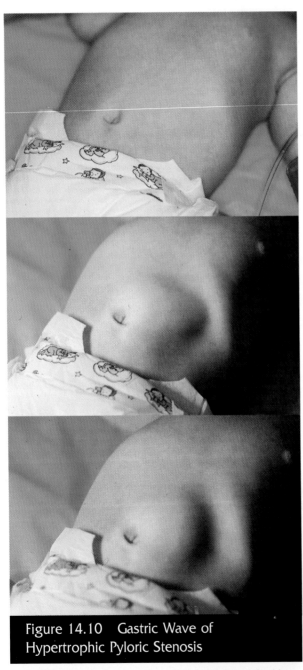

Figure 14.10   Gastric Wave of Hypertrophic Pyloric Stenosis

A gastric wave can be seen traversing the abdomen in this series of photographs of a patient with HPS. (Courtesy of Kevin J. Knoop, MD, MS.)

Differential Diagnosis

Intestinal obstruction, atresia, malrotation with volvulus, hiatal hernia, gastroenteritis, adrenogenital syndrome, increased intracranial pressure, esophagitis, sepsis, gastroesophageal reflux, and poor feeding technique should be considered.

ED Treatment and Disposition

Once the diagnosis is considered, treatment includes correction of fluids and electrolyte imbalance followed by surgical referral for curative pylorotomy. Patients benefit from a nasogastric tube on low intermittent suction.

Clinical Pearls

1. Any infant in the first 2 months of life who presents with postprandial vomiting, some evidence of failure to gain weight, easy refeeding, hunger after vomiting, and infrequent bowel movements should be carefully evaluated to rule out the possibility of HPS.
2. Clinical suspicion can be heightened with serial examinations and observation of the child after oral fluid challenges for persistent projectile vomiting.
3. Correction of any electrolyte imbalance should occur prior to surgery.

Rashes and Lesions

ERYTHEMA INFECTIOSUM (FIFTH DISEASE)

Associated Clinical Features

Erythema infectiosum is a viral infection caused by parvovirus B19. It is characterized by an eruption that presents initially as an erythematous malar blush followed by an erythematous maculopapular eruption on the extensor surfaces of extremities, that evolves into a reticulated, lacy, mottled appearance (Fig. 14.11). It may present with low-grade fever, malaise, general aches, arthritis, or arthralgias.

Differential Diagnosis

Morbilliform eruptions may be caused by viruses such as measles, rubella, roseola, and infectious mononucleosis. Bacterial infections (i.e., scarlet fever), drug reactions, and other skin conditions such as guttate psoriasis, papular urticaria, and erythema multiforme are included in the differential.

ED Treatment and Disposition

There is no specific treatment. Once the rash appears, the patient is no longer contagious. It is important to educate the patient and family about the possible risk of B19 virus as a cause of hydrops fetalis or fetal deaths early in pregnancy and the issue of an aplastic crisis in patients with hematologic problems such as sickle cell disease, hereditary spherocytosis, other hemolytic anemias, or immunosuppressed host.

Clinical Pearl

1. Classically this infection begins with the intense redness of both cheeks ("slapped-cheek appearance"). Although the eruption tends to disappear within 5 days of the initial presentation, recrudescences may occur with exercise, overheating, and sunburns as a result of cutaneous vasodilatation.

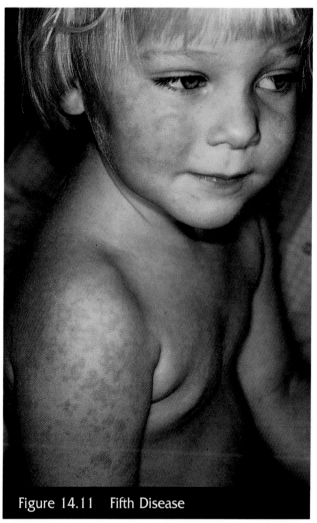

Figure 14.11 Fifth Disease

Toddler with the classic slapped-cheek appearance of fifth disease caused by parvovirus B19. Also note the lacy reticular macular rash on the shoulder and upper extremity. (Courtesy of Anne W. Lucky, MD.)

Associated Clinical Features

The typical presentation of roseola infantum is that of a child with a 2- or 3-day history of fever and irritability. This is followed by rapid defervescence and the appearance of an erythematous morbilliform eruption (Fig. 14.12). It has been associated with various viral agents such as parvovirus, echovirus, and other enteroviruses. Most recently it has been associated with herpesvirus 6.

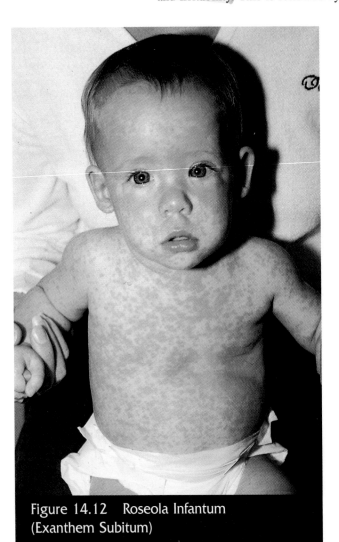

Figure 14.12 Roseola Infantum (Exanthem Subitum)

Toddler with maculopapular eruption of roseola. (Courtesy of Raymond C. Baker, MD.)

Differential Diagnosis

Morbilliform eruptions may be caused by common viruses such as measles, rubella, parvovirus B19, or infectious mononucleosis. Bacterial infections (e.g., scarlet fever), drug reactions, and other skin conditions such as guttate psoriasis, papular urticaria, and erythema multiforme may be included in the differential.

ED Treatment and Disposition

Like most viral infections, only supportive therapy is necessary. Special attention should be paid to maintaining fluid intake, fever control for patient's comfort, and parental education about the benign self-limiting characteristics of this illness.

Clinical Pearls

1. The presence of mild eyelid edema with posterior cervical adenopathy in the febrile child without a source may be early indicators for the diagnosis of roseola. Once the fever ends and the rash appears, the diagnosis is clinically confirmed.

2. Rashes *during* the febrile course of an illness are not roseola.

Associated Clinical Features

Impetigo is a bacterial infection of the skin produced by *Streptococcus pyogenes* and *Staphylococcus aureus*. It begins as small vesicles or pustules with a very thin roof that rupture easily with the release of a cloudy fluid and the subsequent formation of a honey-colored crust (Figs. 14.13 and 14.14). Often the lesions spread rapidly and coalesce to form larger ones.

Differential Diagnosis

Second-degree burns, cutaneous diphtheria, herpes simplex infections, nummular dermatitis, and kerion may present with crusts and be confused with impetigo.

ED Treatment and Disposition

Since these lesions are contagious, good hand washing and personal hygiene should be discussed with the patient and family. Antibiotic coverage should be directed against the organisms mentioned above. Effective oral agents include erythromycin, first-generation cephalosporins, cloxacillin, or amoxicillin with clavulanic acid. Topical agents such as mupirocin ointment have been proved to be as effective as oral antibiotics.

Clinical Pearls

1. A red, weeping surface and the presence of moist, thin vesicles with honey-colored crusts makes the diagnosis of impetigo.
2. Inflicted cigarette burns may resemble the lesions of impetigo.

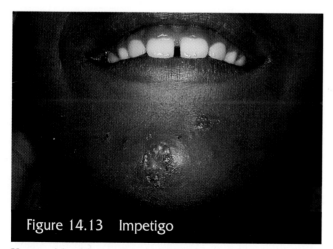

Figure 14.13 Impetigo

Young girl with crusting impetiginous lesions on her chin. (Courtesy of Michael J. Nowicki, MD.)

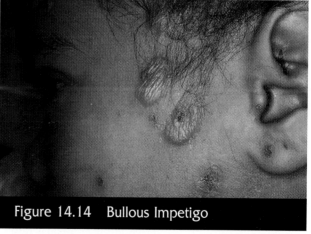

Figure 14.14 Bullous Impetigo

A child with impetiginous lesions on the face. Note the formation of bullae. (Courtesy of Anne W. Lucky, MD.)

Associated Clinical Features

A kerion consists of inflammatory boggy nodules with pustules caused by an exaggerated host delayed hypersensitivity response to infections with either *Microsporum canis* or *Trichophyton tonsurans*. These lesions usually remain localized to one area (Fig. 14.15). It appears 2 to 8 weeks after the initial fungal infection and resolves over 4 to 6 weeks. If untreated, scarring and hair loss may occur.

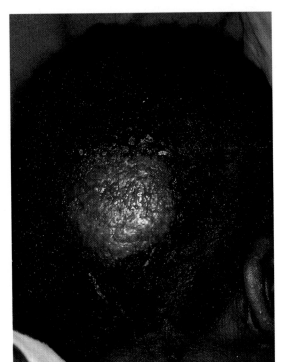

Figure 14.15   Kerion

Occipital boggy swelling with hair loss consistent with kerion. (Courtesy of Anne W. Lucky, MD.)

Differential Diagnosis

Bacterial pyoderma is commonly mistaken for kerion but yields a purulent discharge when aspirated. The diagnosis should be made on clinical appearance.

ED Treatment and Disposition

Topical agents have no role in the treatment of tinea capitis or kerion. Griseofulvin for 4 to 6 weeks is the treatment of choice. Ketoconazole has also been used. Viable spores can be eradicated by adding selenium sulfide shampoo (2.5%) to this therapy. In cases of severe inflammatory reaction, prednisone combined with griseofulvin ensures a rapid resolution of the infection and immunogenic reaction. Incision should be avoided to prevent scar tissue.

Clinical Pearl

1. If a kerion happens to be aspirated or incised, only serosanguineous fluid is obtained.

Associated Clinical Features

Chickenpox results from a primary infection with varicella virus and is characterized by a generalized pruritic vesicular rash (Fig. 14.16), fever, and mild systemic symptoms. The skin lesions have an abrupt onset, develop in crops, and evolve from papules to vesicles (rarely bullae) and finally to crusted lesions within 48 h. The classic lesions are teardrop vesicles surrounded by an erythematous ring (dewdrop on a rose petal) (Fig. 14.17). Secondary bacterial infection of these lesions can occur causing cellulitis, which may be severe. Other complications from varicella include encephalitis, pancreatitis, hepatitis, pneumonia, arthritis, or meningitis. Cerebritis (ataxia) may develop and is usually self-limiting.

Differential Diagnosis

Although several illnesses can present with vesiculobullous lesions, the typical varicella is seldom confused with other problems. Common viral infections that manifest with vesicular rashes include herpes simplex, herpes zoster, coxsackie, influenza, and echovirus infections or vaccinia. On occasions it can be confused with papular urticaria.

ED Treatment and Disposition

Most patients do not develop any complications. Treatment should be symptomatic and directed to pruritus and fever control (avoid salicylates due to association with Reye's syndrome). Oral acyclovir given within 24 h of the onset of the illness may result in a modest decrease in the duration of symptoms and in the number and duration of skin lesions. Acyclovir is not recommended routinely for treatment of uncomplicated varicella in an otherwise healthy child. In the immunocompromised host, VZIG (varicella zoster immunoglobulin) and intravenous acyclovir are effectively used.

Clinical Pearl

1. Skin lesions in varicella present in successive crops so that papules, vesicles, and crusted lesions may be present at any one time. The earliest lesions may begin at the hairline on the nape of the neck.

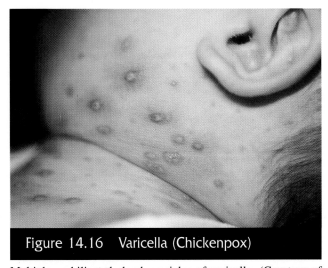

Figure 14.16   Varicella (Chickenpox)

Multiple umbilicated cloudy vesicles of varicella. (Courtesy of Lawrence B. Stack, MD.)

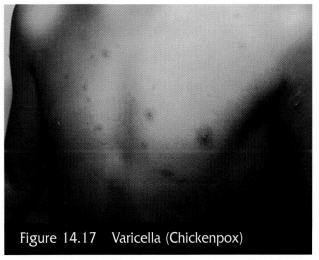

Figure 14.17   Varicella (Chickenpox)

Vesicles in different stages of maturation. Note the clear vesicle on an erythematous base ("dewdrop in a rose petal") in the center of the chest. (Courtesy of Judith C. Bausher, MD.)

Associated Clinical Features

Measles presents as an acute febrile illness with a 3- to 4-day prodromal period characterized by cough, coryza, and conjunctivitis associated with fever (101° to 104°F), chills, and malaise.

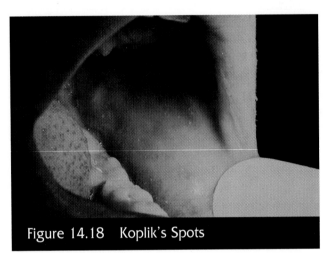

Figure 14.18   Koplik's Spots

Tiny white dots (Koplik's spots) are seen on the buccal mucosa. (Courtesy of Lawrence B. Stack, MD.)

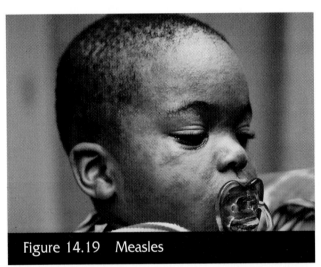

Figure 14.19   Measles

School-age child with morbilliform rash on face consistent with measles. (Courtesy of Javier A. Gonzalez del Rey, MD.)

Koplik's spots, the pathognomonic sign of measles, appear as 1- to 3-mm white elevations on the buccal mucosa (Fig. 14.18, see also Fig. 6.34). They usually present 1 to 2 days before the development of the characteristic erythematous maculopapular rash. This rash appears during the third or fourth day of the illness. It usually begins around the hairline, behind the earlobes, and spreads downward (Fig. 14.19). It tends to fade in the same order it appears. Most cases recover without complications; others may develop otitis media, croup, pneumonia, encephalitis, and rarely subacute sclerosing panencephalitis (SSPE), a very late complication.

Differential Diagnosis

The differential diagnosis of the characteristic rash is vast and includes exanthem subitum; rubella; infections caused by echovirus, coxsackie and adenoviruses; toxoplasmosis; infectious mononucleosis; scarlet fever; Kawasaki disease; drug reactions; Rocky Mountain spotted fever, or meningococcemia.

ED Treatment and Disposition

Supportive therapy includes bedrest, antipyretics, and adequate fluid balance. Complications should be treated according to the presentation. Current available antiviral compounds are not effective. The use of gamma globulins and steroids in SSPE is limited. Passive immunization is effective for prevention and attenuation of measles if given within 5 days of the initial exposure. During outbreaks, measles vaccine (MMR) is given earlier than 15 months and may need to be repeated. A second dose is recommended after the primary series for those born after 1956. This is given at age 11 or 12 years or by entry to junior high school.

Clinical Pearls

1. The classic presentation includes a prodromal phase (fever, hacking cough, coryza, and conjunctivitis), Koplik's spots followed by an abrupt temperature rise, and the rash that spreads in a caudal distribution.
2. Examination of the oral mucosa to identify Koplik's spots may diagnose measles early if performed in all children with an acute febrile illness.

Associated Clinical Features

Hand, foot, and mouth disease is a seasonal (summer-fall) viral infection caused by coxsackievirus A16. It is characterized by fever, malaise, and anorexia over 1 to 2 days, followed by oral lesions (small, red macules that evolve into small vesicles 1 to 3 mm in diameter) in the posterior oropharynx (Fig. 14.20). This enanthem is then followed by a superficial, nonloculated vesicular eruption on the hands and feet (3 to 7 mm) (Figs. 14.21 and 14.22). These may also be present on the buttocks, face, and legs.

Differential Diagnosis

Herpes simplex, varicella, varicella zoster, influenza, echovirus infections, vaccinia, and other coxsackieviruses should all be considered.

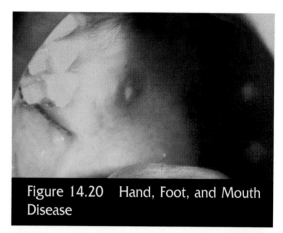

Figure 14.20   Hand, Foot, and Mouth Disease

Discrete vesicular erosions on the posterior oropharynx and soft palate secondary to coxsackievirus. (Courtesy of James F. Steiner, DDS.)

ED Treatment and Disposition

Supportive therapy, especially fluid maintenance and fever control for the patient's comfort are the mainstays of treatment. The duration and characteristics of the illness should be discussed with the parents. In the majority of cases the course is self-limited and the prognosis excellent. On rare occasions, secondary complications such as myocarditis, pneumonia, and meningoencephalitis may occur.

Clinical Pearl

1. The individual lesions are usually seen on the palms, fingertips, and soles. Oral cavity lesions appear as discrete oval erosions and most are classically seen in the posterior oropharynx and soft palate.

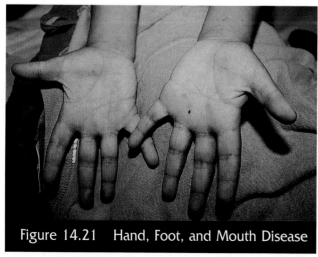

Figure 14.21   Hand, Foot, and Mouth Disease

Erythematous vesicular rash scattered on the palms consistent with coxsackievirus. (Courtesy of Michael J. Nowicki, MD.)

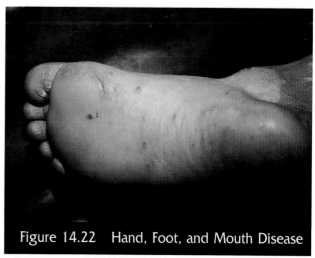

Figure 14.22   Hand, Foot, and Mouth Disease

Vesicular rash of the feet consistent with coxsackievirus. (Courtesy of Raymond C. Baker, MD.)

Associated Clinical Features

Cold panniculitis is an acute cold injury to the fat of the cheeks in infants. It manifests as red, indurated nodules and plaques on exposed skin, especially the face (Fig. 14.23). These lesions appear 1 to 3 days after exposure and gradually soften and return to normal over 1 or more weeks. This phenomenon is caused by subcutaneous fat solidification when exposed to low temperature. It is more frequent in children than adults.

Differential Diagnosis

Facial cellulitis, trauma, pressure erythema, giant urticaria, and contact dermatitis may have a similar presentation.

ED Treatment and Disposition

Treatment is not necessary; parental reassurance is very important.

Clinical Pearl

1. Because these lesions may also be painful, its differentiation from cellulitis may be difficult on occasion. The absence of systemic symptoms, especially fever, and the history of cold exposure, are very suggestive of cold panniculitis.

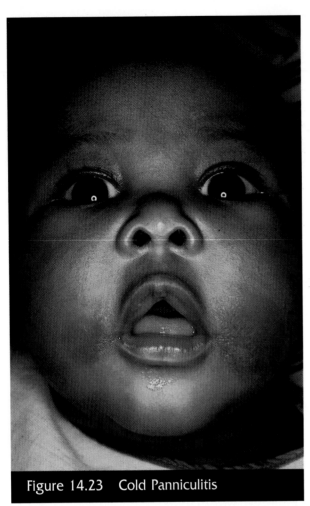

Figure 14.23   Cold Panniculitis

Infant with cheek erythema, swelling, and discoloration consistent with Popsicle panniculitis or cold injury. (Courtesy of Anne W. Lucky, MD.)

Associated Clinical Features

Herpetic gingivostomatitis is a viral infection commonly seen in infants and children caused by herpes simplex. Patients usually present with fever, malaise, cervical adenopathy, and pain in the mouth and throat on attempting to swallow. Vesicular and ulcerative lesions appear throughout the oral cavity. The gingiva becomes very friable and inflamed, especially around the alveolar rim. Increased salivation with foul breath may be present. Although fever disappears in 3 to 5 days, children may have difficulty eating for 7 to 14 days. Sometimes, autoinoculation produces vesicular lesions on the fingers (herpetic whitlow) (Fig. 14.24).

Differential Diagnosis

Vincent's angina, aphthous stomatitis, erythema multiforme, Behçet's disease, and other viral infections such as herpangina and hand, foot, and mouth disease (coxsackieviruses) should be considered.

ED Treatment and Disposition

No specific treatment is available. In immunocompromised patients, acyclovir should be considered. In the normal host, fluid balance should be maintained throughout the illness. Because of ulcerative lesions, avoidance of citrus juices or spicy food prevents pain on swallowing. Clear fluids, ice pops, and ice cream may be used in small children. Not infrequently, admission for IV hydration is necessary. Adequate fever control is also necessary for patient comfort and to avoid an increase in fluid losses. Pain control may be achieved by using mixtures of antihistamine (diphenhydramine elixir) and antacids (1:1) applied to lesion with Q-tips. In small children local application of viscous lidocaine (Xylocaine) should be avoided since patients may develop toxic plasma levels due to an altered absorption from an inflamed oral mucosa.

Clinical Pearl

1. Most of these lesions are in the anterior two-thirds of the oral cavity. Posterior lesions sparing the gingiva are most commonly seen in coxsackie infections.

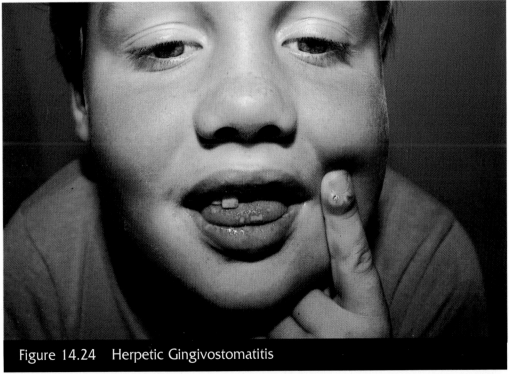

Figure 14.24   Herpetic Gingivostomatitis

Multiple oral vesicular lesions consistent with herpes gingivostomatitis. Vesicular lesions from autoinoculation are present on the finger (herpetic whitlow). (Courtesy of Michael J. Nowicki, MD.)

Associated Clinical Features

Urticaria is a localized, edematous skin reaction from histamine release that usually follows an infection, insect sting or bite, ingestion of certain foods, or medications. It is characterized by a sudden onset of pruritic, transient well circumscribed wheals scattered over the body. These are flat-topped and may vary from pinpoint size to several centimeters in diameter. They usually have a central clearing, peripheral extension, and can have tense edema (Fig. 14.25). Most urticarial reactions last 24 to 48 h; on rare occasions, they may take weeks to resolve. Rarely, there may be systemic reactions such as wheezing, stridor, or angioedema.

Differential Diagnosis

Erythema multiforme, arthropod bites, dermatographism, contact dermatitis, reactive erythemas, allergic vasculitis, juvenile rheumatoid arthritis, mastocytosis, and pityriasis rosea can all present with a similar-appearing rash.

ED Treatment and Disposition

Treatment is symptomatic. Oral antihistamines are useful in the control of pruritus. If a systemic reaction is also part of the initial presentation, epinephrine and steroids should be added to the therapy. In most cases it is very difficult to identify the etiologic factor. Unless there is evidence of acute angioedema, most cases can be discharged home on oral antihistamines.

Clinical Pearl

1. Erythema multiforme can be commonly mistaken for polycyclic urticaria (multiple red wheals of different sizes). Clinicially these two entities can be differentiated by the duration and color of the lesions. In urticaria, the center is clear and each lesion usually lasts a few hours. In erythema multiforme, the center is dusky and the lesion remains in the same place for several days to weeks.

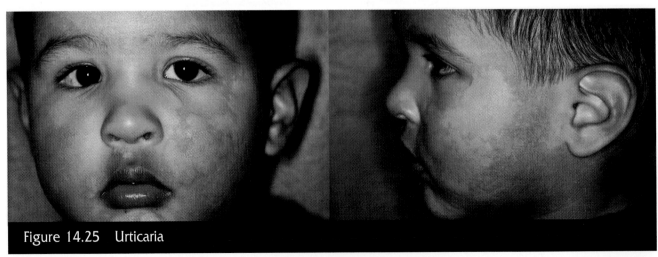

Figure 14.25 Urticaria

Preschool child with annular raised pruritic lesions with central clearing and tense edema of polycyclic urticaria. The lesions had completely disappeared after about 5 min. (Courtesy of Kevin J. Knoop, MD, MS.)

Associated Clinical Features

Staphylococcal scalded skin syndrome is caused by a staphylococcal toxin-producing strain. It may present with fever, malaise, and irritability following an upper respiratory infection. Patients develop a diffuse faint erythematous rash that becomes tender to touch. Crusting around the mouth, eyes, and neck is not uncommon. Within 2 to 3 days the upper layers of dermis may be easily removed; finally a flaccid bulla develops with subsequent exfoliation of the skin (Fig. 14.26). In young patients this exfoliation may involve a large surface area with significant fluid and electrolyte losses.

Differential Diagnosis

Toxic epidermal necrolysis, exfoliative erythroderma, bullous erythema multiforme, bullous pemphigoid, bullous impetigo, sunburn, acute mercury poisoning, toxic shock syndrome, and scarlet fever should be considered.

ED Treatment and Disposition

Treatment is directed at the eradication of the *Staphylococcus,* thus terminating the production of toxin. Synthetic penicillins should be used intravenously. Admission is usually necessary, especially in young infants. This age group requires careful attention to fluid and electrolyte losses and the prevention of secondary infection of the affected skin.

Clinical Pearl

1. The wrinkling or peeling of the upper layer of the epidermis (pressure applied with a Q-tip or gloved finger) that occurs within 2 or 3 days of the onset of this illness is known as the "Nikolsky sign."

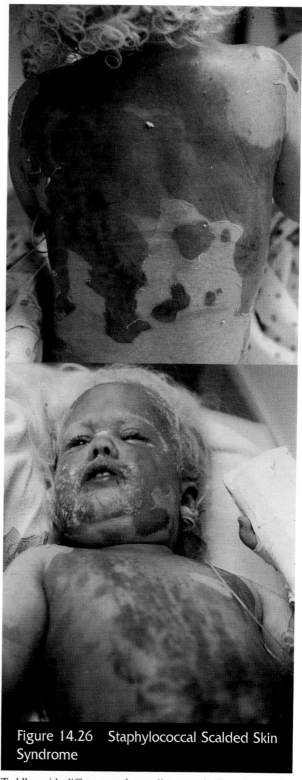

Figure 14.26   Staphylococcal Scalded Skin Syndrome

Toddler with diffuse macular peeling eruption consistent with scalded skin syndrome from *Staphylococcus aureus.* (Courtesy of Judith C. Bausher, MD.)

Associated Clinical Features

Meningococcemia is characterized by an acute febrile illness with generally rapid onset of marked toxicity, purpura, and petechiae (Fig. 14.27). It progresses rapidly to hypotension with multisystem failure. In cases of fulminant disease, this shock stage is accompanied by disseminated intravascular coagulation and massive mucosal hemorrhages. Occasionally there may be a specific prodrome with upper respiratory infection and malaise.

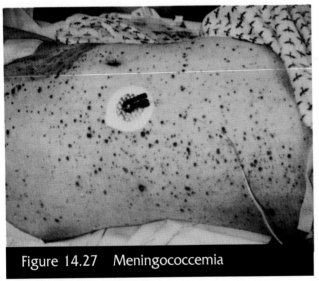

Figure 14.27 Meningococcemia

Diffuse petechiae in a patient with meningococcemia. (Courtesy of Javier A. Gonzalez del Rey, MD.)

Differential Diagnosis

Gonococcemia, *Haemophilus influenzae* infection, pneumococcemia, Rocky Mountain spotted fever, sepsis with thrombocytopenia or disseminated intravascular coagulation (DIC), endocarditis, Henoch-Schönlein purpura, typhoid fever, leukemia, hemorrhagic measles, or hemorrhagic varicella may have a similar appearance.

ED Treatment and Disposition

In stable patients in whom the diagnosis of meningococcemia is entertained, cultures of blood, spinal fluid, nasopharynx, complete blood count, platelet count, and coagulation studies should be obtained. Consider arterial blood gas, liver function tests, and other studies as indicated. These patients should be admitted for close monitoring to institutions capable of delivering critical care services. Broad spectrum parenteral antibiotics should be used in the initial coverage until the organism is identified and sensitivities available. In the unstable septic patient, adequate ventilation and cardiac function must be ensured, in addition to performing the above tests and treatment. Hemodynamic monitoring and support (fluids and vasoactive drugs) are of paramount importance in the management. Peripheral and central venous catheters and urinary and arterial catheters are usually necessary for optimal care of these patients.

Clinical Pearls

1. Skin scraping of the purpuric lesion can be microscopically examined for the presence of gram-negative diplococci and may be cultured for organisms.
2. A child with a fever and a petechial rash must be presumed to have meningococcemia.

Associated Clinical Features

Scarlet fever manifests as erythematous macules and papules that result from an erythrogenic toxin produced by a group A streptococcus. The most common site for invasion by this organism is the pharynx and occasionally skin or perianal areas. The disease usually occurs in children (2 to 10 years of age) and less commonly in adults. The typical presentation of scarlet fever includes fever, headache, sore throat, and malaise followed by the scarlatiniform rash (Fig. 14.28). The rash is typically erythematous, blanches (in severe cases may include petechiae), and owing to the grouping of the fine papules gives to the skin a rough sandpaperlike texture (Fig. 14.29). On the tongue, a thick, white coat and swollen papillae gives the appearance of a strawberry ("strawberry tongue").

Differential Diagnosis

A similar syndrome is caused by staphylococci producing an exfoliative exotoxin which can be differentiated from the streptococcal infection because of the absence of pharyngitis, strawberry tongue, and negative cultures. Enteroviral infections, viral hepatitis, infectious mononucleosis, toxic shock syndrome, drug eruptions, rubella, mercury intoxication, and mucocutaneous lymph node syndrome should be considered.

ED Treatment and Disposition

Penicillin, either benzathine penicillin G or oral penicillin, to maintain levels for 10 days is the key to therapy. Alternatives include erythromycin, or clindamycin in penicillin-allergic patients.

Clinical Pearls

1. Petechiae (commonly found as part of the scarlatiniform eruption) in a linear pattern seen along the major skin folds in the axillae and antecubital fossa are known as "Pastia's lines."
2. In black skin, the rash may be difficult to differentiate and may consist only of punctate papular elevations called "goose flesh."

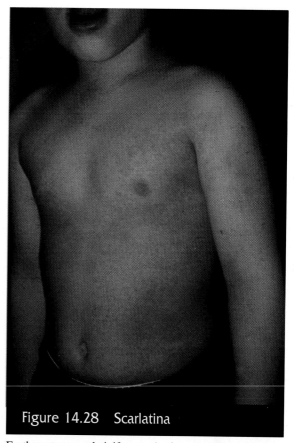

Figure 14.28   Scarlatina

Erythematous scarlatiniform rash of scarlet fever. (Courtesy of Lawrence B. Stack, MD.)

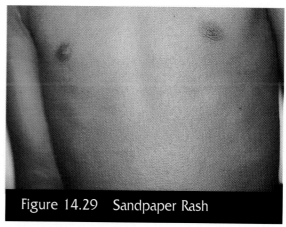

Figure 14.29   Sandpaper Rash

Typical sandpaper rash of scarlet fever. The grouping of the fine papules gives the skin a rough sandpaperlike texture. (Courtesy of Jeffery S. Gibson, MD.)

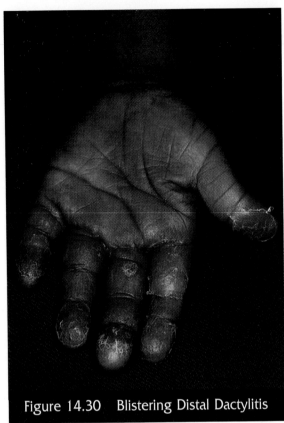

Figure 14.30   Blistering Distal Dactylitis

Blistering rash of the distal fingers with surrounding erythema typically caused by *Streptococcus*. Note the location of the rash over the volar finger pad. (Courtesy of Anne W. Lucky, MD.)

Associated Clinical Features

Blistering distal dactylitis is a cellulitis of the fingertips (Fig. 14.30) caused by beta-hemolytic streptococcal and, in rare occasions, by *Staphylococcus aureus* infections. The typical lesion is a fluid-filled tense blister with surrounding erythema located over the volar fat pad on the distal portion of the fingers. Polymorphonuclear leukocytes and gram-positive cocci can be found in the Gram's stain of the purulent exudate from the lesion.

Differential Diagnosis

Bullous impetigo, burns, friction blisters, and herpetic whitlow should be considered.

ED Treatment and Disposition

There is usually a rapid response to incision and drainage of the blister and a 10-day course of antibiotic therapy (dicloxacillin, cephalexin, or erythromycin).

Clinical Pearl

1. This diagnosis should be entertained in any child presenting with a tender, cloudy fluid-filled blister of the fingertips or toes.

Associated Clinical Features

Strawberry hemangioma often appears as small telangiectatic papules or a patch surrounded by an area of pallor. These lesions grow and become vascularized during the first 2 months of life. The classic lesion is a raised gray to reddish nodule with defined borders (Fig. 14.31). They commonly regress in almost all patients by 2 to 3 years of age. In a few cases, very large vascular lesions can cause platelet trapping or high-output cardiac failure. Localized hemangiomas can affect the airway, eyes, or other areas on which they occur.

Differential Diagnosis

Malignant vascular tumors, pyogenic granulomas, and giant melanocytic birthmarks should be considered.

ED Treatment and Disposition

Most cases require no therapy because strawberry hemangiomas usually regress without residual lesion. Treatment is indicated when there is an obstruction of a vital orifice (i.e., airway, mouth, or nares) or vision (eyelids), or if hematologic or cardiovascular complications are present. Parental reassurance is important because there is great pressure to treat for cosmetic reasons. Steroids, liquid nitrogen, grenz ray therapy, and pulse dye laser are some of the different therapeutic modalities used in its treatment. In complex cases, dermatologic consultation is recommended.

Clinical Pearl

1. The diagnosis of strawberry hemangioma should always be considered in the presence of any purplish, red, raised, tumorlike lesion not present at birth which appears in the first month of life.

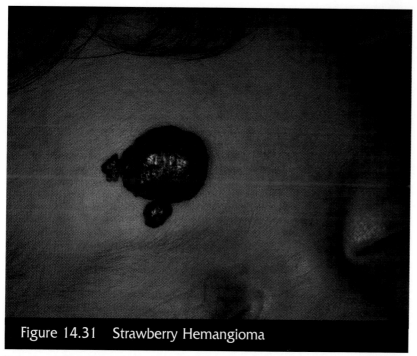

Figure 14.31   Strawberry Hemangioma

Raised umbilicated vascular lesion on the right forehead consistent with strawberry hemangioma. (Courtesy of Anne W. Lucky, MD.)

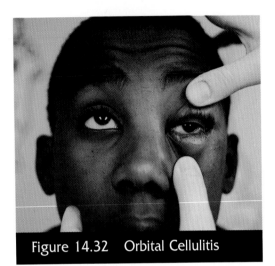

Figure 14.32 Orbital Cellulitis

Left orbital cellulitis with decreased range of motion secondary to edema. Note the infected conjunctiva. (Courtesy of Javier A. Gonzalez del Rey, MD.)

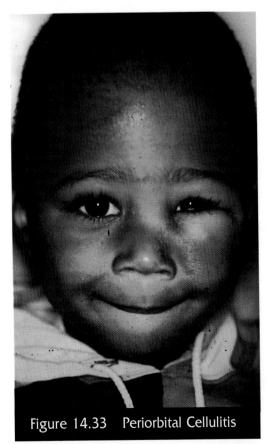

Figure 14.33 Periorbital Cellulitis

Left periorbital cellulitis with edema and erythema of the eyelids. Note that the conjunctiva is clear and not infected. (Courtesy of Kevin J. Knoop, MD, MS.)

Associated Clinical Features

Orbital cellulitis is a serious bacterial infection characterized by painful, purple-red swelling of the eyelids, restriction of eye movement (Fig. 14.32), proptosis, and a variable degree of decreased visual acuity. It may begin with eye pain and low-grade temperature. In general it is caused by *Staphylococcus aureus, Haemophilus influenzae, Streptococcus,* or *Pneumococcus.* It usually follows an upper respiratory tract infection or sinusitis but can occur from local trauma. If not treated promptly, it can lead to abscess formation, blindness, or meningitis. Periorbital (preseptal) cellulitis usually presents with edema and erythema of the eyelids (Fig. 14.33), minimal pain of the affected area, and fever. Proptosis or ophthalmoplegia are not characteristic. Common organisms are *H. influenzae* type B or *Pneumococcus.* In cases of eyelid trauma, *S. aureus* and group A streptococcus are the most common pathogens.

Differential Diagnosis

Erysipelas, allergic reactions, trauma, sunburns, frostbite, chemical burns, subperiosteal abscess, and cavernous sinus thrombosis should be considered.

ED Treatment and Disposition

Parenteral antibiotic coverage with broad spectrum antistaphylococcal coverage, ophthalmologic consultation, and admission are indicated in cases of orbital cellulitis. Computerized tomography of the orbit is necessary in certain cases to rule out the possibility of an abscess that may require surgical drainage. In febrile or ill-appearing patients with periorbital cellulitis, admission is indicated with broad spectrum antibiotic therapy. This coverage can be adjusted once results of cultures are available. Mild cases of preseptal cellulitis (especially those with history of trauma, e.g., abrasion, insect sting) can be treated as outpatients with close follow-up. Adequate coverage for *Staphylococcus* and *Streptococcus* is necessary.

Clinical Pearls

1. Periorbital cellulitis presents with circumferential redness, edema, and tenderness in the febrile toddler. Orbital cellulitis must be considered if there is eye pain or globe motion limitation.
2. The conjunctiva is typically clear with periorbital cellulitis.

Associated Clinical Features

Cystic hygromas are lymphatic tumors found in the head and neck region (Fig. 14.34). They present as nontender or nonpainful, compressible unilocular or multilocular masses with thin, transparent walls and are filled with straw-colored fluid. Unlike hemangiomas, these lesions rarely undergo spontaneous regression. The vast majority tend to grow and infiltrate adjacent structures. In cases in which the tongue is involved, they may produce tracheal compression and respiratory difficulty.

Differential Diagnosis

Cavernous hemangiomas and cavernous lymphangiomas should be considered.

ED Treatment and Disposition

Surgery is the treatment of choice in the vast majority of cases, since they do not regress and may affect local tissues. Extent of the lesion should be evaluated prior to its removal (x-rays and CT). The earlier these lesions can be removed, the better the cosmetic results.

Clinical Pearls

1. The diagnosis of cystic hygroma should be considered in all spongy, soft, tumorlike masses filled with fluid in the neck. They may appear spontaneously during a coughing episode or after Valsalva as a mass in the neck.

2. This "benign" tumor can locally invade adjacent tissues and become life-threatening.

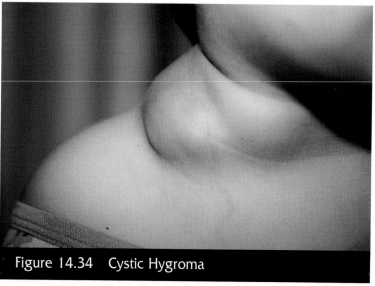

Figure 14.34   Cystic Hygroma

A bright, supraclavicular, soft, boggy, compressible mass consistent with cystic hygroma. (Courtesy of Richard M. Ruddy, MD.)

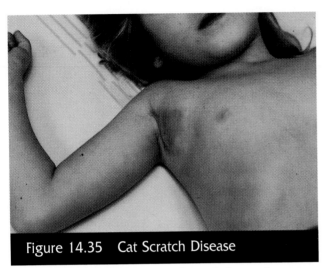

Figure 14.35   Cat Scratch Disease

An erythematous, tender, suppurative node is seen in a young febrile patient with a history of cat scratch on the extremity. The node required drainage 2 days later. (Courtesy of Kevin J. Knoop, MD, MS.)

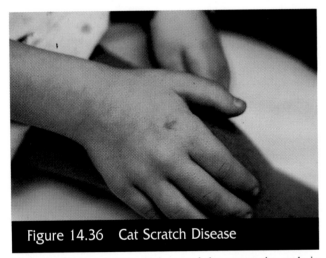

Figure 14.36   Cat Scratch Disease

The precipitating wound which caused the suppurative node in Fig. 14.35. (Courtesy of Kevin J. Knoop, MD, MS.)

Associated Clinical Features

Cat scratch disease is a benign self-limited condition that manifests with regional lymphadenopathy (Fig. 14.35) which usually follows (1 to 2 weeks) a skin papule at the presumed site of bacterial inoculation. A history of contact or scratch from a cat (Fig. 14.36) is usually present. Lymphadenopathy may persist for months, and in rare cases patients may develop complications such as encephalitis, osteolytic lesion, hepatitis, weight loss, fever, and fatigue. A skin test using cat scratch antigen can identify the etiology in suspected patients when confirmation of the diagnosis is needed.

Differential Diagnosis

Lymphogranuloma venereum, bacterial adenitis, sarcoidosis, infectious mononucleosis, tumors (benign or malignant), tuberculosis, tularemia, brucellosis, and histoplasmosis should be considered.

ED Treatment and Disposition

The disease is usually self-limited and management is primarily symptomatic. Parents and patients should be reassured that the nodes are benign and frequently resolve within 2 to 4 months. In cases of painful fluctuant nodes, needle aspiration may be necessary for relief of symptoms. Antibiotic therapy should be considered for acutely or severely ill patients. Several anecdotal reports have suggested that oral antibiotics such as rifampin, trimethoprim-sulfamethoxazole, and ciprofloxacin; or intravenous gentamicin, cefotaxime, and mezlocillin may be effective. Surgical excision of the affected nodes is generally unnecessary.

Clinical Pearl

1. Cat scratch disease is the most common cause of regional adenitis and should be considered in all children or adolescents with persistent lymphadenopathy.

General Conditions

Associated Clinical Features

Epiglottitis is a life-threatening condition characterized by sudden onset of fever, toxicity, moderate to severe respiratory distress with stridor, and variable degrees of drooling. The patient prefers a sitting position, leaning forward in a sniffing position with an open mouth. This symptomatology is the result of a direct infection and subsequent swelling of the epiglottis and aryepiglottic folds (Figs. 14.37 and 14.38) from *Haemophilus influenzae* type B (HIB). On x-ray the epiglottis is seen as rounded and blurred (thumbprint) (Fig. 14.39). Epiglottitis frequently worsens to complete obstruction if not treated with endotracheal intubation and antibiotics. Other causes include staphylococcal or streptococcal disease, thermal epiglottitis, or *Candida* in the immunocompromised host. Adults have a more indolent course and are infrequently protected by the HIB vaccine, which has been in use since its release in 1985.

Differential Diagnosis

Acute infectious laryngitis, acute laryngotracheobronchitis, acute spasmodic laryngitis, membranous tracheitis, diphtheritic croup, aspiration of foreign body, retropharyngeal abscess, and extrinsic or intrinsic compression of the airway (tumors, trauma, cysts) should be considered.

ED Treatment and Disposition

Immediate intervention is required. An artificial endotracheal airway must be established. If time and clinical status permit, this should be done in the operating room or designated area where advance airway management with sedation, but not neuromuscular paralysis, can be performed.

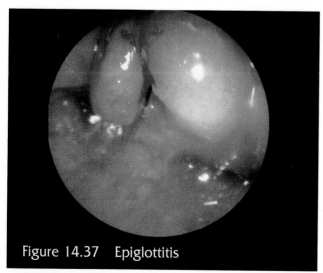

Figure 14.37   Epiglottitis

Endoscopic view of almost complete airway obstruction secondary to epiglottitis. Note the slitlike opening of the airway. (Courtesy of Department of Otolaryngology, Childrens Hospital Medical Center, Cincinnati, Ohio.)

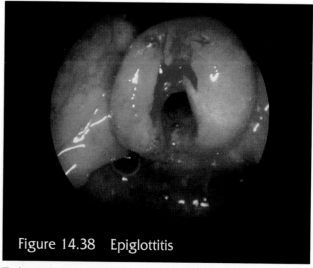

Figure 14.38   Epiglottitis

Endoscopic view of the same patient immediately after extubation. Although erythema and some edema persist, the airway is widely patent. (Courtesy of Department of Otolaryngology, Childrens Hospital Medical Center, Cincinnati, Ohio.)

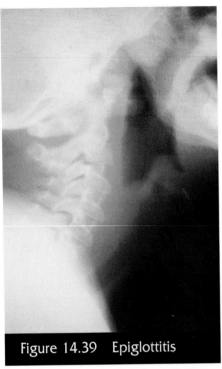

Figure 14.39   Epiglottitis

Lateral soft-tissue x-ray of the neck demonstrating thickening of aryepiglottic folds and thumbprint sign of epiglottis. (Courtesy of Richard M. Ruddy, MD.)

An experienced anesthesiologist and surgeon should be available in case a surgical airway is needed. Once the airway has been protected, the patient should be sedated to avoid accidental extubation, and adequate antibiotic therapy should be immediately instituted (second- or third-generation cephalosporins or ampicillin/chloramphenicol).

Clinical Pearls

1. Children with epiglottitis usually present with respiratory distress of sudden onset with high fever. Because of the inflammation of the epiglottis, they commonly refuse to drink fluids secondary to pain.
2. Every effort should be made to allow the child to remain undisturbed (in mother's lap) in a position of comfort while urgent preparations are made for airway management. An agitated child is at risk for suddenly losing the airway.

DIAGNOSIS	RETROPHARYNGEAL ABSCESS

Associated Clinical Features

Patients with a retropharyngeal abscess usually present with fever, difficulty in swallowing, excessive drooling, sore throat, changes in voice, or neck stiffness. The resultant edema (Fig. 14.40) is the result of a cellulitis and suppurative adenitis of the lymph nodes located in the preverte-

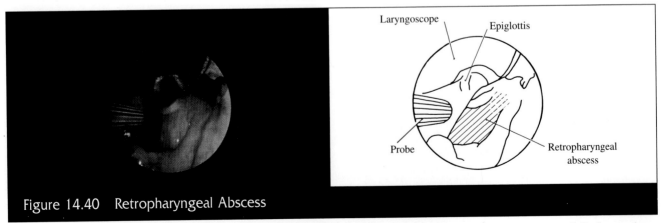

Figure 14.40   Retropharyngeal Abscess

Endoscopic view of a retropharyngeal abscess. Note the massive swelling posteriorly. (Courtesy of Department of Otolaryngology, Childrens Hospital Medical Center, Cincinnati, Ohio.)

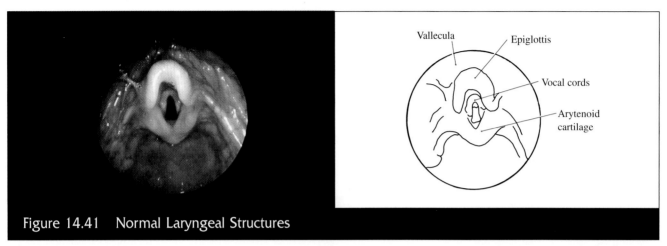

Figure 14.41 Normal Laryngeal Structures

Endoscopic view of a normal epiglottis and surrounding structures. (Courtesy of Department of Otolaryngology, Childrens Hospital Medical Center, Cincinnati, Ohio.)

bral fascia and is seen on a soft-tissue lateral x-ray of the neck as prevertebral thickening (Fig. 14.42). The initial insult may be the result of pharyngitis, otitis media, or a wound infection following a penetrating injury into the posterior pharynx.

Differential Diagnosis

Acute laryngotracheobronchitis, epiglottitis, membranous tracheitis, acute bacterial laryngitis, infectious mononucleosis, peritonsillar abscess, aspiration of foreign body, and diphtheria should be considered. These patients may present with stiff neck mimicking meningitis.

ED Treatment and Disposition

This illness requires immediate intervention to prevent respiratory obstruction. The first step is to evaluate the airway and to establish an artificial one if necessary. Antibiotic coverage should be initiated immediately (semisynthetic penicillin or equivalent). Anal-gesia should be given as needed. If obstruction is present or there is evidence of abscess, immediate incision and drainage should be performed in the operating room. These patients require hospitalization and immediate otolaryngologic or surgical consultation.

Clinical Pearls

1. If the diagnosis of retropharyngeal abscess is considered in a patient with above presentation, a lateral soft-tissue neck x-ray may help to confirm the diagnosis. In these cases, the retropharyngeal soft tissue at the level of C-3 is > 5 mm, or more than 40% of the diameter of the body of C-4 at that level.
2. Neck CT is a useful tool to evaluate the extent of the lesion.

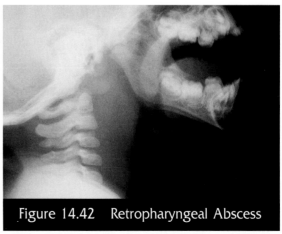

Figure 14.42 Retropharyngeal Abscess

Lateral soft-tissue neck x-ray demonstrating prevertebral soft-tissue density consistent with retropharyngeal abscess. (Courtesy of Richard M. Ruddy, MD.)

Associated Clinical Features

Membranous tracheitis is an acute bacterial infection (*Staphylococcus aureus, Haemophilus influenzae,* streptococci, and pneumococci) of the upper airway capable of causing life-threatening airway obstruction. It is considered a bacterial complication because it almost always follows an apparent upper respiratory tract viral infection. The infection produces marked swelling and thick purulent secretions of the tracheal mucosa below the vocal cords. The secretions form a thick plug that, if dislodged, may ultimately lead to an acute tracheal obstruction. Patients appear toxic, with fever and a crouplike syndrome that can progress rapidly. The usual treatment for croup is ineffective in these patients. The characteristic "membranes" may be seen on x-rays of the airway as edema with an irregular border of the subglottic tracheal mucosa. On direct laryngoscopy, copious purulent secretions can be found in the presence of a normal epiglottis.

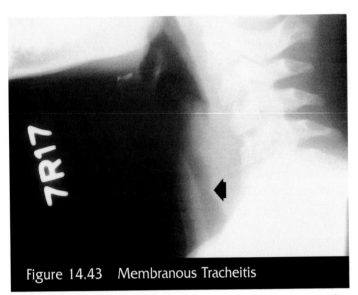

Figure 14.43   Membranous Tracheitis

Lateral soft-tissue x-ray of the neck reveals mild subglottic narrowing (arrow) and membrane consistent with bacterial tracheitis. (Courtesy of Alan S. Brodie, MD.)

Differential Diagnosis

Acute laryngotracheobronchitis, retropharyngeal abscess, peritonsillar abscess, foreign body aspiration, and acute diphtheric laryngitis can present in a similar manner.

ED Treatment and Disposition

Immediate endotracheal intubation is needed to protect the airway and allow for repeated suctioning of the airway. The patient should be sedated and admitted to the intensive care unit for close monitoring. Aggressive management of pulmonary secretions is essential to avoid acute obstruction. Appropriate antibiotic coverage against suspected organisms should be immediately instituted. Otolaryngologic consultation is recommended.

Clinical Pearls

1. Bacterial tracheitis often presents with acute severe airway obstruction after a short prodrome. It should be suspected in all patients with an atypical crouplike presentation: unusual age group, toxicity, not improving with routine croup therapy, and unusual roentgenographic changes.
2. Up to 50% of soft-tissue films may delineate a subglottic membrane (Fig. 14.43).

Associated Clinical Features

There are several fractures unique to children. These include physeal fractures, torus fracture, green stick fractures, avulsion fractures, and bowing fractures or deformities. Physis fractures (growth plate fractures) are relatively common because of weakness of the germinal growth plate. The Salter-Harris (SH) classification was designed to describe each type of physeal fracture, its prognosis, and treatment (Fig. 14.44).

Differential Diagnosis

SH type I: Fracture that extends through the physis. It is a very difficult radiologic diagnosis since it may not be displaced. It is usually a clinical diagnosis, but occasionally there is a physeal widening observed on the x-ray.

SH type II: Oblique fracture extending through the metaphysis into the physis. It is the most common and the prognosis is good.

SH type III: This rare type of fracture goes along the growth plate, then extends through the epiphysis, ossification center, and articular cartilage into the joint.

SH type IV: Fracture that extends from the metaphysis, across the growth plate, and into the joint.

SH type V: Crushing injury to the growth plate.

ED Treatment and Disposition

Immobilization by splinting is the treatment of choice in types I and II (minimum of 3 weeks). In these cases, reduction is easy to achieve and maintain. Growth is unimpaired. Types III and IV may require open reduction to avoid later traumatic arthritis and in some cases growth arrest. Type V fractures are rare and require very close follow-up because of arrest of growth caused by the death of the germinal cells. Types III, IV, and V require immediate orthopaedic consultation.

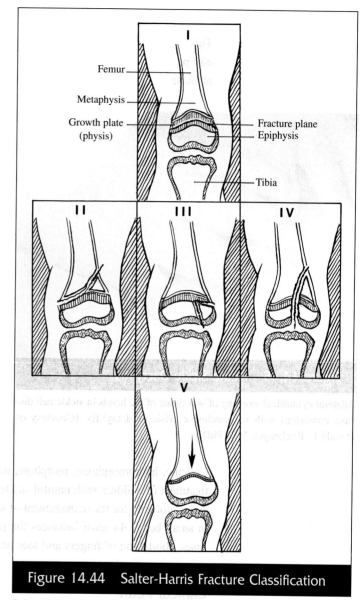

Figure 14.44   Salter-Harris Fracture Classification

Salter-Harris classification for epiphyseal plate fractures.

Clinical Pearl

1. After initial assessment and evaluation, always suspect SH type I if there is evidence of tenderness around the growth plate area despite negative x-rays.

ACUTE SICKLE DACTYLITIS
(HAND-FOOT SYNDROME)

Associated Clinical Features

This painful condition is commonly the first clinical manifestation of sickle cell disease. It usually presents in children younger than 5 years of age. The pain and abnormalities are the result of ischemic necrosis of the small bones caused by the decreased blood supply as the bone marrow rapidly expands. These children present acutely ill, with fever, refusing to bear weight, and have puffy hands and feet (Fig. 14.45). They may have a marked leukocytosis, and the initial x-rays may be normal. It is not until 1 to 2 weeks when subperiosteal new bone, cortical thickening, and even complete bone destruction can be seen.

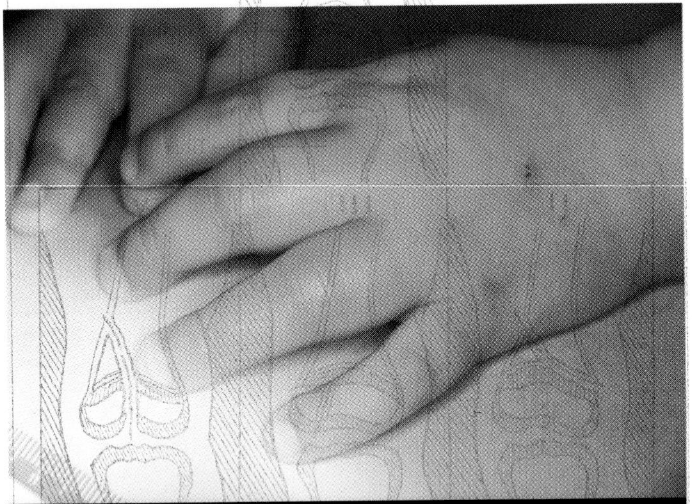

Differential Diagnosis

Osteomyelitis, trauma, cold injuries, acute rheumatic fever, juvenile rheumatoid arthritis, and leukemias should be considered.

ED Treatment and Disposition

The most important aspects in the treatment of vasoocclusive crisis in sickle cell disease (hemoglobin SS) include an adequate fluid balance, oxygenation, and analgesia. Therapy should be individualized. Codeine, hydromorphone, morphine, and ketorolac are analgesic agents commonly used in the treatment of children with painful sickle crisis. In cases of dactylitis, very close follow-up is necessary not only for the management of sickle cell disease but to reevaluate the radiologic changes in small bones. In most instances the previously described changes disappear; however, in rare cases, shortening of fingers and toes have been described as the result of severe bone infarcts.

Figure 14.45   Acute Sickle Dactylitis

Bilateral cylindrical swelling of soft tissue of the hands in sickle cell disease consistent with vasoocclusive crisis or dactylitis. (Courtesy of Donald L. Rucknagel, MD, PhD.)

Clinical Pearl

1. Most clinical manifestations of sickle cell disease occur after the first 5 to 6 months of life. The hemolytic anemia gradually develops over the first 2 to 4 months (changes that follow the replacement of fetal hemoglobin by hemoglobin S) and leads to the clinical syndromes associated with an increased SS hemoglobin.

Associated Clinical Features

A single strand of hair or thread may encircle a finger, a toe, or the penis, leading to constriction (Fig. 14.46). Children in their first year of life are particularly at risk from inadvertent attachment of a parent's hair or loose thread. The digit appears edematous, erythematous, and painful. If not corrected vascular compromise or infection can ensue.

Differential Diagnosis

Insect bites, trauma, or cellulitis of the digit may have a similar appearance.

ED Treatment and Disposition

Visualization of the constricting material may be difficult. Edema, erythema, and periarticular skin folds may hide the hair or thread. It is imperative to carefully retract the skin around the proximal aspect of the edema. A magnifying lens may be helpful in identifying the band. Since the removal can be painful, consider local digital block prior to removal. Using a small hemostat, grasp a portion of the material and then cut it with a surgical blade. On occasions, depilatory agents have been used to remove hair fibers. Elevation of the involved digit after removal of the constricting agent provides resolution of the edema and erythema within 2 to 3 days. In some cases the digit blood supply may have been irreversibly compromised. Subspecialty consultation should be considered whenever neurovascular integrity is in question.

Clinical Pearl

1. In the vast majority of cases, a clear line of demarcation can usually be identified between the normal tissue and the affected area.

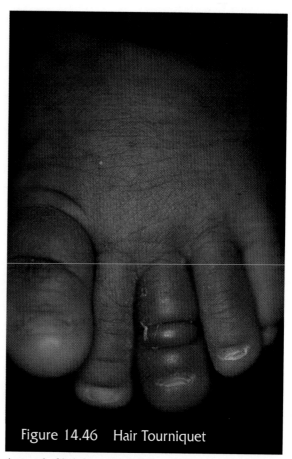

Figure 14.46   Hair Tourniquet

A strand of hair has encircled the middle toe in two places, causing erythema and swelling. (Courtesy of Kevin J. Knoop, MD, MS.)

Associated Clinical Features

Failure to thrive (FTT) is a chronic pattern of inability to maintain normal growth pattern in weight, stature, and occasionally in head growth (Fig. 14.47). It is most common in infancy, and the condition is nonorganic (50%), organic (25%), or mixed (25%) in etiology. The diagnosis is made after complete history and physical examination with comparison of the measurements of length (supine in children <3 years of age), weight, and head circumference (maximal occipital-frontal circumference) to standard measurements. In cases of deficient caloric intake or malabsorption, the patient's head circumference is normal and the weight is reduced out of proportion to height. Subnormal head circumferences with weight reduced in proportion to height and normal or increased head circumferences with weight moderately reduced are usually indicative of an organic problem.

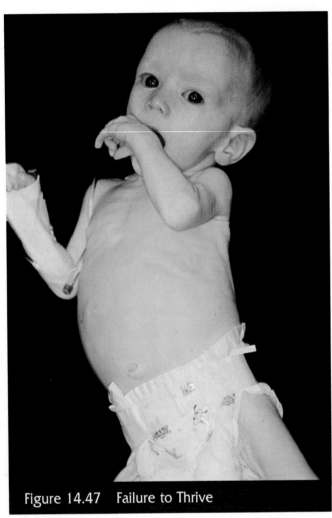

Figure 14.47   Failure to Thrive

This infant has not been able to maintain a normal growth pattern and appears cachectic. (Courtesy of Kevin J. Knoop, MD, MS.)

Differential Diagnosis

The differential diagnosis of failure to thrive is lengthy. Nonorganic disorders include poor feeding technique, disturbed maternal-child interaction, emotional deprivation, inadequate caloric intake, and child neglect. Organic causes are numerous.

ED Treatment and Disposition

Depending on history, physical findings, and the social situation, some cases can be managed as outpatients. The primary care provider can determine whether outpatient management is indicated. For the vast majority of cases, if the diagnosis of failure to thrive is made in the ED, admission is suggested to complete the evaluation. This could be the only indication of a poor social environment or inadequate access to medical care. Initial laboratory investigations should include a complete blood count, eletrolytes, BUN and creatinine urinalysis, and stool examination if stool pattern is abnormal. More specific testing should be used only if clinically indicated and targeted to the possible underlying cause. Early involvement of social services may facilitate the evaluation and follow-up. Treatment will vary according to the underlying disorder.

Clinical Pearl

1. Failure to thrive in neglected children is accompanied by signs of developmental delays, emotional deprivation, apathy, poor hygiene, withdrawing behavior, and poor eye contact.

Associated Clinical Features

Nursemaid's elbow is a condition that occurs commonly in children younger than 5 years of age whom are usually picked up or pulled by the arms while the arm is pronated. The children present unwilling to supinate or pronate the affected elbow (Fig. 14.48). Generally they keep the arm in a passive pronation and develop pain over the head of the radius. Radiographic studies should be considered only in patients with an unusual mechanism of injury or those who do not become rapidly asymptomatic after the reduction maneuvers.

Differential Diagnosis

Radial head fracture or complete dislocation, posterior elbow dislocation, condylar and supracondylar fractures of the distal humerus, or buckle fracture of radius or ulna should be considered.

ED Treatment and Disposition

Carefully palpate for tenderness at all points of the affected arm. (There is no tenderness found when not rotating the involved arm.) Orthopedic consultation is generally not indicated unless an underlying fracture is diagnosed. Reduction is usually achieved by supination of the forearm while applying pressure over the head of the radial head and flexing the elbow. Usually a palpable click can be felt over the area. The patient usually becomes asymptomatic after a few min-

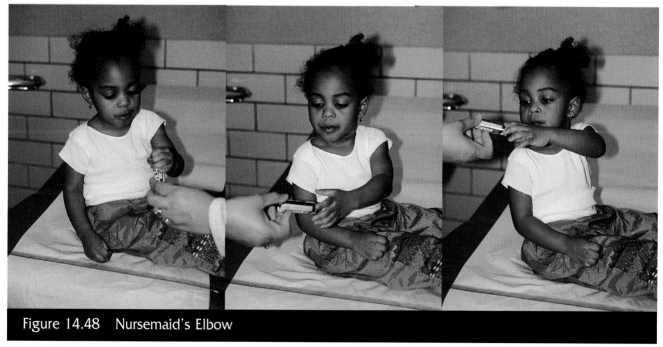

Figure 14.48 Nursemaid's Elbow

This child presents with pseudoparalysis of the right arm after a pulling injury. Note how she avoids use of the affected arm and preferentially uses the other arm. (Courtesy of Kevin J. Knoop, MD, MS.)

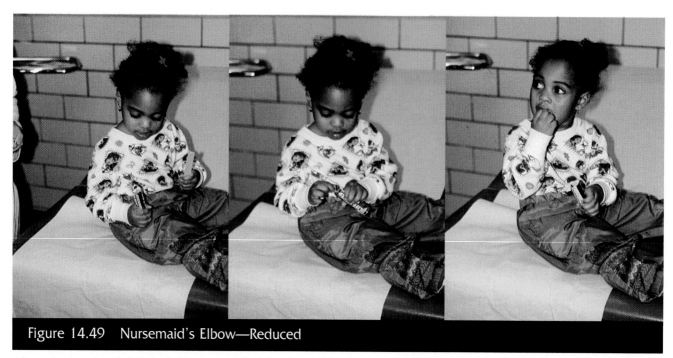

Figure 14.49   Nursemaid's Elbow—Reduced

After reduction, there is initial reluctance to use the injured arm. With distraction and encouragement, the patient demonstrates successful use of the extremity. (Courtesy of Kevin J. Knoop, MD, MS.)

utes (Fig. 14.49). When the injury has been present for several hours, reduction may be difficult and it may take several hours to recover full function of the elbow.

Clinical Pearls

1. In any child (usually between ages 1 to 5 years) who presents with sudden onset of elbow pain and immobility following a traction injury, the diagnosis of nursemaid's elbow should be strongly considered.
2. Nonjudgmental parental education about the mechanism should be an integral part of the visit.

Associated Clinical Features

This extensive form of tooth decay (generally in the necks of the teeth near the gingiva) is the result of sleeping with a bottle containing milk or sugar-containing juices. The condition generally occurs before 18 months of age and it is more prevalent in medically underserved children. Upper central incisors are most commonly involved (Fig. 14.50).

Differential Diagnosis

Less extensive tooth decay (caries) may be seen in some infants who do not sleep with a bottle. Caries can also result from tooth trauma. Dental referral is indicated.

ED Treatment and Disposition

Parental education and immediate referral to a dentist is necessary to prevent complications. If untreated, the caries may destroy the teeth and spread to contiguous tissues. These patients have a high risk for microbial invasion of the pulp and the alveolar bone with the subsequent development of a dental abscess and facial cellulitis. In these cases, aggressive treatment with antibiotics (penicillin) and pain control, with prompt dental referral for definitive care, is necessary.

Clinical Pearl

1. The role of the ED physician is to recognize this pattern of dental decay (upper incisors most commonly) and immediately initiate dental referral and parental education.

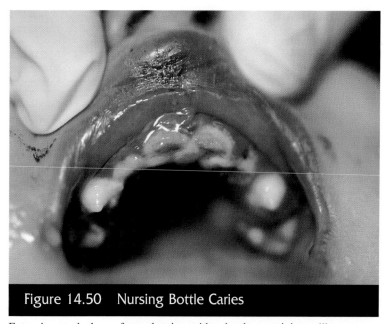

Figure 14.50   Nursing Bottle Caries

Extensive tooth decay from sleeping with a bottle containing milk or sugar-containing juices. (Courtesy of Lawrence B. Stack, MD.)

Associated Clinical Features

Enterobius vermicularis is a 0.5-inch threadlike, white worm that infects the colon and causes intense pruritus of the perianal region where the adult gravid female migrates to deposit eggs (Fig. 14.51). In rare occasions it can cause vulvovaginitis. The diagnosis can be made by direct visualization of the nematode by the parents or by using a transparent adhesive tape touched to the perianal lesion (at night). This tape is then applied to a glass slide for microscopic examination under low power.

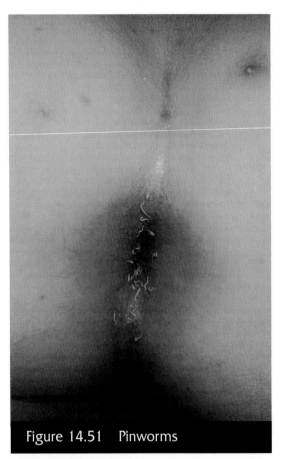

Figure 14.51   Pinworms

Multiple tiny pearly-white worms are seen at the anus. (Courtesy of Timothy D. McGuirk, DO.)

Differential Diagnosis

Perianal irritation, fissures, hemorrhoids, and contact dermatitis should be considered.

ED Treatment and Disposition

The treatment of choice is pyrantel pamoate or mebendazole. Either of these drugs is given as a single dose and repeated in 1 to 2 weeks (to treat secondary hatchings of the organism). Because of the high frequency of reinfections, families should be treated as a group.

Clinical Pearls

1. Reinfection from other infected individuals or autoinfection is necessary to maintain enterobiasis in the individual since these nematodes usually die after depositing the eggs in the perianal region. Good personal hygiene may reduce chances of infection.
2. If there is evidence of cellulitis, antibiotic coverage primarily against *Staphylococcus* is indicated.
3. If infection and point tenderness (in the absence of cellulitis) persist, antipseudomonal coverage should be considered.
4. Pinworms are the most common cause of pruritus in children.

CHAPTER 15
CHILD ABUSE

Robert A. Shapiro
Charles J. Schubert

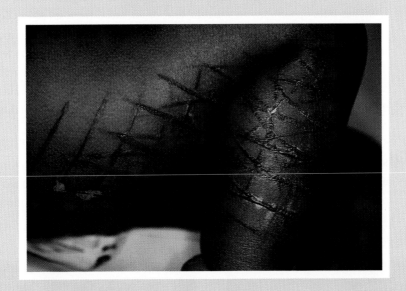

Physical Abuse

Associated Clinical Features

Burns in children are frequently the result of child abuse. The most common types of pediatric burns from abuse are immersion burns and contact burns. Certain clues may assist the physician in differentiating accidental burns from inflicted burns, but often considerable doubt remains even after a careful evaluation.

In an *immersion burn,* a thoughtful assessment of the pattern and location of the burns, as well as of the unaffected areas, helps to differentiate between accidental and inflicted burns. Postulate possible mechanisms for the injury, and correlate the assessment with the given history. A child who is held firmly and deliberately immersed has burn margins that are sharp and distinct. If the child has little opportunity to struggle, few, or no, burns from splashing liquid will occur. In contrast, a child who accidentally comes into contact with a hot liquid will move about in an attempt to escape further injury. This movement causes the burn margins to be less distinct and may result in additional small burns as hot liquid splashes onto the skin. Children who are "dipped" into a bath of hot water often show sparing of their feet and/or buttocks because they are held firmly against the tub's bottom (Fig. 15.1). A child who has a hand dipped and held into hot water may reflexively close the fingers, sparing the palm and fingertips.

Contact burns usually create a burn with a distinct and recognizable shape. Contact burn patterns most commonly associated with abuse include burns from curling irons, hair dryers, heater elements, and cigarettes (Figs. 15.2, 15.3, 15.4, and 15.5). A child who has multiple contact burns or who has burns to areas that are unlikely to come in contact with the hot object accidentally should be evaluated for abuse.

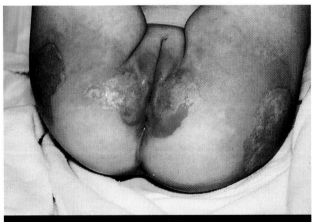

Figure 15.1   Immersion Burns

Immersion burns are often associated with toilet training accidents. This girl was plunged into hot water after soiling herself. She shows sparing of the buttocks, which contacted the surface of the bathtub and avoided being burned. (Courtesy of *The Visual Diagnosis of Child Physical Abuse,* American Academy of Pediatrics, 1994.)

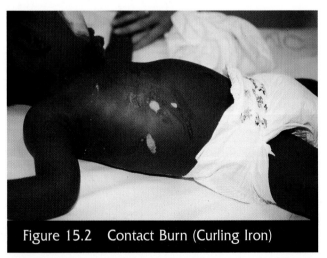

Figure 15.2   Contact Burn (Curling Iron)

Burns on the chest and abdomen from a curling iron. The burn pattern on the injured skin indicates multiple contact burns from an object the size and shape of a curling iron. Accidental curling iron burns occur, but because this infant has so many burns, the injury is suspicious for abuse. Child abuse should be suspected and reported unless the historian can provide a plausible explanation of how these burns occurred accidentally. (Courtesy of Robert A. Shapiro, MD.)

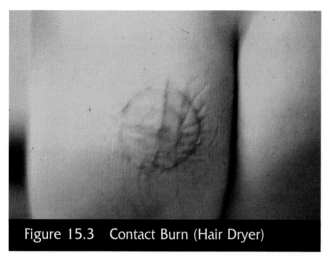

Figure 15.3 Contact Burn (Hair Dryer)

The heated grid from the end of a hair dryer caused this child's burns. The burn size and pattern marks of the burn matched exactly the hair dryer grid that was found in the child's home. The history of accidental injury was thought to be unlikely, and child abuse was suspected. (Courtesy of Robert A. Shapiro, MD.)

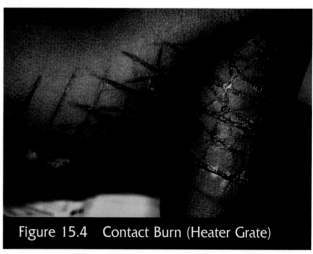

Figure 15.4 Contact Burn (Heater Grate)

This child was held against a heater grate. The pattern became more obvious with the child's knee flexed—the position of the leg at the time of the injury. (Courtesy of David W. Munter, MD.)

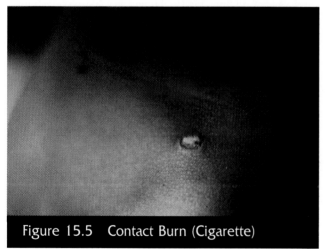

Figure 15.5 Contact Burn (Cigarette)

Cigarette burns are circular injuries with a diameter of about 8 mm. It can be difficult for the clinician to determine if the burn is from an accidental injury or from abuse. Children who accidentally run into a lit cigarette often have burns to the face or distal extremities. Accidental burns may be less distinct and deep compared with inflicted burns. A report of alleged child abuse should be made if there are multiple cigarette burns, burns to locations unlikely to come into contact with a cigarette accidentally, or other signs that suggest abuse. (Courtesy of Robert A. Shapiro, MD.)

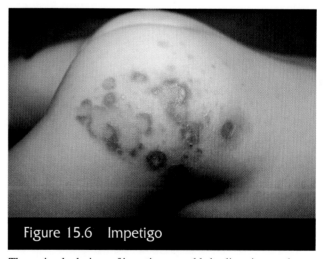

Figure 15.6 Impetigo

These circular lesions of impetigo resemble healing cigarette burns. (Courtesy of Michael J. Nowicki, MD.)

Differential Diagnosis

Some burn look-alikes may be confused with child abuse. Impetigo (Fig. 15.6) may be mistaken for healing cigarette burns, and bullous impetigo can resemble second-degree burns. Contact dermatitis and cellulitis may resemble first-degree burns.

ED Treatment and Disposition

Document thoroughly all burns that may be due to abuse. Draw sketches and take photographs of the injuries. Obtain a skeletal survey in children under the age of 2 years. Report any suspected abuse immediately to the local child protective agency before discharge from the ED. Provide standard burn therapy.

Clinical Pearls

1. Evaluate the alleged history carefully and obtain sufficient details before making any judgment. Assess whether the explanation and history that are given of the alleged episode are inconsistent with the injuries and/or with the child's developmental abilities. Suspect abuse if, without convincing explanation, the historian alters the initial history.
2. Maintain a high index of suspicion whenever caring for a pediatric burn patient. Look carefully for other signs of abuse, such as bruising, fractures, or signs of neglect.
3. Accidental burns from a cigarette are usually single, superficial, and not completely round. Common sites of accidental cigarette burns are the face, trunk, and hands.
4. Report suspicions to the mandated child protection agency whenever a burn may have been deliberately inflicted.
5. Injuries due to suspected child abuse may be photographed without parental consent in most states.

DIAGNOSIS   **INFLICTED BRUISES AND SOFT-TISSUE INJURIES**

Associated Clinical Features

Bruises are the most common manifestation of physical child abuse. Child abuse should be suspected whenever bruises are: (1) over soft body areas, such as the thighs, buttocks, cheeks, abdomen, and genitalia, since common childhood activities do not commonly cause trauma to these areas; (2) more numerous than usual; (3) of different ages (suggests repeated episodes of abuse); (4) the shape of objects such as belts, cords, or hand prints (demonstrates that the injuries were inflicted) (Figs. 15.7, 15.8); or (5) noted in young, nonambulating children (infants are not capable of getting into accidents).

The color of the ecchymosis will change as healing progresses. New injuries are usually red and purple. They may also be tender and swollen. Within a few days, the bruise may turn blue, then green, then yellow, and finally brown. The shape and margins of the bruise become less distinct as it heals. The time period in which these color changes occur is variable. Some bruises

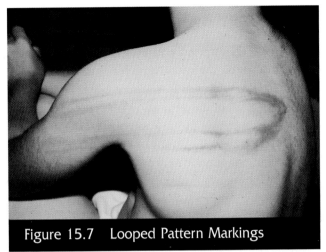

Figure 15.7   Looped Pattern Markings

Loop marks are clearly seen within the bruising on this child's back. The loop marks indicate that an extension cord, a belt, or some similar object was used to punish him. The color of the bruise is red, which indicates that the injury is only a few days old. (Courtesy of Robert A. Shapiro, MD.)

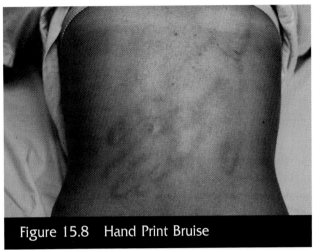

Figure 15.8   Hand Print Bruise

Bruise from a slap showing the outline of her father's hand is clearly seen on the back of this adolescent. (Courtesy of Robert A. Shapiro, MD.)

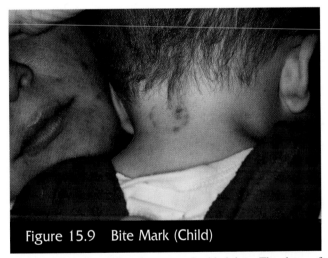

Figure 15.9   Bite Mark (Child)

Distinct impressions of teeth are seen in this injury. The shape of the injury outlines the upper and lower oral arches. Note the size of the mother's mouth in relationship to the size of the bite on the neck, making an adult mouth an unlikely source. (Courtesy of Kevin J. Knoop, MD, MS.)

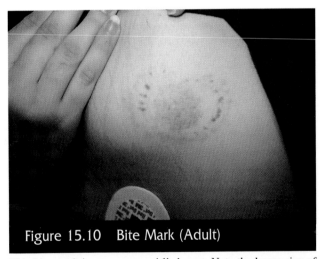

Figure 15.10   Bite Mark (Adult)

This bite mark is on a young girl's breast. Note the larger size of the wound, which is more consistent with an adult bite. (Courtesy of Robert A. Shapiro, MD.)

resolve within a few days, whereas others resolve over weeks. The amount of time until resolution depends on factors such as the location, size, and depth of the injury.

Bite marks (Figs. 15.9, 15.10) have special forensic characteristics that should be recorded. The size, shape, and pattern of the injury can identify a specific perpetrator. Most human bite injuries are caused by children, not adults, but recognition of an adult bite is important because the injury represents abuse. Compared with an adult's, the shape of a child's bite is rounder. If the impressions from the canine's are visible in the bite, the perpetrator's age can be estimated. Most

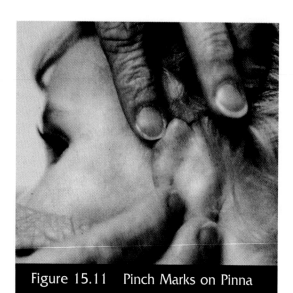

Figure 15.11   Pinch Marks on Pinna

Children may be pulled up or along by their ears, causing this injury. A child's ears should be inspected for this injury whenever abuse is suspected. (Courtesy of Robert A. Shapiro, MD.)

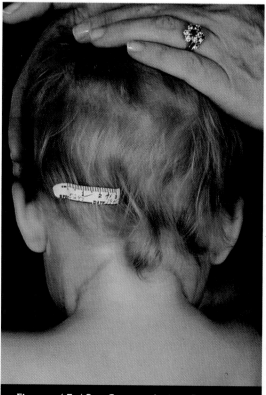

Figure 15.12   Strangulation Bruise

This child was beaten while at the sitter's and suffered circumferential linear neck abrasions consistent with attempted strangulation. There is also occipital ecchymosis from the abuse. (Courtesy of Barbara R. Craig, MD.)

children under 8 years of age have less than 3 cm between their canines. Some bites have saliva within the center of the bite, which also can be used to identify the perpetrator. Although some bite marks are immediately obvious during the initial inspection, others can be difficult to recognize. If an adult bite is suspected but unprovable because distinct impressions of the teeth are absent, reexamination of the injury a few days later may facilitate recognition and documentation.

Bites from animals are usually easy to distinguish from human bites. The size is usually smaller, and shape of the arch mark is narrower than a human's. Sharp animal canines often cause tearing of the skin instead of the crushing seen in human bites.

Differential Diagnosis

Bleeding disorders, such as idiopathic thrombocytopenic purpura (ITP), Henoch-Schönlein purpura, and leukemia, can mimic child abuse. Folk remedies, such as cupping and coining, may result in soft-tissue findings that are not reportable as abuse (see "Lesions Mistaken for Abuse").

ED Treatment and Disposition

Completely undress the child and look for all additional signs of abuse (Figs. 15.11 and 15.12). Obtain a complete history of all injuries. Sketch and photograph the injuries. Obtain a platelet count and bleeding studies [prothrombin time and partial thromboplastin time (PT and PTT)] to rule out a bleeding diathesis as the cause of the findings. For children under 2 or 3 years who have extensive injuries, obtain a skeletal survey, serum glutamic-oxaloacetic transaminase (SGOT), serum glutamic pyruvate transaminase (SGPT), amylase, and urinalysis.

If human bites are found or suspected, consider consultation with a forensic dentist. If appropriate, collect swabs for forensic analysis from the center of unwashed, fresh bites, which may contain saliva from the perpetrator.

Report suspected abuse to the legally mandated child protection agency before the child is discharged from the emergency department.

Clinical Pearls

1. Determination of the age of a bruise is imprecise. Bruises that are "fresh" (< 48 h) are usually recognizable because they are tender, red, and swollen. Occasionally, bruises may not be visible for up to 48 h after an injury.

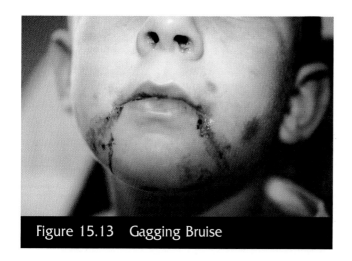

Figure 15.13 Gagging Bruise

This child had a sock stuffed into his mouth and tied around his head. The bruises in the corners of the child's mouth are indicative of gagging. Additionally, there are circular bruises on his left and right cheeks caused from the perpetrator's fingers as he held the child still to insert the sock. Pattern markings within the bruises match the fabric pattern of the sock. Photographs of these patterns should be obtained and provided to the police. The red color of the bruises and the fresh facial excoriations indicate that the injuries are recent. (Courtesy of Robert A. Shapiro, MD.)

2. Children may deny abuse when questioned because of threats made to them. The child in Fig. 15.13 initially denied that he had been gagged. He told the examining physician that he had spilled some cleaning fluid onto his lips.
3. When a parent or caretaker inflicts an injury while disciplining a child, the incident must be reported to the local child protection agency. Even if corporal punishment is lawful in a given state, the infliction of an injury is never lawful.
4. Place a millimeter ruler or coin next to a pattern injury before taking photographs so that measurements can be made.
5. Consent is not required in most states to photograph injuries suspicious for child abuse.

LESIONS MISTAKEN FOR ABUSE

DIAGNOSIS

Associated Clinical Features

Whenever bruising is excessive, is not associated with a compatible history, or occurs in an unusual distribution, seek a specific etiology. It may be appropriate to suspect and report child abuse when these conditions exist, but also consider other diagnoses.

Common Childhood Bruising

Accidental trauma can result in a bruise to any part of the body, but the forehead and the extensor surfaces of the tibia, elbow, and knee are the most common locations. When other areas of the body are bruised, etiologies other than accidental bruising should be considered.

Mongolian Spots

Mongolian spots are bluish, sacral or truncal lesions, most often seen in non-Caucasian infants and young children. They may be mistaken for bruises. Mongolian spots may be limited to only a few lesions, or they may extend up the back and shoulders of the child (Fig. 15.14).

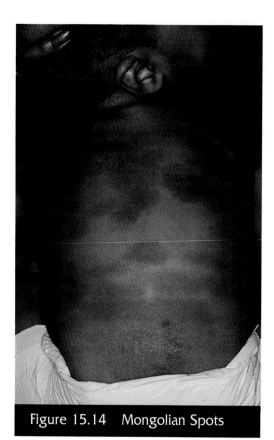

Figure 15.14   Mongolian Spots

Numerous mongolian spots on this youngster extend up the back and shoulders. (Courtesy of Douglas R. Landry, MD.)

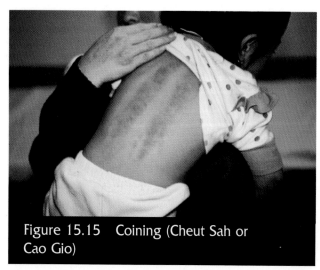

Figure 15.15   Coining (Cheut Sah or Cao Gio)

This child has petechiae and bruising along her spine. Her parents were practicing the Southeast Asian practice of coining, a healing remedy, in which a coin is rubbed along the spine to heal an illness. Coining should not be painful and is not considered abusive. (Courtesy of Robert A. Shapiro, MD.)

Cupping, Coining, and Moxibustion

Asian families sometimes practice traditional cures with their children, such as cupping, coining, and moxibustion. Each of these practices leaves markings on the child's skin, which may be interpreted as child abuse. In cupping, a flammable object is ignited and placed into a cup. After the flames have extinguished, the cup is inverted and placed onto the child's skin. As the warm air within the cup cools, a vacuum is produced. This "cure" leaves circular suction markings on the child's skin but should not be painful to the child. Coining (Fig. 15.15) is done by rubbing a coin up and down the child's back, just lateral to the spine. This results in bilateral ecchymosis and chronic skin changes on the

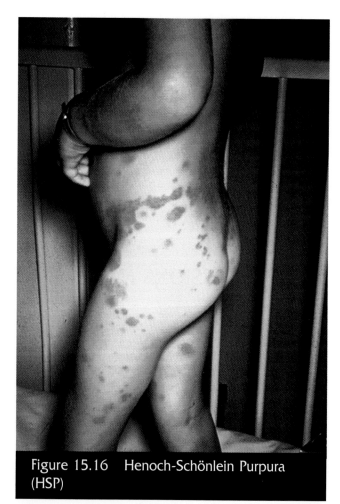

Figure 15.16   Henoch-Schönlein Purpura (HSP)

This child has palpable purpura on the extensor surfaces of the legs. HSP should be considered whenever there is symmetric ecchymosis along the extensor surfaces of the extremities and buttocks. The illness is most often seen in school-age children. Migratory arthritis and abdominal pain may be present. (Courtesy of Ralph A. Gruppo, MD.)

back. Coining should also not be painful to the child. Neither of these practices should be reported as child abuse. In moxibustion, a flammable object, such as a thread, is ignited on or near the child's skin. Moxibustion may cause superficial burns. Whether moxibustion is reported as child abuse would depend on the physical findings and the judgment of the physician.

Henoch-Schönlein Purpura

Henoch-Schönlein purpura (HSP) is a vasculitis of the small blood vessels. The skin lesions are usually small, symmetric, palpable purpuras. They may appear in a linear pattern and are often confined to the lower extremities (Fig. 15.16). Associated symptoms may include joint and abdominal pain.

Idiopathic Thrombocytopenic Purpura

Idiopathic thrombocytopenic purpura (ITP) is an acquired platelet disorder which results in abnormal bleeding. It is most common in 1- to 4-year-old children. The presenting complaint is most often abnormal bruising. The bruises can appear anywhere on the body and are numerous, mimicking child abuse (Fig. 15.17). The child may also have epistaxis, hematuria, or other bleeding.

Hemophilia

Hemophilia is usually diagnosed soon after birth because of abnormal bleeding. The ecchymosis and soft-tissue swelling are greater than would be expected given the history of trauma (Fig. 15.18).

Differential Diagnosis

Diagnostic suspicion and awareness of the above conditions is the most important step leading to the correct diagnosis. HSP, mongolian spots, and cultural practices such as moxibustion and cupping are diagnosed clinically. If ITP or other thrombocytopenic disorders are suspected, a platelet count is diagnostic. Newborns and infants with significant bleeding should have PT, PTT, and bleeding time tests to rule out a coagulopathy.

ED Treatment and Disposition

A hematologist should be consulted for children with platelet disorders and coagulopathies. HSP requires supportive care and close follow-up. The most serious complication of HSP is bowel obstruction from intussusception.

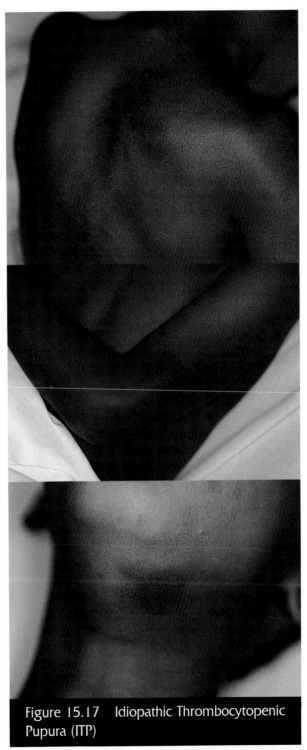

Figure 15.17   Idiopathic Thrombocytopenic Pupura (ITP)

This child has many areas of ecchymoses that appear to be in random areas of his body (back, arm, chin). The child's parent could provide no explanation for the bruising and was concerned that something was wrong with the child. ITP should be suspected in any pre-school-age child who has multiple, unexplained bruises. A platelet count will diagnose ITP. (Courtesy of Kevin J. Knoop, MD, MS.)

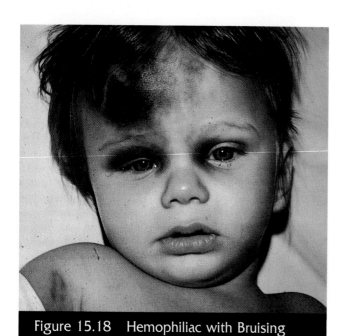

Figure 15.18   Hemophiliac with Bruising

This child's bruising is due to factor VIII deficiency. The degree of bleeding within the ecchymosis is more extensive than that seen in children without coagulopathies. A history of other abnormal bleeding episodes or a history that the child suffers from a coagulopathy is most often obtained at the time of presentation. (Courtesy of Ralph A. Gruppo, MD.)

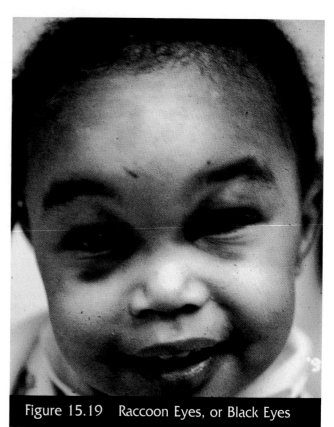

Figure 15.19   Raccoon Eyes, or Black Eyes

The etiology of this child's raccoon eyes was a forehead hematoma. He fell onto his forehead a few days earlier and developed a hematoma, a common accidental injury. As the hematoma healed, blood from the hematoma tracked down along the facial soft tissues and settled under his eyes. The resulting ecchymosis suggests that he was punched, leaving him with two black eyes. The absence of other trauma about the eyes, such as lacerations, abrasions, soft-tissue swelling, or eye injury should cause the examiner to consider a diagnosis other than direct trauma. Observation or palpation of forehead soft-tissue swelling results in the correct diagnosis. (Courtesy of Robert A. Shapiro, MD.)

Clinical Pearls

1. Mongolian spots are noted first in the newborn period.
2. Consider HSP in school-age children with purpura of the lower extremities.
3. Consider ITP in preschool children who have multiple ecchymosis and petechiae without other signs or indications of abuse.
4. Vitamin K deficiency is a cause of bleeding in infancy.
5. Trauma to the forehead may cause bilateral eye ecchymosis (Fig. 15.19) within a few days and can be mistaken for eye trauma.

Associated Clinical Features

Certain fractures should always raise a suspicion of child abuse, such as metaphyseal corner fracture, rib fractures, fractures in a nonambulating child, and untreated healing fractures. Fractures incompatible with the history and those for which no explanation is available are also suspicious of child abuse (Figs. 15.20 to 15.25).

Differential Diagnosis

Normal pediatric radiographic variants, periosteal changes caused by conditions other than healing fractures, and illnesses that cause fragile bones may all be mistaken for fractures due to child abuse. A pediatric radiologist should be consulted if any doubt exists about the radiographic in-

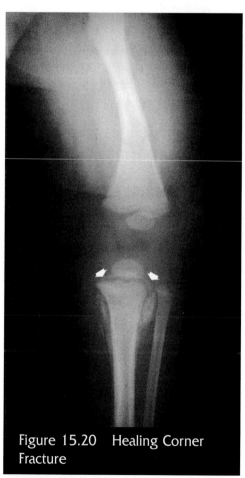

Figure 15.20   Healing Corner Fracture

This radiograph shows a healing metaphyseal corner fracture of the proximal tibia, sometimes referred to as a bucket handle fracture. Arrows point to the impressive periosteal elevation, causing the bucket handle appearance. This fracture is most often seen in children who have been the victims of child abuse, the result of shaking or pulling. (Courtesy of Alan E. Oestreich, MD.)

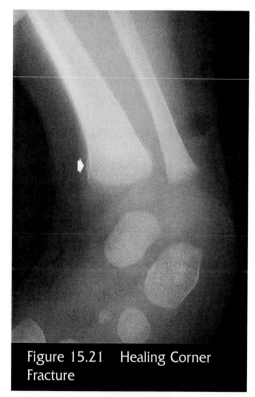

Figure 15.21   Healing Corner Fracture

Periosteal reaction (arrow) of the distal tibia from a corner fracture. (Courtesy of Alan E. Oestreich, MD.)

433

This radiograph shows a displaced spiral femur fracture with faint callus formation. The age of the fracture is just over 10 days. There is also periosteal reaction of the proximal tibia, which is more solid and therefore older than the femur fracture. Spiral femur fractures are caused by trauma that includes a twisting, rotational force to the bone. Accidental falls can result in spiral fractures if the child's foot is fixed while his or her body is rotating. Spiral fractures from abuse are often caused by an angry adult who twists the leg of the child. The radiographic finding in this photograph is almost certainly indicative of child abuse because there are two injuries which occurred at different times and no treatment was obtained when the injuries occurred. (Courtesy of Alan E. Oestreich, MD.)

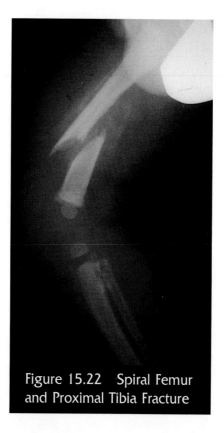

Figure 15.22   Spiral Femur and Proximal Tibia Fracture

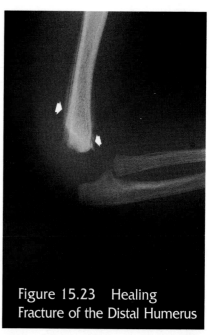

Figure 15.23   Healing Fracture of the Distal Humerus

The periosteal reaction along the distal humerus dates this fracture as older than 10 days. No treatment was obtained for the acute injury. (Courtesy of Alan E. Oestreich, MD.)

There are healing rib fractures of the right posterior fifth, sixth, and seventh ribs, the right lateral sixth rib, the left posterior fourth rib, and the right proximal humerus. The surrounding callus indicates the fractures are older than 10 days. Rib fractures must always raise a suspicion of child abuse since accidental rib fractures are unusual. Rib fractures are usually due to very firm squeezing and may be seen with shaken baby syndrome. Normal handling of infants or playful activities do not cause rib fractures. (Courtesy of Alan E. Oestreich, MD.)

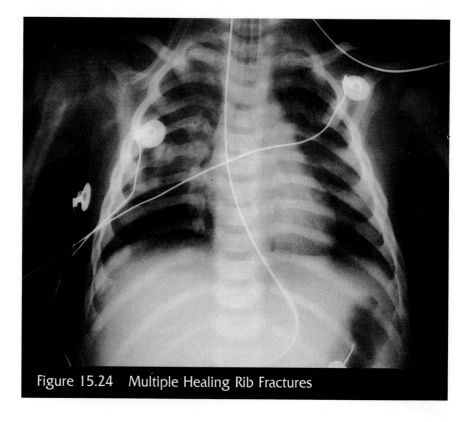

Figure 15.24   Multiple Healing Rib Fractures

terpretation. Specific disorders that can be mistaken for child abuse include osteogenesis imperfecta, copper deficiency, osteopetrosis, rickets, scurvy, hypervitaminosis A, osteomyelitis, tumors, leukemia, prostaglandin E overdose, and Caffey's infantile cortical hyperostosis.

Conditions that cause "brittle bones" must be considered when unexpected fractures are discovered, even though such cases are rare. The most frequently discussed brittle bone disorder is osteogenesis imperfecta (OI), a rare inherited connective-tissue disorder. Associated features seen in some children with OI include blue sclerae, wormian bones (seen on the skull x-ray), and osteopenia. A family history of bone fragility, hearing loss, and short stature is often present. In rare instances, children with OI lack these associated features.

ED Treatment and Disposition

If abuse is suspected in a child under 2 or 3 years of age, obtain a skeletal survey. The skeletal survey should include at least one view of each extremity and single views of the chest, abdomen, entire lateral spine, anteroposterior (AP) spine, and lateral skull. Consider a head CT or MRI in infants with skull fractures, if abuse is suspected. Suspected abuse must be reported immediately to the appropriate child protection agency. Fractures should be managed appropriately.

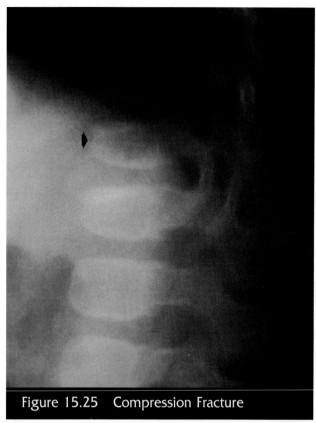

Figure 15.25 Compression Fracture

The wedging of T-12 (arrow) and probably L-1 indicates vertebral compression fractures. These fractures are the result of significant forces applied to the spinal column and are often indicative of child abuse. (Courtesy of Alan E. Oestreich, MD.)

Clinical Pearls

1. Suspect abuse when a child has multiple fractures, fractures of different ages, unsuspected (occult) fractures, fractures without a consistent trauma history.
2. Accidental trauma that includes rotational forces can result in a spiral fracture.
3. Obtain a skeletal survey in any child under 2 years of age who has injuries suspicious of abuse.
4. Radiographic signs of healing are typically first seen 10 days after a fracture.
5. Fractures that are not immobilized have a larger callous compared with immobilized fractures.

Associated Clinical Features

Infants who are violently shaken may suffer intracranial injury, commonly referred to as "shaken baby syndrome". Typically, the infant is held by the chest and violently shaken back and forth. This shaking results in subdural hemorrhages and cerebral contusions (Figs. 15.26 to 15.28). Most of the victims are under 1 year of age. Some investigators believe that shaking alone is insufficient to cause these injuries, and that therefore some blunt head trauma must also occur. The name "shaken impact syndrome" has been suggested to include this mechanism. There are usually no external signs of trauma, although infants who are shaken may also have fractures, abdominal trauma, bruises, and other injuries. Neurologic symptoms, such as apnea, seizures, irritability, or altered mental status are commonly seen, but may be absent. Flame-shaped hemorrhages (Fig. 15.29) are seen in the retina in 80% of shaken babies. The hemorrhages may be unilateral or bilateral. Shaken baby syndrome should be ruled out when retinal hemorrhages are found in any child under 2 years of age.

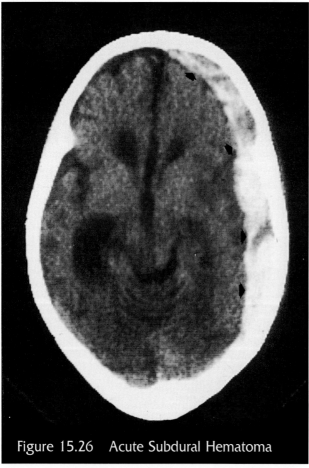

Figure 15.26 Acute Subdural Hematoma

There is a crescentic-shaped, hyperdense collection, indicating an acute subdural hematoma over the left cerebral hemisphere (*arrows*). In addition, the brain demonstrates chronic injury from a previous insult, which left the child severely impaired. (Courtesy of William S. Ball, MD.)

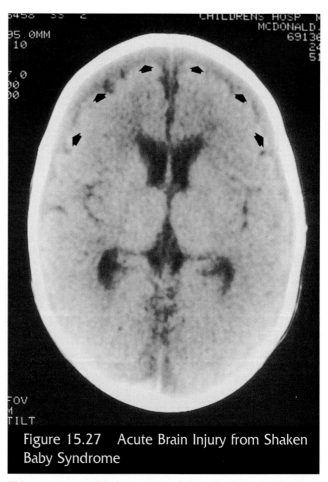

Figure 15.27 Acute Brain Injury from Shaken Baby Syndrome

This noncontrast CT demonstrates bilateral subdural collections over the frontal convexity (*arrows*). (Courtesy of William S. Ball, MD.)

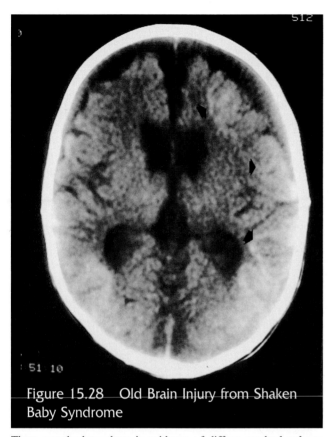

Figure 15.28 Old Brain Injury from Shaken Baby Syndrome

Three months later there is evidence of diffuse cerebral volume loss with multifocal areas of increased density (*arrows*), representing diffuse cortical and subcortical injury. (Courtesy of William S. Ball, MD.)

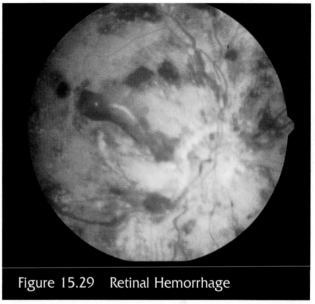

Figure 15.29 Retinal Hemorrhage

Multiple retinal hemorrhages are present. (Courtesy of Rees W. Shepherd, MD.)

Differential Diagnosis

Intracranial injury is most often the result of significant head trauma. Shaken baby syndrome is one of the most common causes of intracranial injury in infants. Relatively minor trauma, such as a fall off a couch or bed, should not cause intracranial damage unless there are predisposing conditions such as a bleeding disorder or a preexisting intracranial vascular disorder. Retinal hemorrhages have not been associated with intracranial trauma other than shaken baby syndrome.

Retinal hemorrhages may be caused by birth trauma, blunt eye trauma, meningitis, severe hypertension, sepsis, and coagulopathies. The hemorrhages that result from birth usually resolve within 3 weeks. There have been a few reports of CPR causing retinal hemorrhages, although this mechanism is not universally accepted.

ED Treatment and Disposition

Head CT or MRI should be obtained and the patient treated in the usual fashion. A report of suspected child abuse must be made to the child protective agency. A skeletal survey should also be obtained and other injuries noted. There is no specific treatment needed for retinal hemorrhages.

Clinical Pearls

1. Child abuse should be suspected in any child with retinal hemorrhages.
2. Young infants with shaken baby syndrome may have no external signs of trauma and minimal neurologic deficits.
3. When retinal hemorrhages are present, an ophthalmologist should be consulted to assist with the differential diagnosis and for medicolegal documentation in abuse cases.
4. Shaken baby syndrome is most common in children under 1 year of age.

Sexual Abuse

DIAGNOSIS

EXAMINATION TECHNIQUES AND NORMAL FINDINGS

Associated Clinical Features

The genital examination of prepubertal girls is usually limited to inspection of the external genitalia and hymen for injury and infection. An internal inspection is rarely required. The child can lie on the examination table or sit on a parent's lap (Fig. 15.30), whichever makes her most comfortable. Position that patient in a supine position with her knees flexed and out. The soles of her feet should be opposed ("frog-leg" position, Fig. 15.30). Alternatively, the child can be placed in a knee-chest position.

First, examine the perineum for trauma, condylomata, herpetic lesions, or discharge. Then examine the hymen. To visualize the hymen, hold the labia majora between the thumb and index fingers of each hand. Apply lateral and posterior traction to the labia while pulling the labia outward (Fig. 15.31). When done properly, this procedure is not painful and provides excellent visualization of the hymen (see Figs. 15.32 to 15.34). If the hymen cannot be visualized in the supine frog-leg position, the knee-chest position should be attempted. Examine the hymen for indications of trauma, such as swelling, ecchymoses, tears, scars, or thinning.

ED Treatment and Disposition

If sexual abuse is suspected, a report of alleged sexual abuse must be made to the child protective agency.

Clinical Pearls

1. Allow the child to sit on her mother's lap during the examination if this makes her more cooperative and less afraid.
2. Speculum examinations are rarely indicated in prepubertal girls and are reserved for removal of an intravaginal foreign body or evaluation of intravaginal trauma. General anesthesia is often required before inserting a speculum into a prepubertal child.

3. Apply caudal traction to the labia during examination to prevent a superficial tear of the posterior fourchette.

4. If a portion of the hymen cannot be visualized because it is adherent to the adjacent labia or to itself, gently touch the adherent tissue with the contralateral labia to pull it free. A drop of saline placed onto the posterior hymen may also separate adherent tissues without causing discomfort to the child.

5. The inner hymenal ring is usually smooth and uninterrupted. Notches at 3 and 9 o'clock are normal.

6. The shape and appearance of the normal prepubertal hymen is variable. Annular (Fig. 15.35) and crescentic (Fig. 15.36) configurations are the most common. Normal hymens may also be septate (Fig. 15.37), imperforate (no central opening), or cribriform (multiple small openings).

7. A normal examination does not exclude sexual abuse. The majority of prepubertal girls with alleged sexual abuse have normal genital examinations. Examination findings specific for sexual abuse are found in approximately 10% of girls who allege abuse.

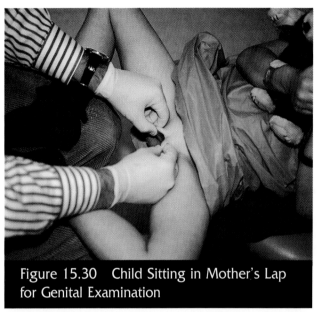

Figure 15.30 Child Sitting in Mother's Lap for Genital Examination

This young girl is being examined while she sits in her mother's lap. Many young children are less fearful of the examination if they are held by a parent during the examination. Her legs are held in the "frog-leg" position as labial traction is applied. (Courtesy of Robert A. Shapiro, MD.)

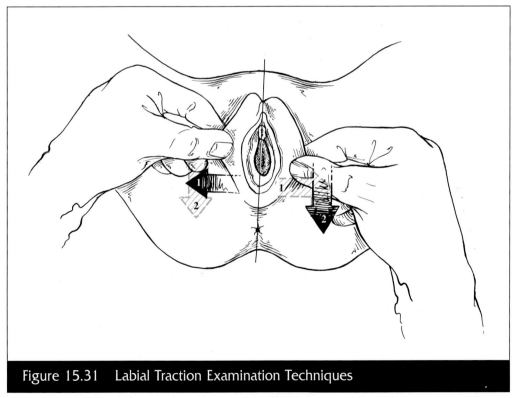

Figure 15.31 Labial Traction Examination Techniques

Hymenal inspection in prepubertal girls is best accomplished in the supine position when lateral (1) and posterior (2) traction to the labia is applied as shown here. (Adapted from Giandino, AP et al, *A Practical Guide to the Evaluation of Sexual Abuse in the Prepubertal Child.* Sage Publications, 1992.)

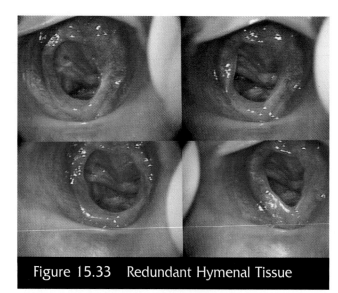

Figure 15.33   Redundant Hymenal Tissue

These photographs show the genitalia of the same patient. Because of redundant hymenal tissue, the introitus appears abnormal in the top two photos as well as the bottom left. The text describes methods to handle redundant hymen. *A. Top left and right:* The hymenal ring appears to have a defect (injury) from 7 to 10 o'clock. *B. Bottom left:* Introitus appears to be enlarged with a loss of hymen at 3 o'clock. *C. Bottom right:* When the hymen is no longer adherent to itself, the introitus appears symmetric and normal. (Courtesy of Robert A. Shapiro, MD.)

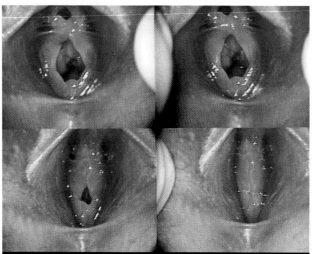

Figure 15.32   Effect of Labial Traction on the Appearance of the Prepubertal Introitus

These photographs demonstrate how the appearance of the introitus changes using different examination techniques in a prepubertal girl. Each photograph shows the introitus of the same child as different types of labial traction are used. *A. Bottom right:* Lateral labial traction only. The hymenal introitus is closed and the hymenal margins cannot be visualized. *B. Bottom left:* More aggressive lateral traction is applied. The introitus is now partially visible. *C. Top right and left:* Lateral, posterior, and caudal labial traction (as illustrated in 15.31). The introitus is now clearly seen, and the hymen can be adequately inspected for signs of injury. (Courtesy of Robert A. Shapiro, MD.)

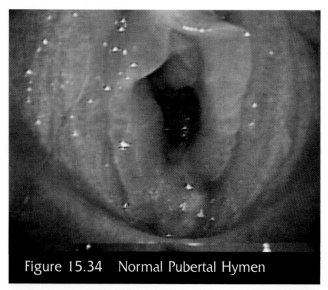

Figure 15.34   Normal Pubertal Hymen

The hymen is thicker and more redundant in this pubertal child compared with a prepubertal girl owing to the effect of estrogens. These effects are part of the changes seen during Tanner stage III development. (Courtesy of Robert A. Shapiro, MD.)

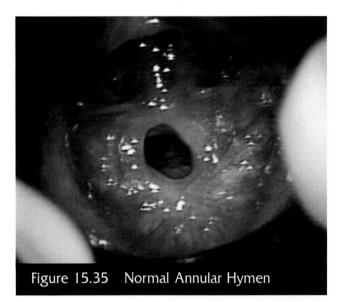

Figure 15.35   Normal Annular Hymen

The hymen in this prepubertal girl is annular in shape, extending completely around the vaginal opening. The inner hymenal ring (introitus) is smooth and free of any defects, such as lacerations or scars. The color of the hymen is more deeply red than seen in pubertal women and does not necessarily indicate infection or trauma. (Courtesy of Robert A. Shapiro, MD.)

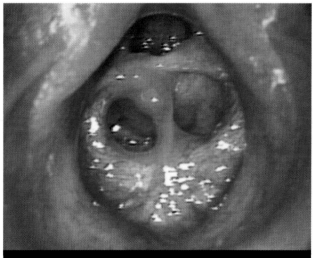

Figure 15.37   Normal Septate Hymen

This prepubertal girl has a septum in the center of her introitus. Hymenal septa are rarely seen after puberty. If the septum breaks down from the superior attachment during growth and sexual maturity, it may appear as a bump on the lower hymenal rim. (Courtesy of Robert A. Shapiro, MD.)

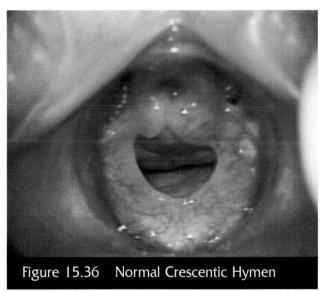

Figure 15.36   Normal Crescentic Hymen

The hymen in this prepubertal girl extends from 2 to 10 o'clock and is absent beneath the urethra between 10 and 2 o'clock. This annular shape is very common and should not be mistaken for trauma or rupture of the superior (2 to 10 o'clock) section. The inner hymenal ring (the introitus) is smooth and free of any defects, such as lacerations or scars. (Courtesy of Robert A. Shapiro, MD.)

Associated Clinical Features

Sexual abuse must be considered in any child with a genital or rectal injury, a sexually transmitted infection, a history of alleged abuse, or symptoms or behaviors seen in abused children.

Acute injuries include lacerations, bruises, abrasions, swelling, and redness (Figs. 15.38 to 15.41). Acute injuries heal quickly, often within a few days to a week. Nonacute findings of trauma secondary to sexual abuse can be more difficult to recognize. These include hymenal thinning and scars, absent hymen (Fig. 15.42), decreased rectal tone, and anal changes. Accurate interpretation of genital findings are dependent on examination technique (see section above for examination technique suggestions).

Sexually transmitted infections, when diagnosed in a young person, may be an indication of sexual abuse. Children infected with *Neisseria gonorrhoeae, Chlamydia trachomatis, Trichomonas,* and syphilis (Fig. 15.43), who did not become infected through perinatal transmission, have almost certainly been infected through sexual contact. Condylomata acuminata (genital warts) (Fig. 15.44) and herpes simplex may be transmitted through sexual or nonsexual contact, so that sexual abuse, as well as other mechanisms, should be considered.

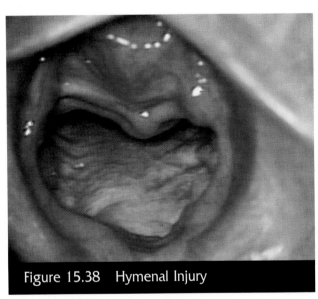

Figure 15.38 Hymenal Injury

The posterior hymen in this prepubertal girl has a defect between 5 and 7 o'clock, the result of vaginal penetration. In addition, there is minimal hymenal tissue along the lateral walls, which may be another indication of trauma. (Courtesy of Robert A. Shapiro, MD.)

An acute laceration with bruising of the posterior fourchette. The nearby hymen is edematous and ecchymotic. This injury is most likely less than 72 h old. Injuries to the hymen and posterior fourchette are usually indicative of sexual assault. Forensic specimens should be collected after acute sexual assault if semen, saliva, hair, or blood from the perpetrator might be recovered from the victim. (Courtesy of Robert A. Shapiro, MD.)

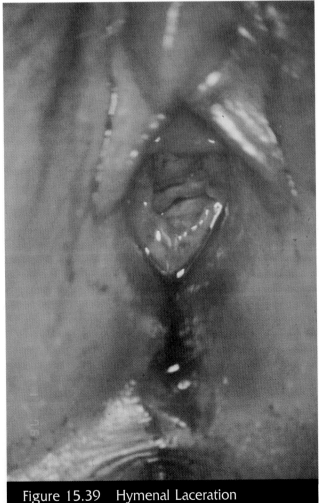

Figure 15.39 Hymenal Laceration

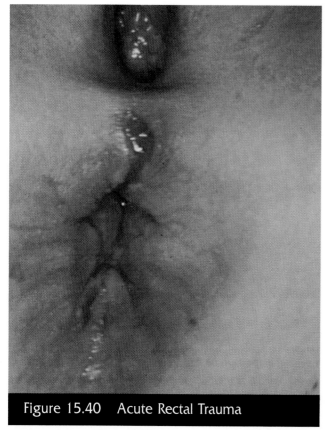

Figure 15.40   Acute Rectal Trauma

An acute rectal injury is visible at 12 o'clock. The perianal skin may normally be darker with red or blue coloration compared to the surrounding skin. (Courtesy of Robert A. Shapiro, MD.)

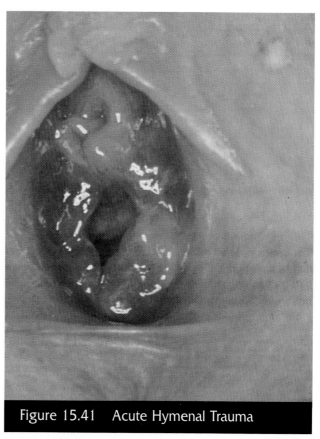

Figure 15.41   Acute Hymenal Trauma

There is a deep laceration of the hymen at 7 o'clock and ecchymosis of the hymen at 6 o'clock after recent sexual assault. (Courtesy of Robert A. Shapiro, MD.)

All children who allege sexual abuse should be evaluated, treated, and protected from the alleged perpetrator. Because of threats by family members or the perpetrator, it is not unusual for a child to recant initial allegations of sexual abuse. Although uncommon, some children falsely allege sexual abuse. The determination of whether allegations are false or of the significance of recantation should be made by the child protective services worker or by law enforcement, not by the emergency physician.

Behaviors or symptoms of abuse are frequently absent at the time of diagnosis, but can include fear or avoidance of an individual, genital or rectal pain, sleep disorders, regression, enuresis, encopresis, sexual acting out or promiscuity, depression, decrease in school performance, and perpetration of sexual abuse on younger victims.

Differential Diagnosis

Injury to the hymen from an event other than sexual abuse is possible, though unusual. Masturbation and self-exploration do not cause vaginal injury in the vast majority of children. Subtle findings of hymenal trauma are difficult to recognize. Normal hymenal anatomy may be misdiagnosed as trauma by inexperienced examiners. Other genital findings mistaken for sexual abuse are listed in the next section.

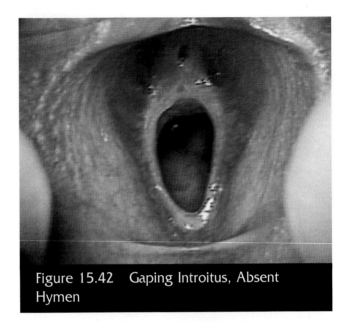

Figure 15.42   Gaping Introitus, Absent Hymen

The hymen is almost totally absent in this prepubertal girl. There may be a slight rim of hymen at 6 o'clock. The hymen in young girls is often very thin and may be totally destroyed after vaginal penetration. (Courtesy of Robert A. Shapiro, MD.)

ED Treatment and Disposition

Report suspected or alleged sexual abuse to the appropriate child protection agency. Clearly document all examination findings. If injuries require repair, appropriate consultation with surgery or gynecology should be made. Culture for sexually transmitted infections if there is a vaginal or urethral discharge. If the history of abuse suggests a risk for infection, obtain cultures from the genitalia, rectum, and pharynx. Consider syphilis and HIV testing. Obtain forensic specimens if the alleged abuse occurred within the previous 72 h, and the examination findings or history suggests that blood, semen, saliva, or hair of the perpetrator might be found on the victim's body. Offer sexually transmitted disease (STD) and pregnancy prophylaxes when indicated. Make discharge plans in consultation with the child protection worker so that the child is not returned to the abusive environment.

Clinical Pearls

1. It is not necessary to measure the vaginal opening of prepubertal girls. The size of the introitus is dependent on examination technique, degree of patient relaxation, patient age, and other variables. Although there is no consensus of normal introitus size among experts, a hymenal opening of greater than 1 cm in a prepubertal girl should raise questions about sexual abuse.
2. Small hymenal notches at 3 and 9 o'clock are normal.
3. Changes to the posterior hymen, such as narrowing and notching, may be indicative of penetrating injury.
4. Rectal abuse often results in no visible trauma. When trauma does occur, healing may be complete within 1 to 2 weeks, leaving no visible indication of the injury.

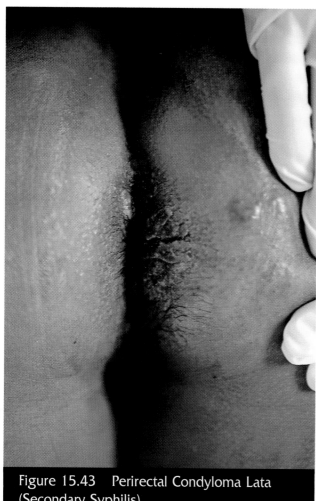

Figure 15.43   Perirectal Condyloma Lata (Secondary Syphilis)

Perirectal condyloma lata are visible around the rectum. (Courtesy of Robert A. Shapiro, MD.)

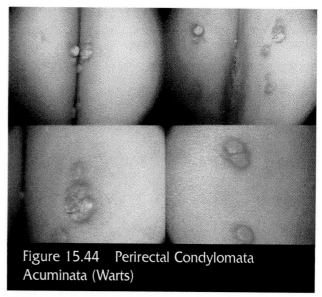

Figure 15.44   Perirectal Condylomata Acuminata (Warts)

Multiple condylomata acuminata near the rectum are visible in this photograph. Both individual and multidigitated lesions are seen. (Courtesy of Robert A. Shapiro, MD.)

5. The external anus is darker in color than the rest of the skin and should not be mistaken for erythema from abuse or infection.

6. Consider sexual abuse when anal fissures are present on examination.

7. Condyloma lata (syphilis) can be mistaken for condylomata acuminata (warts).

8. Vaginal discharge in a prepubertal child should always be cultured for *Neisseria gonorrhoeae* and *Chlamydia.*

STRADDLE INJURY

Associated Clinical Features

Straddle injuries are a frequent cause of genital trauma and most often result in unilateral abrasions, bruising, and hematomas of the labia majora and clitoral hood (Fig. 15.45). A clear history describing the straddle injury should be given by the caretaker.

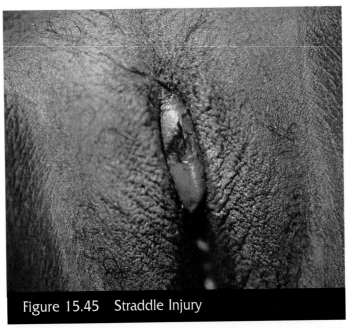

Figure 15.45   Straddle Injury

Laceration of the clitoral hood resulted after a fall onto the bar of a bicycle. (Courtesy of Robert A. Shapiro, MD.)

Differential Diagnosis

Sexual abuse must be considered in all children with genital injuries. Injuries involving the hymen are not typical of straddle injuries and are usually the result of sexual abuse or assault.

ED Treatment and Disposition

Check for urethral injury. Sitz baths and Polysporin ointment promote healing and minimize discomfort. If the child has difficulty voiding, she should be encouraged to void in a bath of warm water.

Clinical Pearls

1. Straddle injuries usually present with a clear mechanism of injury and a physical examination that supports the history.
2. Straddle injuries rarely involve the hymen or internal vaginal mucosa.

LABIAL ADHESIONS

Associated Clinical Features

Adhesions of the labia minora occur in young girls and may persist until puberty. A thin translucent line is seen where the labia meet (Fig. 15.46). The extent of the adhesions vary from child to child. Involvement is often limited to the posterior portion of the labia, but some children have more extensive adhesions completely obscuring the introitus. It is postulated that vulvar irritation and poor hygiene contribute to the etiology of labial adhesions.

Differential Diagnosis

The hymen and introitus may be obscured by the adhesions. If the adhesions are unrecognized, a diagnosis of hymenal trauma and "gaping" introitus may be incorrectly made. Adhesions may be mistaken for vaginal scars.

ED Treatment and Disposition

Prescribe estrogen creme (Premarin) to be applied gently over the adhesions twice daily for 2 to 4 weeks. Recurrence is not uncommon.

Clinical Pearls

1. Adhesions may be congenital or acquired.
2. It is possible that vulvar irritation from sexual abuse may cause labial adhesions, but clear supporting evidence is lacking.

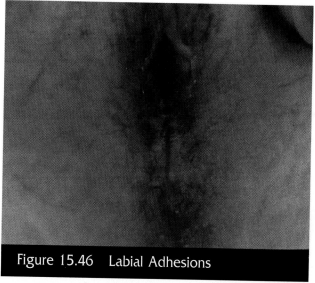

Figure 15.46   Labial Adhesions

Labial adhesions obscure the hymen in this prepubertal girl. (Courtesy of Robert A. Shapiro, MD.)

URETHRAL PROLAPSE

DIAGNOSIS

Associated Clinical Features

Prepubertal girls with urethral prolapse present with vaginal bleeding, vaginal mass, or urinary complaints. On examination, an annular, erythematous vaginal mass is seen (Fig. 15.47). Upon close examination, the mass can be seen to originate from the urethra. If necrotic, the mass is friable.

Differential Diagnosis

Urethral prolapse may be mistaken for vaginal injury, sexual abuse, or vaginal mass.

ED Treatment and Disposition

The prolapse may resolve within a few weeks with conservative medical management consisting of daily sitz baths and topical antibiotics. Topical estrogen cream and oral antibiotic therapy have

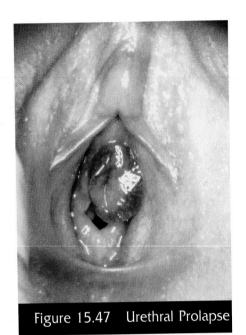

Figure 15.47   Urethral Prolapse

A round reddish-purple mass is seen in this child's introitus. Careful examination reveals the mass originates from the urethra. (Courtesy of Michael P. Poirier, MD.)

also been used with some success. Surgical repair is usually not required but may be indicated if necrosis is present or conservative management fails.

Clinical Pearls

1. Urethral prolapse often presents with painless genital bleeding of unknown etiology.
2. Prolapse is more common in African American girls.

DIAGNOSIS   TOILET BOWL INJURY

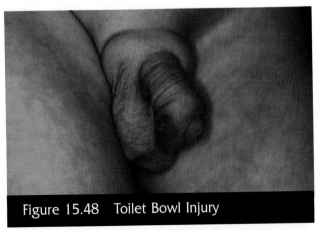

Figure 15.48   Toilet Bowl Injury

This toddler presented with a straightforward history of the toilet seat falling onto his penis during voiding. Despite the swelling and ecchymosis, he was able to void without difficulty. (Courtesy of Kevin J. Knoop, MD, MS.)

Associated Clinical Features

Acute bruising to the glans and corona of the penis can occur if the toilet seat falls onto the penis during voiding, trapping the penis between the seat and toilet bowl (Fig. 15.48). This injury is not uncommon in boys of about 3 years of age who are both inexperienced at voiding while standing and are short enough for this injury to occur.

Differential Diagnosis

Genital trauma is always suspicious for sexual abuse. The mechanism of injury may be difficult to determine if the injury was unwitnessed.

ED Treatment and Disposition

No specific treatment is needed unless the child is unable to void. If the child cannot void, a retrograde urethrogram and urologic consult are indicated.

Clinical Pearl

1. Genital injuries are suspicious of sexual abuse if no appropriate history of accidental trauma is given.

PERIANAL STREPTOCOCCAL INFECTION

DIAGNOSIS

Associated Clinical Features

Presenting complaints are often rectal pain, itching, bleeding, and rash. Symptoms may be present for months prior to the diagnosis. The child may be constipated because of stool retention and may have recently been given laxatives because of these symptoms. Systemic symptoms are absent. The perianal area is erythematous and tender (Fig. 15.49). The involved area is well demarcated from the uninfected skin. Anal fissures and bleeding may be seen.

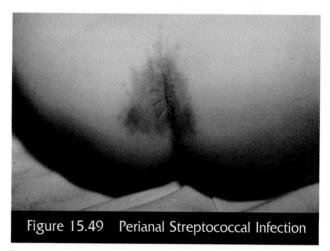

Figure 15.49 Perianal Streptococcal Infection

Intense erythema around the anus consistent with perianal streptococcal infection. (Courtesy of Raymond C. Baker, MD.)

Differential Diagnosis

Sexual abuse is often misdiagnosed because of the child's complaints of rectal pain and bleeding and the above findings on examination. This infection can also be mistaken for poor hygiene, dermatitis, nonspecific irritation, and constipation.

ED Treatment and Disposition

Culture or obtain direct antigen studies for group A beta-hemolytic streptococci. Treat with oral penicillin for 10 days. Substitute erythromycin for patients allergic to penicillin. Treatment failures should be treated with IM penicillin and/or oral clindamycin.

Clinical Pearls

1. Direct antigen studies are sensitive (89%) and specific (100%) for perianal group A streptococci infection.
2. Examine the pharynx for streptococcal infection when considering perianal strep infection.
3. Infection is unusual in children older than 10 years.

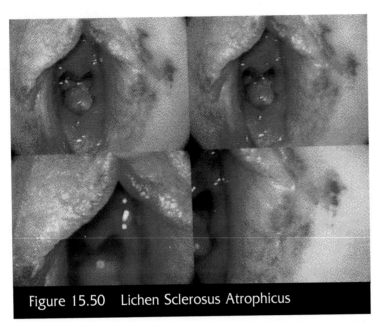

Figure 15.50   Lichen Sclerosus Atrophicus

The perineum surrounding the vagina has a bruised appearance. Atrophic skin is also evident. (Courtesy of Robert A. Shapiro, MD.)

Associated Clinical Features

Lichen sclerosus atrophicus (LSA) is an unusual dermatitis which affects the anogenital area. The diagnosis should be suspected whenever an area of hypopigmentation in the shape of an hourglass is seen around the child's anus and genitalia. The hypopigmented area is caused by small white or yellowish papules which coalesce into large plaques. The affected skin is atrophic and bleeds easily after minor trauma. The hemorrhagic form of LSA includes subepithelial hemorrhagic lesions to the labia and affected skin, which can be mistaken for traumatic lesions (Fig. 15.50). Children may complain of pruritus and dysuria.

Differential Diagnosis

The findings of hemorrhage around the genitalia and rectum are often mistaken for signs of sexual abuse.

ED Treatment and Disposition

Use symptomatic treatment if needed; 1% hydrocortisone cream can be prescribed. Refer to dermatologist for treatment.

Clinical Pearl

1.   Lichen sclerosus atrophicus is the most common dermatitis mistaken for sexual abuse.

CHAPTER 16
ENVIRONMENTAL CONDITIONS

Ken Zafren, Alan B. Storrow,
Joseph C. Schmidt, Lawrence B. Stack

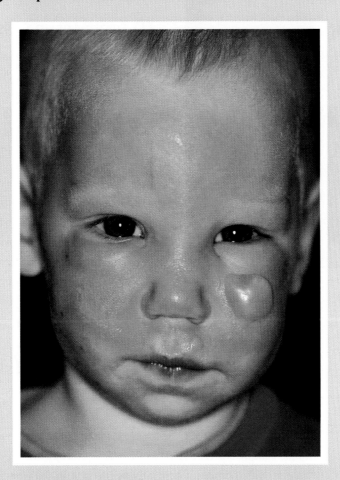

Associated Clinical Features

Retinal hemorrhages (Fig. 16.1) are common above 5200 m and at these high altitudes need not be associated with acute mountain sickness (AMS). Below 5200 m there is an association with altitude illness. High-altitude retinal hemorrhages (HARH) are rarely symptomatic, but if found over the macula, these hemorrhages may cause temporary blindness.

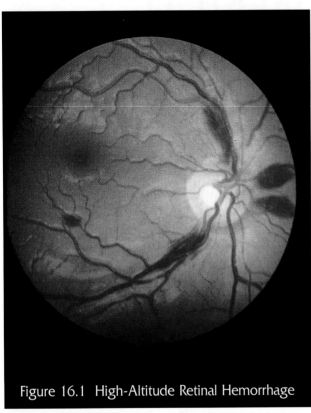

Figure 16.1 High-Altitude Retinal Hemorrhage

(Courtesy of Peter Hackett, MD.)

Differential Diagnosis

The diagnosis can be established by ophthalmoscopy. Without visualization of the lesion, the differential diagnosis of unilateral decreased vision or blindness at high altitude would include high-altitude cerebrovascular accident as well as all conditions found at sea level.

ED Treatment and Disposition

High-altitude retinal hemorrhages generally resolve spontaneously after descent to lower altitudes. No treatment is necessary for asymptomatic HARH. Patients with HARH that has been associated with a decrease in vision should be referred to an ophthalmologist for follow-up.

Clinical Pearls

1. Patients with blurred vision and unilateral mydriasis at a high altitude should be asked about use of medications, including transdermal scopolamine patches.
2. As with almost all altitude-related problems, descent is the primary treatment.

Associated Clinical Features

High-altitude pulmonary edema (HAPE) is a noncardiogenic form of pulmonary edema (Fig. 16.2) found at high altitude. It generally begins within the first 2 to 4 days after ascent above 2500 m. The earliest symptoms are fatigue, weakness, dyspnea on exertion, and decreased exercise performance. Symptoms of acute mountain sickness (AMS) such as headache, anorexia, and

The authors acknowledge the special contributions of: Peter Hackett, MD, FACEP, St. Mary's Hospital, Grand Junction, Colorado; and James O'Malley, MD, Alaska Regional Hospital, Anchorage, Alaska.

lassitude may also be present. If untreated, a persistent dry cough develops followed by tachycardia and tachypnea at rest with cyanosis. HAPE generally begins and is worse at night. Eventually the victim develops dyspnea at rest with audible crackles in the chest and orthopnea. Pink frothy sputum is a grave sign. There may be mental changes and ataxia due to hypoxemia or associated high-altitude cerebral edema (HACE).

Differential Diagnosis

Cardiogenic pulmonary edema is rare at high altitude. Respiratory infections may also be present; distinction is made difficult by the fact that fever up to 38.5°C is common with HAPE.

ED Treatment and Disposition

Mild cases (oxygen saturation in the 90s on low-flow oxygen) at moderate altitudes (below 3500 m) may be treated at altitude with bedrest and oxygen. If home oxygen and a reliable person are available, the patient may be discharged for oxygen therapy and bedrest at home or, more often, in lodgings. More severe cases should descend immediately and may require admission to a hospital at a lower altitude. These patients may require intubation and mechanical ventilation. Nifedipine may be of some benefit, but is not a substitute for altitude or descent. Hyperbaric therapy, especially with a portable hyperbaric chamber (Fig. 16.3), has an efficacy equal to oxygen and is mainly helpful in prehospital settings where oxygen availability is limited.

Clinical Pearls

1. Crackles may be unilateral or bilateral, but usually start in the right middle lobe and are therefore heard first in the right axillary (right auscultatory) area.
2. HAPE limited to the left lung in association with a small right hemithorax without pulmonary markings is pathognomonic for unilateral absent pulmonary artery syndrome. These patients develop HAPE at relatively low altitudes, sometimes below 2500 m.

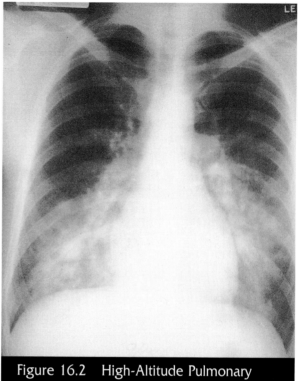

Figure 16.2   High-Altitude Pulmonary Edema

Chest x-ray in patient with HAPE. Note normal heart size with bilateral "patchy" pulmonary infiltrates. (Courtesy of Peter Hackett, MD.)

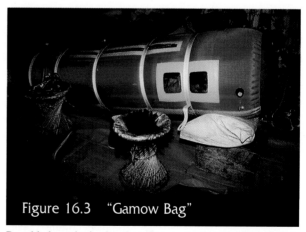

Figure 16.3   "Gamow Bag"

Portable hyperbaric chamber (Gamow bag). A HAPE patient is being treated at 4300 m at Pheriche, Nepal. Due to orthopnea, the patient was unable to tolerate lying flat, so the bag was propped up immediately after inflation. A French-made portable fabric hyperbaric chamber (CERTEC) is also available, and a lighter version with some technical improvements (H.E.L.P. system) has also been developed. (Courtesy of Ken Zafren, MD.)

Associated Clinical Features

Accidental hypothermia is an unintentional decline in core temperature below 35°C. Presentation may be obvious, as in an avalanche victim, or subtle, especially in urban settings. Symptoms vary from vague complaints to altered levels of consciousness, and physical findings include progressive abnormalities of every organ system. Following initial tachycardia there is progressive bradycardia (50% decrease in heart rate at 28°C) with decline in blood pressure and cardiac output. All cardiac cycles are prolonged, first the PR, then the QRS, and then especially the QTc. A J wave (Osborn wave; hypothermic "hump"; Fig. 16.4) may be seen. It is neither pathognomonic nor prognostic. The hump is present at the junction of the QRS complex and the ST segment.

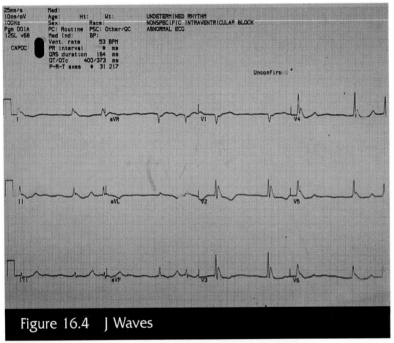

Figure 16.4   J Waves

J waves in a hypothermic patient with core temperature (rectal probe) of 25.5°C. J waves may be seen at any temperature below 32.2°C, most frequently in leads II and V$_6$. Below a core temperature of 25°C, they are most commonly found in the precordial leads (especially V$_3$ and V$_4$) and their size increases. J waves are usually upright in aVL, aVF, and the left precordial leads. (Courtesy of Alan B. Storrow, MD.)

Differential Diagnosis

J waves may also be associated with central nervous system lesions, with focal cardiac ischemia, in young normal patients, and in sepsis. In mildly hypothermic patients, invisible preshivering muscle tone may obscure P waves.

ED Treatment and Disposition

Core temperature measurement (using low-reading thermometers), gentle handling, and appropriate warming methods are the mainstays of ED treatment. Cardiovascular instability often complicates rewarming; Advanced Cardiac Life Support (ACLS) guidelines for hypothermia provide guidance. If not obvious, a cause should be sought (e.g., hypothyroidism, sepsis), as should associated pathology. Except for previously healthy patients with acute mild hypothermia, most patients require admission for observation or to treat associated diseases or injuries.

Clinical Pearls

1. The most common problems with diagnosis of hypothermia in the ED stem from incomplete vital signs.
2. Low-reading thermometers, accurate core temperatures, averaging of respirations over several minutes, and Doppler location of pulses are crucial to appropriate management.

Associated Clinical Features

Frostbite is true tissue freezing resulting from heat loss sufficient to cause ice formation in superficial or deep tissue. Frostbite may affect the extremities, nose, or ears (and the scrotum and penis in joggers). Severity of symptoms is usually related to the severity of the injury. A sensation of numbness with accompanying sensory loss is the most common initial complaint. Usually, by the time the patient arrives in the ED, the extremity has been thawed. The initial appearance in the ED may be deceptively benign (Fig. 16.5). Frozen tissue may appear mottled blue, violaceous, yellowish-white, or waxy. Following rapid rewarming, there is initial hyperemia, even in severe cases.

Favorable signs include return of normal sensation, color, and warmth. Edema should appear within 3 h of thawing; lack of edema is an unfavorable sign. Vesicles and bullae appear in 6 to 24 h. Early formation of large clear blebs that extend to the tips of digits is a good indicator as opposed to small dark blebs that do not extend to the tips, which indicate damage to subdermal plexi.

Differential Diagnosis

Seen early, frostbite may be indistinguishable from non-freezing cold injury such as immersion foot. Mixed injury is common.

ED Treatment and Disposition

If other injuries are ruled out by history and physical examination, rewarm frostbitten areas in warm water bath (37 to 41°C). If associated with severe hypothermia, active core rewarming should precede frostbite rewarming. If swelling occurs, measure compartment pressures (including hands and feet) to determine the need for fasciotomy. Admit all patients with associated hypothermia or in whom swelling occurs. Superficial frostbite (minimal skin changes and erythema) may be treated by home care with nursing instructions. Deep superficial frostbite (clear, fluid-filled blebs, swelling, pain; Fig. 16.6) may be treated by home care in a reliable patient. Deep frostbite (proximal hemorrhagic blebs, no swelling, no pulses; Figs. 16.7 to 16.9) mandates hospital admission.

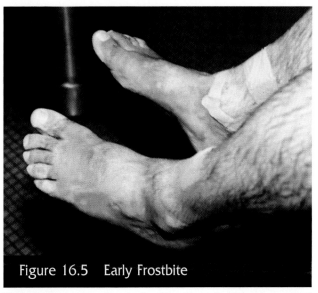

Figure 16.5   Early Frostbite

Typical appearance of early frostbite. Deep frostbite was caused by wearing mountaineering boots that were too tight in extreme cold at high altitude. Note deceptively benign appearance of this devastating injury. (Courtesy of James O'Malley, MD.)

Clinical Pearls

1. Early transfer of the patient to a center experienced in the care of frostbite injuries (even if hundreds of miles away) should be considered. On the other hand, transfer of the patient to a major medical center that does not generally manage frostbite is seldom in the patient's best interest.
2. Treatment of clear versus hemorrhagic blisters is controversial; it has been suggested to debride clear blisters and use topical aloe vera, while leaving hemorrhagic blisters intact.

455

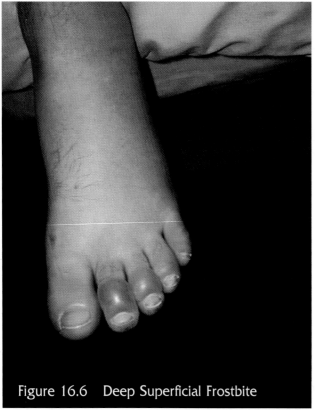

Figure 16.6   Deep Superficial Frostbite

Clear blebs extending distally are indicators for favorable out-come. (Courtesy of James O'Malley, MD.)

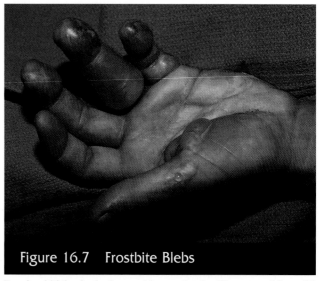

Figure 16.7   Frostbite Blebs

Proximal blebs, both clear and hemorrhagic. (Courtesy of Scott W. Zackowski, MD.)

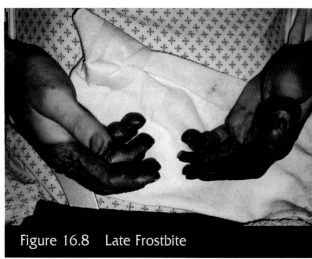

Figure 16.8   Late Frostbite

Late appearance of frostbite with demarcation starting to occur. Early surgery should be avoided in favor of autoamputation, un-less infection supervenes. (Courtesy of James O'Malley, MD.)

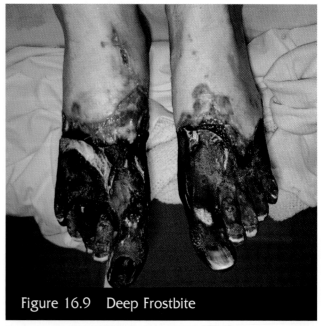

Figure 16.9   Deep Frostbite

Late appearance of deep frostbite with clear demarcation. (Courtesy of James O'Malley, MD.)

Associated Clinical Features

Immersion injury is a peripheral nonfreezing cold injury resulting from exposure to water, usually at temperatures near, but above freezing. However, it can occur during prolonged exposure to any wet environment cooler than body temperature. Dependency and immobility predispose to immersion injury. The degree of injury seems to depend on time and temperature. The first symptoms appear in hours; tissue loss may require many days of exposure. Prior to rewarming, the distal extremities are numb and swollen. The skin is first red, then changes to pale or mottled or black (Figs. 16.10 and 16.11). Cramping of the calves may occur.

Differential Diagnosis

Immersion injury is also known as trench foot, peripheral vasoneuropathy, shelter foot, sea boot foot, and foxhole foot. It is distinct from tropical immersion foot or warm water immersion foot as seen in the Vietnam conflict. Tropical immersion foot was typically seen after 3 to 7 days of exposure to water at 22 to 32°C. Warm water immersion foot was seen after 1 to 3 days at 15 to 32°C. These syndromes were characterized by burning in the feet, pain on walking, pitting edema, and erythema, with wrinkling and hyperhydration of the skin. They resolved completely after rest and removal from the wet environment.

ED Treatment and Disposition

Hypovolemia, hypothermia, and associated injuries are the rule and should be treated first. General treatment of immersion foot (or hand) is the same as that for frostbite that has been rewarmed. Swelling may produce compartment syndrome and require fasciotomy. Most patients require admission to hospital.

Clinical Pearls

1. Pulses may be difficult to feel, but may be found by Doppler.
2. Mixed injuries (frostbite and immersion) are common.

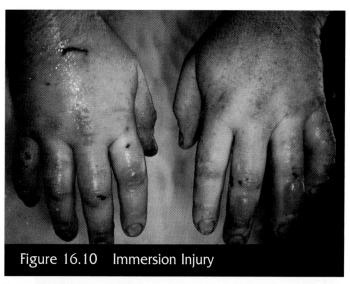

Figure 16.10   Immersion Injury

Immersion injury to hands (unusual location), several hours after rewarming. The patient spent 18 h bailing out a boat in waters just above freezing in Alaska. (Courtesy of James O'Malley, MD.)

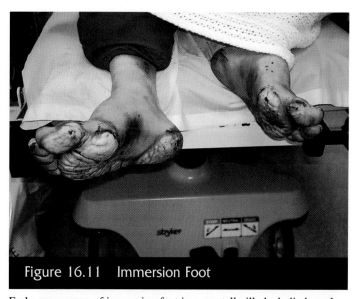

Figure 16.11   Immersion Foot

Early appearance of immersion foot in a mentally ill alcoholic homeless patient. (Courtesy of Ken Zafren, MD.)

Associated Clinical Features

Ultraviolet (UV) radiation causes both acute and chronic skin changes. Sunburn is a partial-thickness burn (Fig. 16.12), which may become full thickness if infected. "Sun poisoning" is a severe systemic reaction to UV radiation. Patients complain of nausea, vomiting, headache, fever, chills, and prostration. Excessive UV radiation may cause injury to the cornea and conjunctiva, termed ultraviolet keratitis (photokeratitis, snow blindness).

Photosensitivity reactions (photodermatoses) are of several types. Phototoxic reactions are an abnormal response to UV radiation caused by a substance that is ingested (prescription or over-the-counter medications) or applied to the skin (even seemingly innocuous perfumes or shampoos); there is a direct relation between the amount of UV exposure and severity. Photoallergic reactions are clinically similar to contact dermatitis and, like phototoxic reactions, may be precipitated by ingested or applied drugs. Unlike phototoxic reactions, photoallergies may be precipitated by a small amount of light. Phytophotodermatitis (Fig. 16.13, see also Fig. 13.61) is precipitated by skin contact with certain plants followed by exposure to UV radiation. It can resemble either phototoxic or photoallergic reactions.

Differential Diagnosis

Phototoxicity should be suspected in any patient with a severe or exaggerated sunburn. Photoallergy is easily misdiagnosed as allergic eczema or contact dermatitis, especially since onset is often delayed up to 2 days after exposure. Phytophotodermatitis may mimic severe sunburn or contact

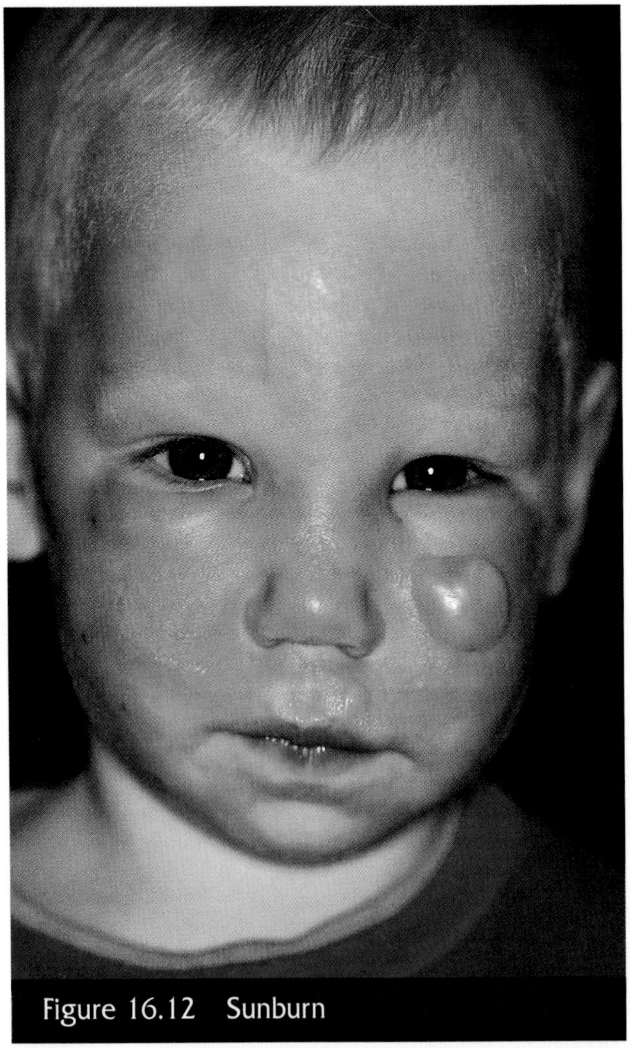

Figure 16.12   Sunburn

Sunburn is characterized by erythema, edema, warmth, tenderness, and blisters. (Courtesy of Kevin J. Knoop, MD, MS.)

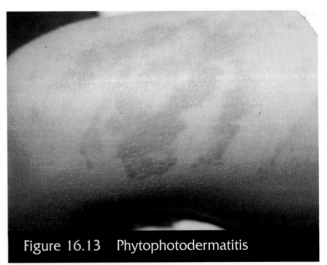

Figure 16.13   Phytophotodermatitis

This severe reaction may require aggressive systemic steroid therapy. The case illustrated is a mild one caused by exposure to limes and UVA. A clue to the diagnosis is the patchy distribution with linear edges. More severe reactions resemble rhus dermatitis. (Courtesy of Lee Kaplan, MD.)

dermatitis, especially rhus (poison ivy, sumac, or oak) dermatitis. Endogenous photosensitizers (endogenous photodermatoses) include solar urticaria, porphyria cutanea tarda, polymorphous light eruption, and systemic lupus erythematosus. These may be provoked by visible light as well as by UV radiation.

ED Treatment and Disposition

Treatment of sunburn and sun poisoning involves standard burn and supportive care. Sunburn is usually a self-limited problem. Cool compresses and nonsteroidal anti-inflammatory drugs may be beneficial. Steroids may be useful for sun poisoning. Ultraviolet keratitis is treated with mydriatic-cycloplegic eyedrops to decrease pain. Severe cases may require bilateral eye patches with antibiotic ointment, and patients may also need narcotic analgesics. These patients require 24- to 48-hour follow up, and ophthalmology referral is indicated to rule out retinal damage.

Treatment of photosensitivity reaction has two components: treatment of the sunburn and recognition of the sensitizing agent or endogenous medical condition. Topical steroids and oral analgesics and antipruritics may be helpful. Systemic steroids may be required. Patients with severe reactions should be referred to a dermatologist for possible photo patch testing.

Clinical Pearls

1.   Even *para*-aminobenzoic acid (PABA) in sunscreens may be a photosensitizer and cause a photoallergic reaction.
2.   The unique properties of individual skin types produce marked differences in response to UV radiation.

LIGHTNING INJURIES   DIAGNOSIS

Associated Clinical Features

Lightning produces injury by means of high voltage, heat production, and explosive shock waves. Indirect injuries may also be produced by lightning-set fires or explosions and by falling objects. Direct injuries include cardiopulmonary arrest and other cardiac arrhythmias and neurologic abnormalities such as seizures, deafness, confusion or amnesia, blindness, and paralysis. The patient may suffer contusions from the shock wave or from opisthotonic muscle contractions. Chest pain and muscle aches are common. One or both tympanic membranes are ruptured in more than 50% of victims. Cataracts are usually a delayed occurrence. Hematologic abnormalities including disseminated intravascular coagulation (DIC) have been described. Fetal demise may occur.

Burns may result from vaporization of sweat or moist clothing, heating of clothing and metal objects such as belt buckles, and direct effects of the strike. Linear burns and punctate burns

(Figs. 16.14 and 16.15) are thermal burns. Feathering burns (Fig. 16.16) are not actually burns but are skin markings caused by electron showers. They are pathognomonic of lightning injury.

Differential Diagnosis

Diagnosis is easy when there is a thunderstorm, witnesses to the strike, and typical physical findings. Lightning on relatively sunny days (without loud thunder) striking a lone victim may produce a confusing picture. The scattering of clothing and belongings may mimic an assault. Side flashes from metal objects and wiring may produce indoor victims during storms. Differential diagnosis of lightning injury includes cerebrovascular accident or intracranial hemorrhage, seizure disorder, spinal cord injury, closed head injury, hypertensive encephalopathy, cardiac arrhythmias, myocardial infarction, or toxic ingestions (especially heavy metals).

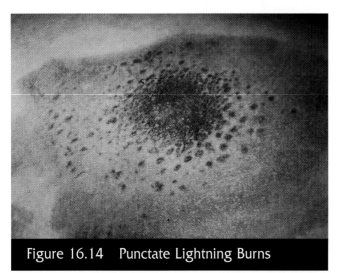

Figure 16.14   Punctate Lightning Burns

Punctate burns due to lightning are partial- or full-thickness thermal burns which range from a few millimeters to a centimeter in diameter. They are multiple and closely spaced. (Courtesy of Arthur Kahn, MD.)

ED Treatment and Disposition

History and physical examination to rule out associated injuries and standard ED care for critical patients, including cardiac enzymes, urinalysis, and ECG, are necessary. All patients, even those apparently well, require admission for observation since their condition may change over several hours following the lightning strike.

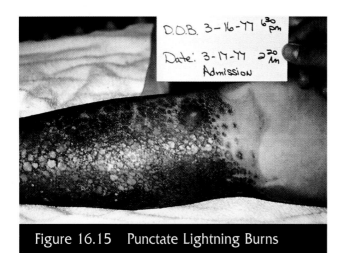

Figure 16.15   Punctate Lightning Burns

More extensive punctate burns from lightning. (Courtesy of Arthur Kahn, MD.)

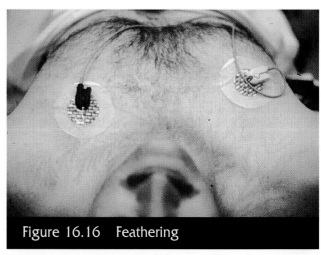

Figure 16.16   Feathering

Feathering burns (Lichtenberg's flowers, filigree burns, arborescent burns, ferning, or keraunographic markings) are pathognomonic of lightning injury. They are not true burns but are imprints on the skin of electron showers. Note the typical pattern over and around both shoulders. (Courtesy of Marco Coppola, DO., and Margaret J. Karnes, DO.)

Clinical Pearls

1. The amount of damage to the exterior of the body does not predict the amount of internal injury.
2. Since lightning most commonly produces cardiac standstill by means of massive direct current countershock, prompt, spontaneous return of normal heart rhythm (by virtue of cardiac automaticity) is the rule. However, respiratory arrest is often more prolonged. In a triage situation, the normal rules do not apply since victims breathing spontaneously are already recovering. The rule in lightning strikes is to resuscitate the dead, since ventilatory support is often all that is required.

TICKS

DIAGNOSIS

Associated Clinical Features

Ticks are blood-sucking parasites of people and animals. Ticks cause human diseases by acting as vectors for pathogens or by secreting toxins or venoms.

Tick paralysis develops 5 to 6 days after an adult female tick attaches. Over the next 24 to 48 h an ascending symmetric flaccid paralysis develops. Ataxia and associated cerebellar findings without muscle weakness or isolated facial paralysis are alternative presentations. Resolution of the paralysis after removal of the tick establishes the diagnosis.

Ticks carry more types of infectious diseases than any other arthropods except mosquitoes. The most important of these are *Borrelia* infections (including Lyme disease and relapsing fever), rickettsial diseases (e.g., Rocky Mountain spotted fever), viral illnesses (e.g., Colorado tick fever), and babesiosis. Rashes are prominent in Lyme disease and Rocky Mountain spotted fever, sometimes present in relapsing fever, uncommon in Colorado tick fever, and absent in babesiosis. The first two are covered in Chap. 13.

Clinically important ticks in North America include *Ixodes dammini,* the deer tick (Lyme disease and babesiosis; Fig. 16.17); *Dermacentor andersonii,* the wood tick (Rocky Mountain spotted fever and Colorado tick fever; Fig. 16.18); and *Amblyomma americanum,* the Lone Star tick (a very widespread tick which is implicated in transmission of Lyme disease outside of the range of *I. dammini;* Fig. 16.19). More than 40 species of ticks can cause tick paralysis. In North America the most common cause is *D. andersonii,* but *A. americanum* and *Ixodes* species have also been reported.

Differential Diagnosis

Tick paralysis should be considered in any patient provisionally diagnosed with Guillian-Barré syndrome, Eaton-Lambert syndrome, myasthenia gravis, poliomyelitis, botulism, diphtheric polyneuropathy, or any disease producing ascending flaccid paralysis or acute ataxia. The main point of differential diagnosis of tick-borne illnesses is to consider these diseases in the differential of ill patients, especially those who have been outdoors in rural areas during seasons when ticks are active.

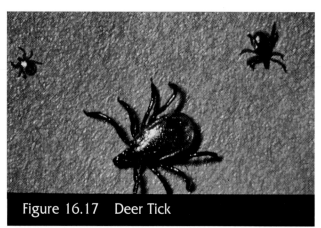

Figure 16.17   Deer Tick

Ixodes dammini, the deer tick, is a vector of Lyme disease and babesiosis. (Courtesy of the Centers for Disease Control and Prevention, Atlanta, GA.)

ED Treatment and Disposition

If still embedded, the tick should be removed promptly by grasping it as close to the skin surface as possible using blunt curved forceps or tweezers. Specialized tick removers are also commercially available. The tick should be pulled out with slow, gentle traction, taking care not to crush or squeeze the body, which may result in injection of contaminated tick fluids. Gloves should be worn for this procedure.

Patients with tick paralysis may require supportive care, including mechanical ventilation. Most patients likely require admission. Patients with tick-borne illnesses may require admission for supportive care or intensive antibiotic treatment.

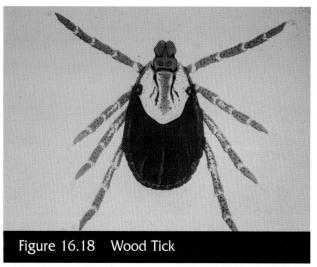

Figure 16.18   Wood Tick

Dermacentor andersonii, the wood tick, is a vector of Rocky Mountain spotted fever and Colorado tick fever. (Courtesy of the Centers for Disease Control and Prevention, Atlanta, GA.)

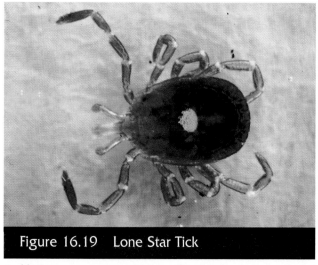

Figure 16.19   Lone Star Tick

Amblyomma americanum, the Lone Star tick, has been implicated as a vector in Lyme disease. (Courtesy of Sherman Minton, MD.)

Clinical Pearls

1. In North America, tick paralysis resolves rapidly after removal of the tick, with improvement in hours and complete recovery in days; in Australia, progression may continue for 48 h after tick removal, and recovery may be prolonged.
2. A pruritic eschar may form at the site of the tick bite in relapsing fever, but is usually gone by the time symptoms appear.
3. A clear history of tick bite is present in less than one-third of Lyme disease cases.
4. Unusual neurologic presentations, particularly bilateral peripheral seventh-nerve palsies, should prompt consideration of Lyme disease.

Associated Clinical Features

The pit vipers (Crotalidae family) indigenous to the United States consist of multiple rattlesnake species, cottonmouths, and copperheads. Pit viper venom is complex and produces hematologic, cardiovascular, and neuromuscular effects. Clinically, envenomation can be divided into four categories. The category of no envenomation consists of only fang marks. Minimal envenomation (Fig. 16.20) consists of fang marks, local swelling, but no systemic symptoms. Moderate envenomation (Fig. 16.21) includes the above with the addition of nausea, vomiting, and mild changes in coagulation parameters. Severe envenomation (Figs. 16.22 and 16.23) includes all the above with marked local swelling and signs of significant coagulopathy to include subcutaneous ecchymosis and hematuria.

Differential Diagnosis

Bites by nonpoisonous snakes frequently present to the ED. However, unless clear identification of the snake is possible, all bites should be considered venomous. Physical characteristics of pit vipers include a triangular head, heat-sensing pits, elliptical pupils, and a single row of ventral scales (Figs. 16.24 and 16.25).

ED Treatment and Disposition

Initial field management of pit viper bites should include immobilization and rapid transport. Application of lymphatic constriction bands and use of extractor devices may be helpful but are controversial. Tourniquets and local incision are most likely ineffective and may do more harm than good. Electric shock or cryotherapy are not recommended. ED management includes resuscitation, establishing a physiologic baseline, and determining the need for antivenin. Pit viper antivenin carries all the risks of any horse serum product. Recommendations for antivenin therapy vary for mild or moderate envenomation. The dose of antivenin increases with the severity of envenomation. The

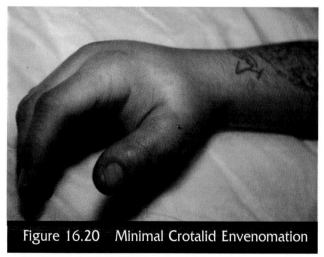

Figure 16.20 Minimal Crotalid Envenomation

Note puncture from a northern copperhead at the base of patient's thumb. (Courtesy of Edward J. Otten, MD.)

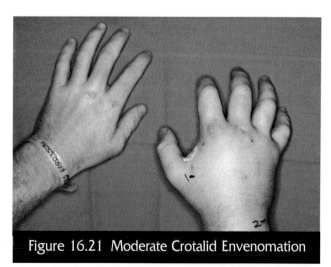

Figure 16.21 Moderate Crotalid Envenomation

Patient was bitten by a rattlesnake on the dorsal aspect of the right hand and presented with edema extending to the wrist. (Courtesy of Edward J. Otten, MD.)

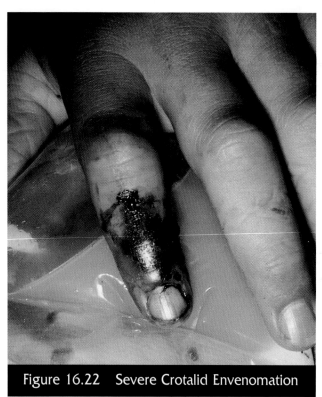

Figure 16.22   Severe Crotalid Envenomation

Despite lack of impressive local swelling, this patient presented with severe coagulopathy after a rattlesnake bite on the index finger. (Courtesy of Lawrence B. Stack, MD.)

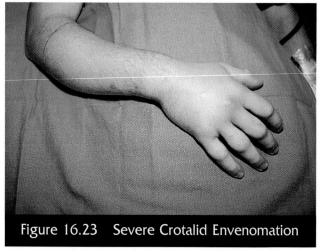

Figure 16.23   Severe Crotalid Envenomation

Patient was bitten on the dorsal aspect of the right hand and presented with progressive swelling of the forearm and systemic symptoms. (Courtesy of Edward J. Otten, MD.)

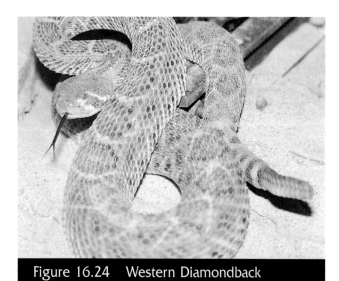

Figure 16.24   Western Diamondback Rattlesnake (Crotalus atrox)

Note characteristic triangular head, elliptical pupils, and rattle. (Courtesy of Edward J. Otten, MD.)

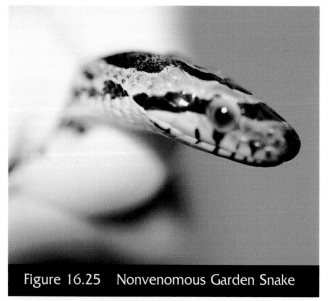

Figure 16.25   Nonvenomous Garden Snake

Note characteristic rounded head and circular pupils. (Courtesy of Steven Holt, MD.)

package insert details the current recommendations for antivenin administration and allergy testing. Compartment syndrome is a possible complication; however, prophylactic fasciotomy is not recommended. Patients who do not develop evidence of envenomation after 6 h of observation may be safely discharged home with close follow-up.

Clinical Pearls

1. Approximately one-fourth of all pit viper bites are "dry" (without any injection of venom).
2. In cases of severe envenomation, antivenin should not be withheld, even in individuals with a history of horse serum allergy. Bedside vasopressors (e.g., epinephrine) and a separate intravenous line for their administration should be available.
3. Allergy testing should be performed only in patients who need antivenin therapy.

CORAL SNAKE ENVENOMATION   DIAGNOSIS

Associated Clinical Features

The United States is home to two members of the Elapidae, or coral snake, family. Coral snakes have small mouths, and bites are usually limited to fingers, toes, or folds of skin. The bite typically produces minimal local inflammation or pain. Paresthesia and muscle fasciculation are common. Systemic symptoms can include tremors, drowsiness, euphoria, and marked salivation. Cranial nerve involvement represented by slurred speech and diplopia may be followed by bulbar paralysis with dysphagia and dyspnea. Deaths occur as a result of respiratory and cardiac arrest. Onset of severe symptoms may be delayed up to 12 h.

Differential Diagnosis

The diagnosis of coral snake bites is more difficult than pit viper bites because the fang marks are small and hard to visualize. The identification of coral snakes is complicated because many nonpoisonous snakes mimic their markings. The adage "red on yellow, kill a fellow; red on black, venom lack" (Fig. 16.26) applies to all coral snakes found in the United States but does not hold true in other parts of the world.

ED Treatment and Disposition

Severe systemic symptoms following Elapidae envenomation may be delayed and cannot be accurately predicted by local wound reactions. It is therefore recommended that

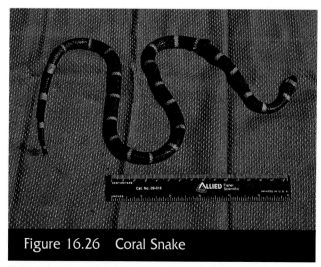

Figure 16.26   Coral Snake

United States coral snake with typical coloring and red on yellow bands. (Courtesy of Steven Holt, MD.)

four to six vials of antivenin be administered for all suspected Elapidae envenomations. Treatment of western coral snake bites is purely supportive because no antivenin is currently available.

Clinical Pearls

1. Treatment with antivenin should be initiated early in cases of eastern coral snake bites since symptoms are often delayed and severe.
2. Coral snake venom is a potent neurotoxin, in contrast to snakes of the Crotalidae family.

DIAGNOSIS   BROWN RECLUSE ENVENOMATION

Associated Clinical Features

The brown recluse spider (*Loxosceles reclusa*) is the prototypical member of the genus *Loxosceles*, which as a group can produce the typical necrotic arachnidism following envenomation. These spiders have a worldwide distribution and are identified by the striking fiddle-shaped markings on their anterodorsal cephalothorax (Fig. 16.27). Initial envenomation may be painful, although patients often report no recollection of being bitten. Initial stinging gives way to aching and pruritus. The wound then becomes edematous with an erythematous halo surrounding a violaceous center (Fig. 16.28). The erythematous margin often spreads in a pattern influenced by gravity, leaving the necrotic center near the top of the lesion (Fig. 16.29). Bullae may erupt, and over a period of 2 to 5 weeks the eschar sloughs, leaving a deep, poorly healing ulcer (Fig. 16.30). In unusual cases systemic symptoms (loxoscelism) may present with hemolytic anemia as a predominant feature. Children are at higher risk of systemic disease. Other symptoms include fever, chills, nausea, vomiting, rash, arthralgia, weakness, and leukocytosis.

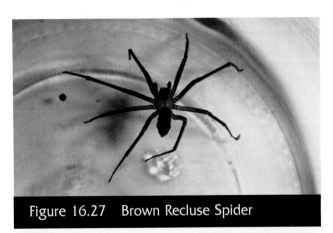

Figure 16.27   Brown Recluse Spider

Brown recluse spider with characteristic fiddle marking on the anterodorsal aspect of the cephalothorax. (Courtesy of Alan B. Storrow, MD.)

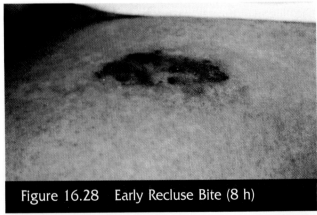

Figure 16.28   Early Recluse Bite (8 h)

Early brown recluse bite (approximately 8 h) with a violaceous center surrounded by faint spreading erythema. (Courtesy of Curtis Hunter, MD.)

Differential Diagnosis

The diagnosis of brown recluse envenomation is based on typical history, clinical features, and possible exposure to the offending species. The local wound can be confused with cellulitis, decubitus ulcer, burns, and pyoderma gangrenosum. Systemic involvement may present as an isolated hemolytic anemia, thrombocytopenia, jaundice, or hemoglobinuria.

ED Treatment and Disposition

Most cutaneous lesions secondary to brown recluse bites can be managed with cold compresses, elevation, loose immobilization, and attention to tetanus immunization. Severe lesions may require reconstructive plastic surgery several weeks after wound stabilization. The use of dapsone to prevent lesion progression is controversial. Any systemic reaction with evidence of hemolysis, hemoglobinuria, or coagulopathy should prompt admission. Hyperbaric oxygen (HBO) therapy and antivenin have been suggested as possible adjuncts, but no clear consensus of preferred treatment has been established.

Clinical Pearls

1. If dapsone therapy is to be administered, screening for glucose-6-phosphate dehydrogenase (G6PD) deficiency should be considered.
2. Prophylactic antibiotics have been suggested to lessen the chance of secondary infection.
3. Field use of suction devices has been suggested to decrease the local reaction, if used early, and may actually be successful in removing small amounts of venom.

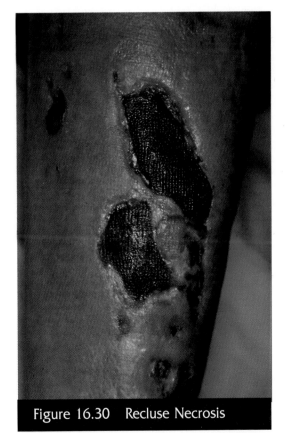

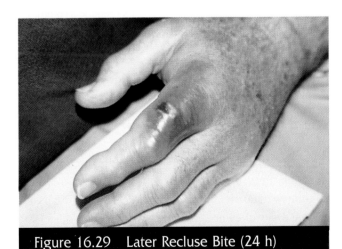

Figure 16.29   Later Recluse Bite (24 h)

Brown recluse bite at approximately 24 h. Note asymmetric spread of erythema and early central ulcer formation. (Courtesy of Edward Eitzen, MD, MPH.)

Figure 16.30   Recluse Necrosis

This plaque from a brown recluse bite is at least 1 week old. The initial, tender, localized erythema became ulcerated, then necrotic. (Courtesy of Christopher R. Sartori, MD.)

Associated Clinical Features

The black widow spider (*Latrodectus mactans*) is the prototype for the genus *Latrodectus,* several members of which cause human disease. Members of this genus are common worldwide. The clinical presentation of severe and sustained muscle spasm is produced by a neurotoxic protein, which causes the release of acetylcholine and norepinephrine at the presynaptic junction. The initial bite is mild to moderately painful and is often missed. Within approximately 1 h, local erythema and muscle cramping begin, followed by generalized cramping involving the large muscle groups such as thighs, shoulders, abdomen, and back. Associated clinical features can include fasciculations, weakness, fever, salivation, vomiting, and diaphoresis. Rare cases of seizure, uncontrolled hypertension, and respiratory arrest have occurred.

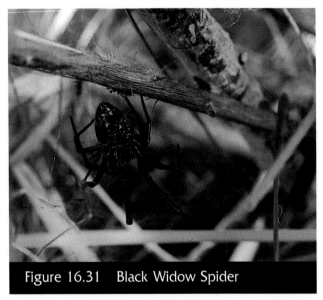

Figure 16.31   Black Widow Spider

Latrodectus mactans with characteristic hourglass marking on abdomen. (Courtesy of Alan B. Storrow, MD.)

Differential Diagnosis

The black widow spider is relatively aggressive and will defend her web, which is often found in wood piles, basements, and garages. Most envenomation occurs between April and October and is located on the hand and forearm. In cases where no history of spider bite can be elicited, a wide differential diagnosis including causes of acute abdominal pain, muscle spasm, or possible toxic ingestion must be entertained.

ED Treatment and Disposition

Treatment of the local wound should include cleansing and tetanus prophylaxis. Severe pain and spasm may require intravenous benzodiazepines and narcotics. Calcium gluconate infusion has long been recommended to reduce symptoms, although evidence for its efficacy is lacking or contradictory. Antivenin exists and carries the same risk as all horse serum products. Antivenin should be strongly considered in cases of respiratory arrest, seizures, uncontrolled hypertension, and pregnancy.

Clinical Pearls

1. Of the five *Latrodectus* species indigenous to the United States, only three are black and only one has the orange-red hourglass marking (Fig. 16.31).
2. Calcium gluconate infusion is controversial for the treatment of muscle spasm. Benzodiazepines have replaced it as the drugs of choice.
3. Envenomation by *L. mactans* can mimic an acute abdomen.

Associated Clinical Features

The order Hymenoptera includes wasps, bees, and ants. Envenomation is usually manifested by local pain, mild erythema, swelling, and pruritus. However, the possibility of more severe reactions make this subgroup the most important venomous insects in terms of human envenomation. A systemic or toxic reaction may occur from one or multiple stings. This may manifest as gastrointestinal symptoms, headache, pyrexia, muscle spasms, or seizure. Anaphylaxis may occur within minutes and may cause death. A serum sickness type reaction may occur 7 to 14 days after envenomation.

Differential Diagnosis

Other arthropod envenomation or plant exposures must be considered.

ED Treatment and Disposition

Anaphylaxis is treated with conventional therapy. Typical bites may be treated with ice packs, steroid cream, and oral antihistamines.

Clinical Pearls

1. Honeybee stings are usually apparent since the stinger apparatus, including barb and venom sac, are often detached and present on the patient's skin (Figs. 16.32 and 16.33).
2. "Brazilian killer" or "Africanized" bees are now present in Texas, Arizona, and California. Their venom is not known to be more toxic; however, their aggressiveness, tendency to swarm in large numbers, and ability to travel long distances make them potentially more dangerous to humans.

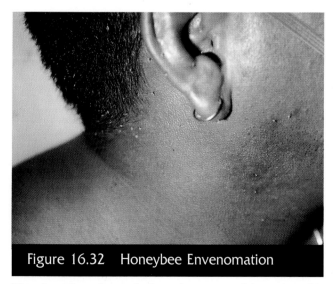

Figure 16.32   Honeybee Envenomation

Many honeybee stingers (barbs and venom sacs) located on this patient's cheek and ear and along the hairline. (Courtesy of Alan B. Storrow, MD.)

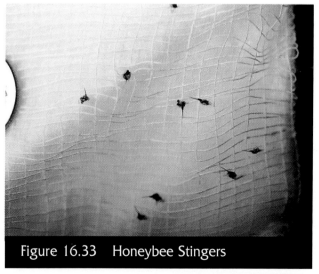

Figure 16.33   Honeybee Stingers

The barbs and attached venom sacs (stinger apparatus) after removal from the patient. (Courtesy of Alan B. Storrow, MD.)

Associated Clinical Features

The order Lepidoptera contains several families of caterpillars that are venomous to humans. The venom apparatus typically consists of barbed spines arranged in clumps or scattered about the dorsal surface of the insect (Fig. 16.34). They may contain venom or serve as a mechanical irritant. The venoms, of which little is known, are purely defensive in nature. Patients who are stung are often gardening or outdoors and come in contact with the caterpillar.

The puss caterpillar, or woolly slug (*Megalopyge opercularis*), is perhaps the most famous and important United States venomous caterpillar (Fig. 16.35). It is found throughout the United States, perhaps with the exception of the Northwest and Central Northern states. It is very hairy, flat, and may reach a length of 4 cm. It lives within and feeds on vegetation from shade trees.

Typical envenomation consists of acute pain, usually mild, followed by erythema and mild swelling (Fig. 16.36). Caterpillars with a less sophisticated venom apparatus, or less toxic venom, may cause simple pruritus or urticaria. Systemic symptoms have been reported, but are very rare.

Differential Diagnosis

Other arthropod envenomations or plant exposures must be considered.

ED Treatment and Disposition

Treatment is purely symptomatic and consists of appropriate pain control, a topical antipruritic cream, and basic wound care. Systemic antihistamines may be useful.

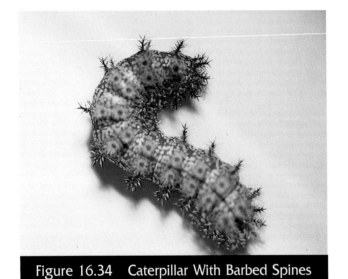

Figure 16.34   Caterpillar With Barbed Spines

Typical garden caterpillar with barbed spines arranged in clumps. (Courtesy of Alan B. Storrow, MD.)

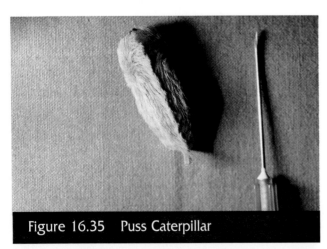

Figure 16.35   Puss Caterpillar

The "puss caterpillar" or "wooly slug" is likely the most important venomous caterpillar in the United States. The hairy appearance and small hair tail is characteristic. (Courtesy of Alan B. Storrow, MD.)

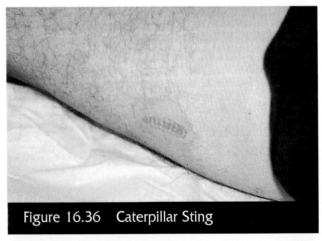

Figure 16.36   Caterpillar Sting

Appearance at 2 h of the sting produced by the above caterpillar. The patient presented with moderate pain and severe itching. Note how the lesion erythema follows the pattern of the caterpillar. (Courtesy of Alan B. Storrow, MD.)

Clinical Pearls

1. Envenomation by the Lepidoptera order are usually from a caterpillar, and not from a cocoon or adult stage.
2. Some caterpillars are capable of producing a fairly painful sting and may require opiate pain control.
3. Attached spines may be removed with adhesive tape.

MIDDLE EAR SQUEEZE

DIAGNOSIS

Associated Clinical Features

Middle ear squeeze (barotitis media) results from relative decreased pressure in the middle ear produced as a diver descends. It can occur in as little as 2 to 3 ft of water. The tympanic membrane (TM) bulges inward, causing discomfort. At a depth of approximately 4 ft, the pressure difference is great enough to collapse the eustachian tube and cause obstruction. If attempts to equalize the pressure (e.g., Valsalva or Frenzel maneuver) fail, ascent is necessary. If a diver continues to descend, TM rupture may occur. The influx of water into the middle ear may cause extreme vertigo and lead to a diving disaster.

Barotitis media may present with pain only (grade 0), TM erythema (grade 1), erythema and mild TM hemorrhage (grade 2, Fig. 16.37), gross TM hemorrhage (grade 3), free middle-ear blood (grade 4), or free blood with TM perforation (grade 5).

Differential Diagnosis

The differential diagnosis of diving-related ear pain includes otitis externa, otitis media, and ear canal squeeze.

ED Treatment and Disposition

Treatment includes ascent, decongestants, and analgesia. Antihistamines may be of use for allergic-related eustachian tube dysfunction. Antibiotics are recommended for preexisting infections or for TM rupture. Most cases resolve spontaneously within hours to days. The patient should not resume diving until the condition has resolved or the TM is completely healed.

Clinical Pearls

1. Barotitis media is the most common medical problem in diving.
2. Associated barotrauma should be investigated in cases of barotitis media.

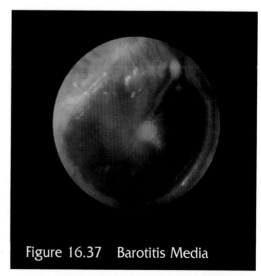

Figure 16.37   Barotitis Media

Tympanic membrane erythema and mild hemorrhage consistent with barotitis media. (Courtesy of Richard A. Chole, MD, PhD.)

Associated Clinical Features

Stingray envenomation involves a forceful thrust of the caudal spine or spines of the animal that produces a puncture wound (Fig. 16.38) or laceration. Since the animal commonly burrows in sand, they may be accidently stepped on. The stingray has a barbed tail that reflexively impacts the victim, usually in the lower extremity. The force of injection causes the integumentary sheath covering the spine to rupture, potentially releasing venom, mucus, pieces of the sheath, and spine fragments. The wound usually produces immediate intense pain, edema, and bleeding. The initially dusky or cyanotic wound may progress to erythema with rapid fat and muscle hemorrhage. Systemic symptoms may include nausea, vomiting, diarrhea, diaphoresis, muscle cramps, fasciculations, weakness, headache, vertigo, paralysis, seizures, hypotension, syncope, arrhythmias, and death.

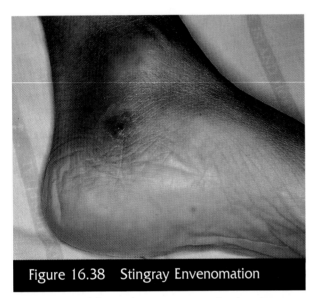

Figure 16.38   Stingray Envenomation

Puncture wound from stingray envenomation in a lower extremity. (Courtesy of Daniel L. Savitt, MD.)

Differential Diagnosis

All marine envenomations, specific to the particular environment, must be considered, since visualization of the offending creature is rare. Nonvenomous stings and simple trauma with infection must also be considered.

ED Treatment and Disposition

Rapid attention to a stingray envenomation is the key to successful treatment. The wound should be irrigated immediately and a primary exploration accomplished to remove visible debris. The use of local suction and proximal constriction bands may be useful but is controversial. Irrigation should be promptly followed by immersion in hot water, to tolerance, for 30 to 90 min. Wounds should be further explored and debrided during soaking. Pain relief should be initiated early, and narcotics may be needed. After soaking, wounds should be formally explored, debrided, and dressed for delayed primary closure or primary closure with drainage. Prophylactic antibiotics are recommended. Patients usually may be discharged home after a 3- to 4-h observation period if no systemic symptoms arise. Tetanus prophylaxis should be addressed.

Clinical Pearls

1. Application of cryotherapy to stingray envenomations may prove disastrous.
2. Retained foreign bodies are a common problem in stingray wounds.
3. Bacteria cultured from marine envenomations are extremely diverse. Antibiotics chosen should include coverage of *Vibrio* species.

Associated Clinical Features

Sea urchins belong to the phylum Echinodermata and are nonaggressive, slow-moving creatures. Envenomation usually occurs after intentional or accidental handling. Long, brittle, venom-filled spines or the three-jawed globiferous pedicellariae are responsible for the injury. The spines frequently break and pedicellariae can remain attached and active for several hours. They may advance into muscle or joint spaces and cause infection (Fig. 16.39). The usual presentation is burning pain evolving into local muscle aching. Erythema and edema may be present. Multiple envenomations may produce systemic symptoms including nausea, vomiting, abdominal pain, paresthesia, numbness, paralysis, hypotension, syncope, and respiratory distress.

Differential Diagnosis

The differential diagnosis of sea urchin envenomation includes other marine envenomations and local trauma. Delayed presentations can mimic a host of local inflammatory reactions, and a careful history of exposure is critical.

ED Treatment and Disposition

Following envenomation, the affected area should be submersed in nonscalding hot water for 30 to 90 min. Pedicellariae may be removed by applying shaving cream and gently scraping with a razor. Obvious embedded spines should be removed. Hand wounds often require surgical debridement. Retained spines often dissolve spontaneously; however, granulomas may form, producing locally destructive inflammation.

Clinical Pearls

1. Sea urchin envenomation involving a joint may produce severe synovitis.
2. Some species of sea urchin contain dye which may give the false impression of a retained spine.

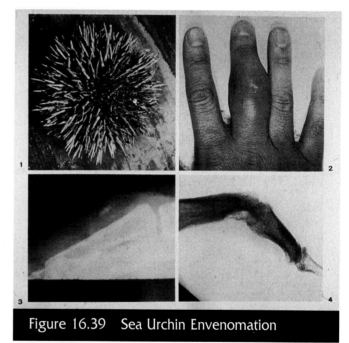

Figure 16.39   Sea Urchin Envenomation

Four images representing: (1) a living sea urchin with characteristic spines; (2) puncture wound of the right middle finger revealing swelling during the chronic phase; (3) radiograph taken shortly after sea urchin injury revealing the calcified sea urchin spine; and (4) osteolytic process of the right middle phalanx caused by an embedded sea urchin spine. (From Halstead BH: *Venomous Marine Animals of the World.* US Government Printing Office, 1965.)

Associated Clinical Features

The phylum Coelenterata contains approximately 10,000 different species, of which several hundred are a danger to humans. This diverse group includes hydrozoans (e.g., Portuguese man-of-war), scyphozoans (i.e., "true" jellyfish), and anthozoans (i.e., soft corals, stony corals, and anemones). They account for more marine envenomations than any other phylum. The important species involved in human injuries share sharp stinging cells called nematocysts. Nematocysts are enclosed in venom sacs and are present in tentacles that hang from air-filled structures. After external contact, the nematocysts are discharged from their sacs, often penetrate the skin, and release their venom. Nematocyst venom is an extremely complex substance containing numerous proteins and enzymes. Clinical presentation following envenomation ranges from the mild dermatitis to cardiovascular and pulmonary collapse. Mild envenomations usually result in a self-limited papular inflammatory eruption associated with burning and limited to areas of contact. Moderate to severe envenomations produce a spectrum of neurologic, cardiovascular, respiratory, and gastrointestinal symptoms. Anaphylactoid reactions, including hypotension, dysrhythmias, bronchospasm, and cardiovascular collapse, may play a role.

Differential Diagnosis

Coelenterate stings often produce a telltale linear pattern corresponding to the shape of tentacles (Figs. 16.40 and 16.41). Coelenterate envenomation must also be considered as a potential contributing cause in unexplained cases of collapse while swimming, diving, or in near-drowning incidents.

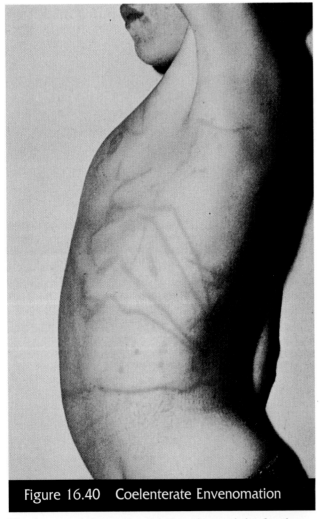

Figure 16.40   Coelenterate Envenomation

The sharp angulations and undulations characteristic of coelenterate envenomation. (From Halstead BH: *Venomous Marine Animals of the World.* US Government Printing Office, 1965.)

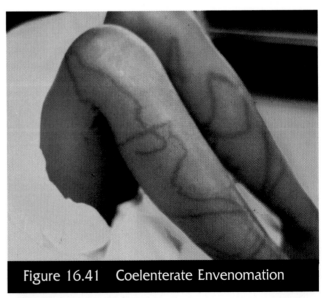

Figure 16.41   Coelenterate Envenomation

Coelenterate envenomation on the lower extremities. (Courtesy of Dept. of Dermatology, Naval Medical Center, Portsmouth.)

ED Treatment and Disposition

Concurrently with primary resuscitation, nematocyst decontamination should be accomplished beginning with sea water flushing. The hypotonic nature of fresh water, as well as isopropyl alcohol, may cause additional nematocysts to fire and should be avoided. A 5% solution of acetic acid (vinegar) applied for at least 30 min is the most widely accepted detoxicant. It has been suggested to remove tentacles with the application of shaving cream, followed in 5 min by a careful scraping with a firm, dull object (e.g., tongue blade, credit card). Pruritus may be treated with antihistamines. Pain may be addressed with immersion in hot water or with systemic analgesics. Any victim with systemic symptoms requires at least 6 to 8 h of observation because rebound phenomena are common.

Clinical Pearls

1. The box jellyfish (*Chironex fleckeri*) is generally considered the most deadly of marine animals and is most predominant in Australian and Southeast Asian waters. It may produce severe systemic symptoms hours after exposure. A sheep-derived antivenin (Commonwealth Serum Laboratory, Australia) is available.
2. The detached tentacles of some species may contain active nematocysts for months, even when fragmented on the beach or floating in water.
3. The Portuguese man-of-war is present in the Floridian Atlantic coast and the Gulf of Mexico. It is known to have a neurotoxin that may cause severe pain and death.

SEA BATHER'S ERUPTION   DIAGNOSIS

Associated Clinical Features

Sea bather's eruption refers to a pruritic dermatitis commonly mislabeled *sea lice*. Symptoms usually occur a few minutes to 12 h after exposure. The offending organisms are probably numerous and include the larval form of the thimble jellyfish and the planula form of the sea anemone *Edwardsiella lineata*. The rash consists of erythematous wheals and papules, which may be extremely pruritic (Fig. 16.42). Systemic manifestations include fever, malaise, headache, conjunctivitis, and urethritis.

Differential Diagnosis

Sea bather's eruption should be considered when a pruritic dermatitis follows sea water exposure. The incidence increases significantly during the late summer and fall off Long Island and in the late spring and early summer in south Florida. Contact dermatitis and some fungal skin disorders may present in a similar fashion.

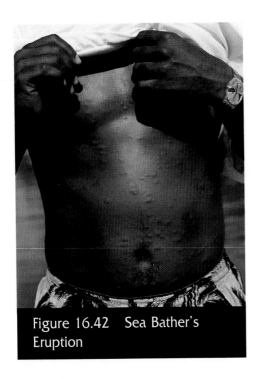

Figure 16.42　Sea Bather's Eruption

ED Treatment and Disposition

Sea bather's eruption is self-limited, rarely persisting beyond 10 days to 2 weeks. The dermatitis may be partially prevented by a vigorous soap and water scrub after saltwater bathing. Treatment is symptomatic, and calamine lotion with 1% menthol may bring relief. Topical steroids may provide additional relief. In severe cases oral antihistamines and corticosteroids may be necessary.

Clinical Pearls

1. Sea bather's eruption primarily affects areas covered by caps, fins, and bathing suits.
2. Individual lesions may appear like insect bites.

Typical appearance of sea bather's eruption. (Courtesy of Richard A. Clinchy III, PhD.)

DIAGNOSIS　　TOXICODENDRON EXPOSURE

Associated Clinical Features

Poison ivy, oak, and sumac (Figs. 16.43 and 16.44) cause more cases of allergic contact dermatitis than all other allergens combined. At least 70% of the U.S. population is sensitive to the *Toxicodendron* species.

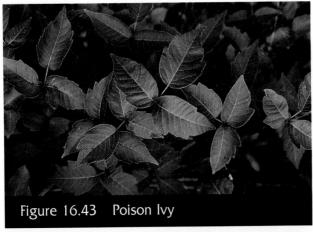

Figure 16.43　Poison Ivy

The dermatitis begins as pruritus and redness (Fig. 16.45), usually within 2 days of exposure in susceptible persons. The degree of dermatitis depends on the patient's degree of sensitivity, amount of allergen exposed, and the reactivity of the skin at the exposed body location. The dermatitis may vary from erythema, to erythema with papules, to erythema with vesicles and bullae. A linear distribution of the cutaneous lesions is strongly suggestive of *toxicodendron* dermatitis. This distribution occurs from contaminated fingernails scratching the skin or plant parts rubbing against the skin.

Differential Diagnosis

Medical problems which may appear like a *Toxicodendron* rash include photodermatitis, cellulitis, thermal burns, and other causes of contact dermatitis.

Toxicodendron radicans (poison ivy—shrub or climbing vine). Note that the leaves of poison ivy have three leaflets. Poison ivy occurs throughout the United States. (Courtesy of Lawrence B. Stack, MD.)

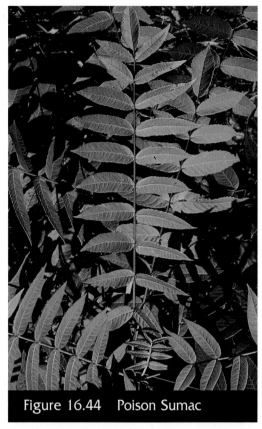

Figure 16.44   Poison Sumac

Toxicodendron vernix (poison sumac). Note that the leaves of poison sumac have 7 to 13 leaflets. It grows as a tree or woody coarse shrub. Only one species of poison sumac is found in the United States. (Courtesy of Lawrence B. Stack, MD.)

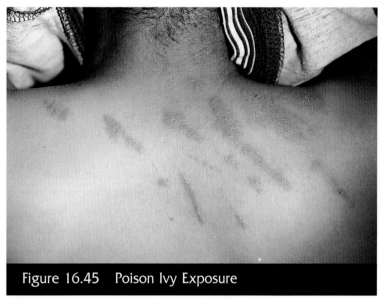

Figure 16.45   Poison Ivy Exposure

Erythematous papules and vesicles in a linear distribution consistent with *Toxicodendron* dermatitis. (Courtesy of Alan B. Storrow, MD.)

ED Treatment and Disposition

If symptoms are limited to erythema and papules and a small surface area, calamine lotion or topical steroid sprays provide adequate symptomatic relief. Pruritus can be treated with antihistamines. Vesicles and bullae require Domeboro compresses (for 60 min, three times daily) to help dry these lesions and relieve pruritus. Systemic corticosteroids tapered over 3 weeks are used in severe reactions. Secondary infection should be treated with systemic antibiotics against staphylococcal and streptococcal species.

Clinical Pearls

1. Fluid from the vesicles or bullae does not contain any allergen.
2. Removal of the allergen from the skin within 30 min of exposure may prevent dermatitis.
3. Deliberate removal of allergen from under the fingernails may prevent dermatitis spread.
4. Treatment with systemic steroids for less than 2 or 3 weeks may result in rebound exacerbations of the dermatitis.

Associated Clinical Features

Cardiac glycosides (CG) are found in the leaves of the *Nerium oleander* (Fig. 16.46), *Digitalis purpurea* (foxglove, Fig. 16.47), and *Convallaria majalis* (lily of the valley) and, if ingested, produce clinical findings similar to digoxin toxicity. Toxicity can also occur if smoke from burning plants is inhaled. Foxglove and oleander tea may be a cause of cardiac glycoside toxicity. Therapeutic effects occur from inhibition of the cardiac cell membrane sodium-potassium adenosine triphosphate pump. These effects result in increased automaticity, improved conduction, and improved inotropy.

Toxic effects are an exaggeration of therapeutic effects. Bradydysrhythmias may result from excessive pacemaker function. Tachydysrhythmias may occur from increased automaticity. Nausea, vomiting, confusion, depression, and fatigue may be present. Headaches, paresthesias, weakness, scotoma, and color disturbance (yellow vision) may also be seen.

Differential Diagnosis

Conditions that may mimic cardiac glycoside plant ingestion include cardiac medication overdose, cardiac ischemia, myocardial infarction, pulmonary embolus, and any condition associated with cardiac condition disturbances.

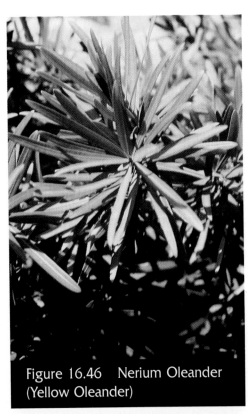

Figure 16.46   Nerium Oleander (Yellow Oleander)

A common decorative plant in subtropical climates often seen lining roads and highways. Flowers may be white, yellow, red, or purple. Plants may grow to heights of 15 ft. (Courtesy of Lawrence B. Stack, MD.)

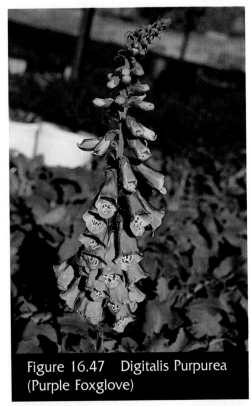

Figure 16.47   Digitalis Purpurea (Purple Foxglove)

The ornamental plant. (Courtesy of Lawrence B. Stack, MD.)

ED Treatment and Disposition

Atropine should be initially given for bradydysrhythmias. Refractory bradydysrhythmias require pacing. Ventricular tachydysrhythmias usually respond to phenytoin or lidocaine. Activated charcoal is the preferred method of decontamination. Cardioversion should be avoided in CG toxicity. Digoxin-specific Fab fragments are the treatment of choice for life-threatening dysrhythmias that fail conventional therapy.

Clinical Pearls

1. Treat cardiac glycoside overdose from plant exposure the same as an acute digoxin overdose.
2. Fab fragments have been used successfully to treat CG overdose from plant ingestion.

AMANITA PHALLOIDES INGESTION

DIAGNOSIS

Associated Clinical Features

Mushrooms are the fruit of certain fungi. *Amanita phalloides* (the "death cap," Fig. 16.48) and *Amanita virosa* (the "destroying angel") species produce amantoxins and account for most fatalities due to mushroom ingestion. Mushroom poisoning commonly occurs in the early fall when wild mushrooms are abundant and amateur foragers mistake poisonous mushrooms for edible ones.

Amantoxin poisoning results in abrupt onset of nausea, vomiting, diarrhea, and abdominal pain 6 to 24 h after ingestion. Hematemesis, hematochezia, and severe dehydration resulting in hypotension may occur. Metabolic acidosis and electrolyte loss may be found on laboratory evaluation in severe poisoning. Gastrointestinal symptoms may last 12 to 24 h and are followed by a latent period of apparent improvement. This period is followed by a rise in liver enzymes and bilirubin and elevations in the PT and PTT. Liver and renal failure may become apparent.

Differential Diagnosis

The large differential surrounding acute abdominal pain and gastrointestinal bleeding should be entertained. Acute viral hepatitis may present similar to mushroom ingestion.

ED Treatment and Disposition

Once the ABCs have been stabilized, gastric decontamination and activated charcoal administration are recommended. Specific interventions that may be helpful, but are yet unproved, include forced diuresis, charcoal hemoperfusion, high-dose cimetidine, high-dose penicillin, high-dose ascorbic acid, *N*-acetylcysteine, and hyperbaric oxygen therapy.

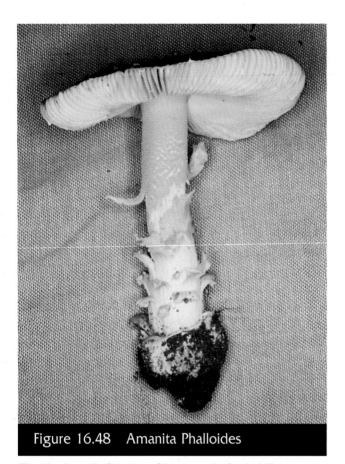

Figure 16.48   Amanita Phalloides

The "death cap." (Courtesy of Lawrence B. Stack, MD.)

Clinical Pearls

1. A history of wild mushroom ingestion by less than experts in identification should prompt suspicion of this problem.
2. A single "death cap" may contain enough toxin to kill an adult.
3. Cooking these mushrooms does not substantially alter their toxicity.

CHAPTER 17
MICROSCOPIC FINDINGS

Diane M. Birnbaumer

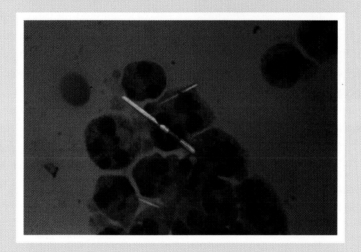

Uses

To evaluate for the presence of cells, casts, and crystals. See Figs. 17.1 to 17.5.

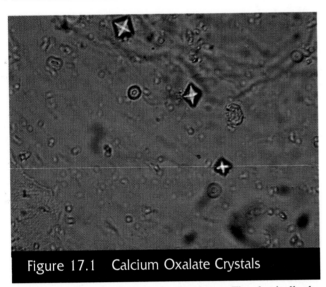

Figure 17.1   Calcium Oxalate Crystals

Calcium oxalate crystals come in two shapes. The classically described octahedral, or envelope-shaped, crystals are made of calcium oxalate dihydrate. Calcium oxalate monohydrate crystals are needle-shaped. They are seen in acid or neutral urine. They may be found in the urine of patients with ethylene glycol ingestion. In addition, the urine of patients with ethylene glycol ingestion may also fluoresce under a Wood's lamp. (From Susan K. Strasinger: *Urinalysis and Body Fluids*, ed. 3, F. A. Davis, 1994.)

Materials

Freshly collected urine specimen, centifuge, graduated centrifuge tubes, glass microscope slide, coverslip.

Method

1. Pour 10 mL of freshly collected urine into a graduated centrifuge tube.
2. Centrifuge at $400 \times$ to $450 \times$ gravity for 5 min.
3. Decant 9 mL of supernatant, leaving 1 mL in the tube.
4. Resuspend the centrifuged pellet in the remaining 1 mL of urine by stirring with a pipet.
5. Place one drop of resuspended urine on a glass microscope slide.
6. Overlay with a coverslip.
7. Examine initially using scanning $10 \times$ power, emphasizing the periphery of the coverslip, since urinary elements tend to gather at the edges.
8. Switch to $40 \times$ power to focus on specific urinary elements such as cells, casts, and crystals. Use $100 \times$ power as needed for specific identification.

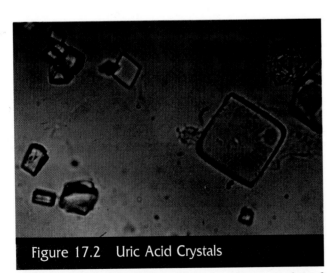

Figure 17.2   Uric Acid Crystals

Uric acid crystals often have a yellow hue and have a variety of sizes and shapes. They are found in acidic urine. (From Susan K. Strasinger: *Urinalysis and Body Fluids*, ed. 3, F. A. Davis, 1994.)

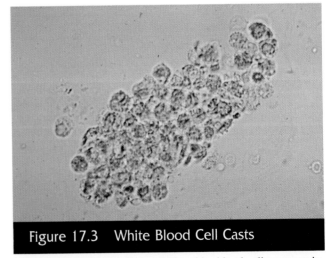

Figure 17.3   White Blood Cell Casts

Usually two to three cells in width, white blood cell casts are indicative of upper urinary tract infection such as pyelonephritis. (Courtesy of American Society of Clinical Pathologists.)

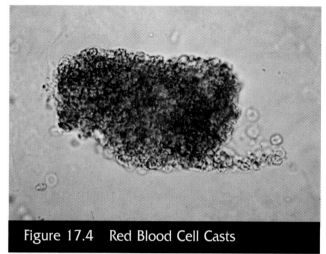

Figure 17.4   Red Blood Cell Casts

Red blood cells casts range from 3 to 10 cells in width and are seen in glomerulonephritis. (Courtesy of American Society of Clinical Pathologists.)

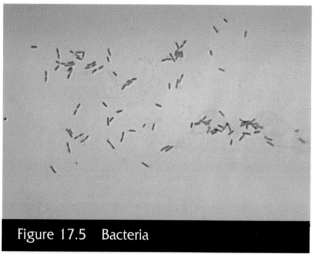

Figure 17.5   Bacteria

Bacteria are often seen in urine specimens and either can be consistent with infection or may result from local contamination from surrounding skin during specimen collection. (Courtesy of Roche Laboratories, Division of Hoffman-LaRoche Inc. Nutley, NJ.)

SYNOVIAL FLUID ANALYSIS FOR CRYSTALS   TECHNIQUE

Uses

To determine the presence of uric acid crystals (in patients with gout) or calcium pyrophosphate crystals (in patients with pseudogout) in joint fluid. See Figs. 17.6 and 17.7.

Materials

Freshly collected joint fluid, glass microscope slide, coverslip, polarizer.

Method

1. To prevent interference from polarizing artifacts, clean the slide and coverslip with alcohol prior to using them.
2. Using freshly collected unspun joint fluid, place a drop of joint fluid on the glass microscope slide.
3. Overlay coverslip.
4. View the slide using the polarizer.
5. Scan at 10 × power; 100 × power is needed to see intracellular crystals.

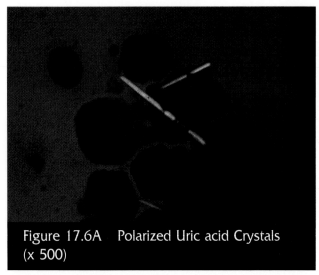

Figure 17.6A   Polarized Uric acid Crystals (x 500)

Intracellular needlelike uric acid crystals are seen within the poly-morphonuclear cells from the joint fluid in a patient with gout using a direct polarizing light. (From Susan K. Strasinger: *Urinalysis and Body Fluids*, ed. 3, F. A. Davis, 1994.)

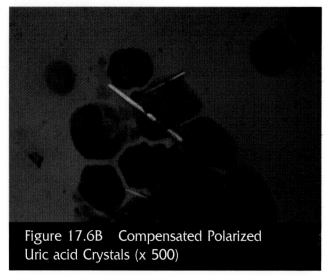

Figure 17.6B   Compensated Polarized Uric acid Crystals (x 500)

Once crystals are found with a direct polarizing light, identification is made by using a compensated polarized light. The yellow crystal is aligned parallel to the slow vibration component of the compensator (negatively birefringent). The blue crystal is perpendicular (Crossed Urate Blue). (From Susan K. Strasinger: *Urinalysis and Body Fluids*, ed. 3, F. A. Davis, 1994.)

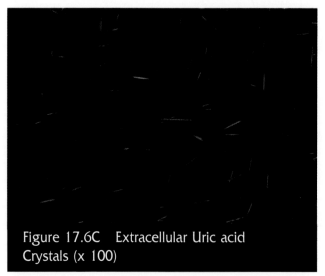

Figure 17.6C   Extracellular Uric acid Crystals (x 100)

Extracellular uric acid crystals are seen under compensated polarized light. Notice the change of color with crystal alignment. (From Susan K. Strasinger: *Urinalysis and Body Fluids*, ed. 3, F. A. Davis, 1994.)

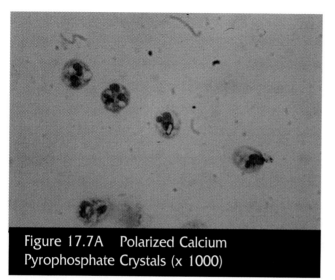

Figure 17.7A Polarized Calcium Pyrophosphate Crystals (x 1000)

Intracellular rhomboid shaped crystals in the joint of a patient with pseudogout. They may also appear as rods. (From Susan K. Strasinger: *Urinalysis and Body Fluids*, ed. 3, F. A. Davis, 1994.)

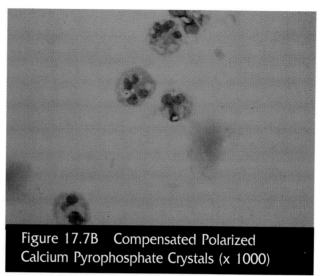

Figure 17.7B Compensated Polarized Calcium Pyrophosphate Crystals (x 1000)

The blue calcium pyrophosphate crystal is aligned parallel to the slow vibration component of the compensator (positively birefringent). (From Susan K. Strasinger: *Urinalysis and Body Fluids*, ed. 3, F. A. Davis, 1994.)

GRAM'S STAIN   TECHNIQUE

Uses

To determine adequacy of specimen (e.g., sputum); to determine the morphology of predominant organisms in a specimen. See Figs. 17.8 to 17.11.

Materials

Freshly collected specimen to be examined, glass microscope slide, crystal violet, Gram's iodine, acetone-alcohol (acetone, 30 mL, and 95% alcohol, 70 mL), safranin, Bunsen burner.

Method

1. Put specimen on dry, clean glass microscope slide and allow to air dry.
2. Heat fix specimen by gently passing over flame.
3. Cover specimen with crystal violet for 1 min.
4. Rinse off completely with water; do not blot.
5. Cover specimen with Gram's iodine for 1 min.
6. Rinse off completely with water; do not blot.
7. Decolorize for 30 s with gentle agitation in acetone-alcohol.
8. Rinse off completely with water; do not blot.
9. Cover with safranin for 10 to 20 s.
10. Rinse off completely with water and let air dry.

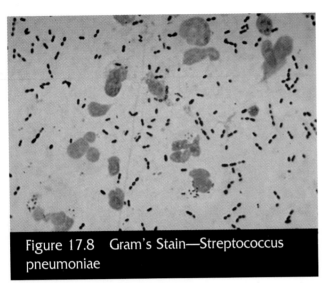

Figure 17.8   Gram's Stain—Streptococcus pneumoniae

Gram-positive, kidney-shaped diplococci of *S. pneumoniae*. (Courtesy of Roche Laboratories, Division of Hoffman-LaRoche Inc. Nutley, NJ.)

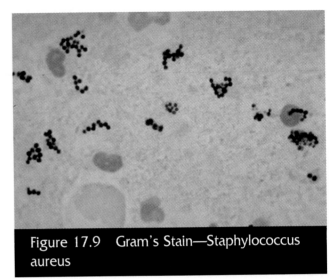

Figure 17.9   Gram's Stain—Staphylococcus aureus

Small clusters of gram-positive cocci seen in *S. aureus* infection. (Courtesy of Roche Laboratories, Division of Hoffman-LaRoche Inc. Nutley, NJ.)

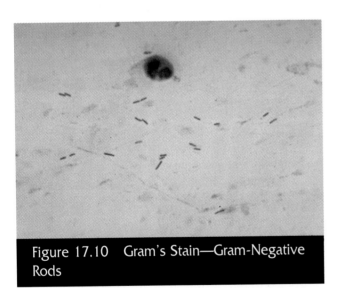

Figure 17.10   Gram's Stain—Gram-Negative Rods

Gram-negative rods of *Pseudomonas aeruginosa*. (Courtesy of Roche Laboratories, Division of Hoffman-LaRoche Inc. Nutley, NJ.)

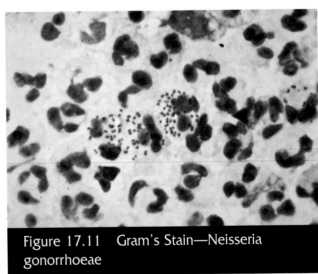

Figure 17.11   Gram's Stain—Neisseria gonorrhoeae

Multiple gram-negative, intracellular diplococci from a patient with *N. gonorrhoeae*. (Courtesy of Morse, Moreland, Thompson: *Atlas of Sexually Transmitted Diseases*. London, Mosby-Wolfe, 1990.)

Uses

To examine lesions (chancres, mucous patches, condyloma lata, skin rash) for the presence of Treponema pallidum. See Fig. 17.12.

Materials

Compound microscope with dark-field condensor (dark-field microscope), glass microscope slide, coverslip, physiologic saline.

Method for Obtaining and Viewing the Specimen

1. From chancre or condyloma lata:
   a. Gently abrade the lesion with a dry gauze.
   b. Dab away any bleeding.
   c. Touch slide to exudative fluid in base of lesion.
   d. Overlay coverslip and view immediately under dark-field microscope using 40 × and 100 × objectives.
2. From mucous patch:
   a. Touch slide to mucous patch.
   b. Overlay coverslip and view immediately under dark-field microscope using 40 × and 100 × objectives.
3. From skin lesion:
   a. Gently scrape surface of skin lesion with edge of a 15-blade scalpel blade.
   b. Dab away any bleeding.
   c. Touch slide to exudative fluid rising from skin lesion.
   d. Overlay coverslip and view immediately under dark-field microscope using 40 × and 100 × objectives.

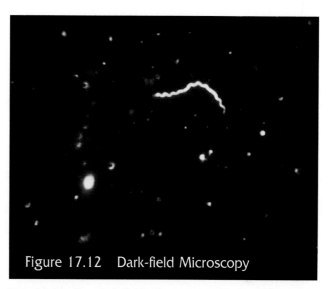

Figure 17.12   Dark-field Microscopy

Examined under a dark-field microscope at 40 × or 100 × power, spirochetes appear as motile, bright corkscrews against a black background. (Courtesy of Morse, Moreland, Thompson: *Atlas of Sexually Transmitted Diseases*. London, Mosby-Wolfe, 1990.)

Uses

To examine for clue cells, *Trichomonas,* and sperm. See Figs. 17.13 to 17.15.

Materials

Aqueous sodium chloride, glass microscope slide, coverslip.

Method

1. Place a drop of saline onto the middle of the glass slide. (Alternative Method: Place several drops of saline in a small glass test tube and place the swab in the tube. The swab can then be wiped onto a slide at a later time.)
2. Mix a small amount of vaginal fluid to be examined into the saline drop.
3. Overlay a coverslip.
4. Examine directly through microscope at 40 X and 100 X (oil immersion).

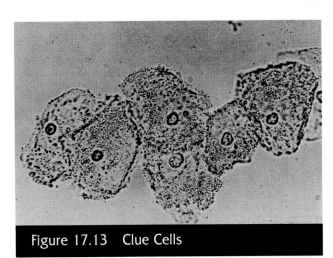

Figure 17.13   Clue Cells

"Glitter cell," or "clue cell": Epithelial cell covered with adherent bacteria in a wet mount of a vaginal specimen from a patient with *Gardinerella vaginalis* (also known as nonspecific vaginitis or bacterial vaginosis). Note the refractile appearance, indistinct borders, and ragged edges of the epithelial clue cell. (Courtesy of Curatek Pharmaceuticals.)

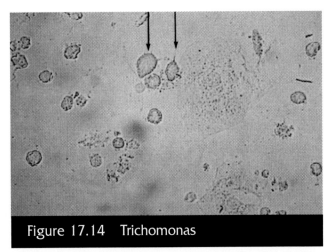

Figure 17.14   Trichomonas

Saline wet mount demonstrating oval-bodied, flagellated trichomonads. They are similar in size to leukocytes and can be distinguished from them by their motility and presence of flagella. (Courtesy of H. Hunter Hansfield: *Atlas of Sexually Transmitted Diseases.* New York, McGraw-Hill, 1992.)

Uses

To examine for yeast and fungus. See Fig. 17.16.

Materials

Ten percent aqueous potassium hydroxide (KOH), glass microscope slide, coverslip.

Method

1. Place a drop of KOH onto the middle of the glass slide.
2. Suspend a small amount of vaginal fluid into the drop of KOH.
3. Overlay a coverslip.
4. Let sit at room temperature for 30 min; as an alternative, gently heat the slide over a Bunsen burner but do not boil.
5. Examine under microscope for hyphae and spores.

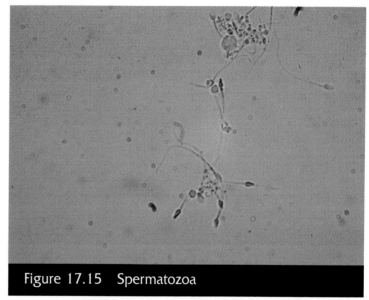

Figure 17.15   Spermatozoa

Spermatozoa may be motile or immotile. (From Susan K. Strasinger: *Urinalysis and Body Fluids*, ed. 3, F. A. Davis, 1994.)

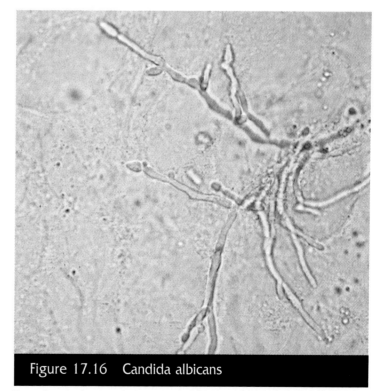

Figure 17.16   Candida albicans

Potassium hydroxide preparation of vaginal secretions from a patient with vaginal candidiasis due to *Candida albicans*. Note the pseudohyphae characteristic of this organism. (Courtesy of H. Hunter Hansfield: *Atlas of Sexually Transmitted Diseases*. New York, McGraw-Hill, 1992.)

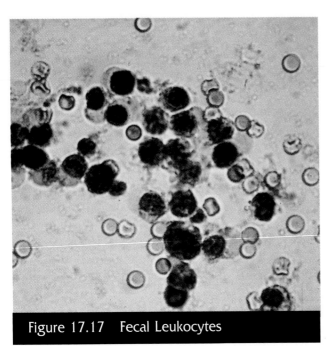

Figure 17.17   Fecal Leukocytes

Multiple white cells in the stool specimen from a patient with bacterial diarrhea. (Courtesy of Herbert L. DuPont, MD.)

Uses

To evaluate a patient for the presence of fecal leukocytes. See Fig. 17.17.

Materials

Freshly collected liquid stool specimen, glass microscope slide, coverslip, methylene blue.

Method

1. Place a drop of liquid stool onto the glass slide.
2. Add two drops of methylene blue to the stool specimen.
3. Mix thoroughly.
4. Overlay with a coverslip.
5. Place the edge of a piece of filter paper adjacent to the coverslip to absorb any excess methylene blue.
6. Examine using $10 \times$ objective to scan specimen and $40 \times$ and $100 \times$ to identify specific leukocytes.

TECHNIQUE | **SKIN SCRAPING FOR DERMATOSES AND INFESTATIONS**

Uses

To determine fungal dermatoses or skin infestations. See Figs. 17.18 to 17.21.

Materials

Fresh skin scraping, glass microscope slide, coverslip, potassium hydroxide (10%).

Method

1. Specimen collection:
   a. Gently scrape skin lesion with edge of a 15-blade scalpel.
2. Slide preparation:
   a. Place a drop of KOH onto the middle of the glass slide.
   b. Suspend a small smount of skin scraping into the drop of KOH.
   c. Overlay a coverslip.

d. Let sit at room temperature for 30 min; as an alternative, gently heat the slide over a Bunsen burner but do not boil.

e. Examine under microscope for hyphae, spores, or infestations.

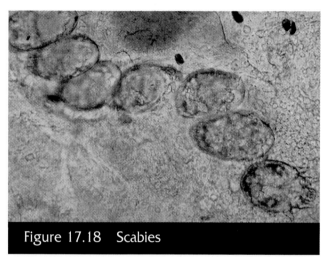

Figure 17.18   Scabies

Skin scraping from a patient with scabies. Note the intact mite at the lower right of the photograph, and the ova and fecal pellets. (Courtesy of Dept. of Dermatology, Naval Medical Center, Portsmouth, VA.)

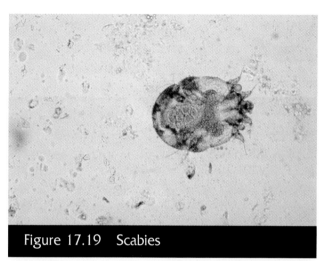

Figure 17.19   Scabies

Adult female scabies mite. (Courtesy of Morse, Moreland, Thompson: *Atlas of Sexually Transmitted Diseases.* London, Mosby-Wolfe, 1990.)

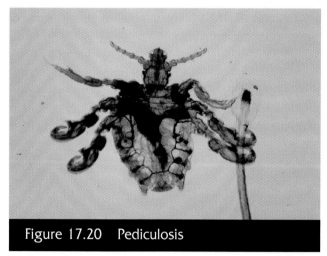

Figure 17.20   Pediculosis

Phthirus pubis, the crab louse. Note the short body and clawlike legs, which are ideally suited for clinging to the hair shaft. (Courtesy of Dept. of Dermatology, Naval Medical Center, Portsmouth, VA.)

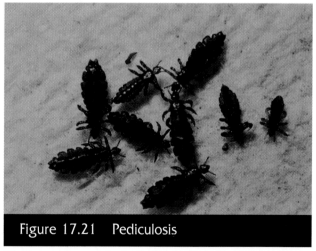

Figure 17.21   Pediculosis

Phthirus corporus, the body louse. Note the elongated body. (Courtesy of Dept. of Dermatology, Naval Medical Center, Portsmouth, VA.)

Cerebrospinal Fluid Examination

INDIA INK PREPARATION

Materials

India ink, glass microscope slide, coverslip. See Fig. 17.22.

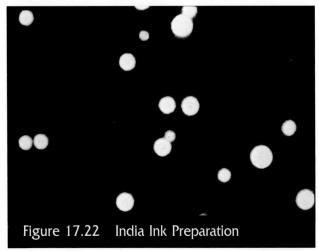

Figure 17.22   India Ink Preparation

Budding yeast with prominent capsule on india ink preparation from a patient with *Cryptococcus neoformans* meningitis. (Courtesy of Morse, Moreland, Thompson: *Atlas of Sexually Transmitted Diseases*. London, Mosby-Wolfe, 1990.)

Uses

To examine cerebrospinal fluid for organisms with capsules, particularly *Cryptococcus neoformans.*

Method

1. Lightly centrifuge cerebrospinal fluid to concentrate cells at bottom of tube (1 to 2 min).
2. Pour off excess fluid (retain if further testing may be necessary).
3. Take a drop from the bottom of the centrifuge tube and place it in the middle of a glass microscope slide.
4. Place a drop of india ink into the specimen drop; gently mix.
5. Overlay a coverslip.
6. Examine at 10 × to screen specimen, use 40 × objective to confirm findings.

INDEX

Note: Page numbers followed by f indicate figures; page numbers followed by t indicate tables.

ISBN 0-07-035202-X

90000>